CANCER CONTROL OPPORTUNITIES
IN LOW- AND MIDDLE-INCOME COUNTRIES

Committee on Cancer Control in Low- and Middle-Income Countries
Board on Global Health

Frank A. Sloan and Hellen Gelband, *Editors*

INSTITUTE OF MEDICINE
OF THE NATIONAL ACADEMIES

THE NATIONAL ACADEMIES PRESS
Washington, D.C.
www.nap.edu

THE NATIONAL ACADEMIES PRESS 500 Fifth Street, N.W. Washington, DC 20001

NOTICE: The project that is the subject of this report was approved by the Governing Board of the National Research Council, whose members are drawn from the councils of the National Academy of Sciences, the National Academy of Engineering, and the Institute of Medicine. The members of the committee responsible for the report were chosen for their special competences and with regard for appropriate balance.

This study was supported by Contract No. NOI-OD-4-2139 between the National Academy of Sciences and the National Cancer Institute and Grant No. 71685 between the National Academy of Sciences and the American Cancer Society. Any opinions, findings, conclusions, or recommendations expressed in this publication are those of the authors and do not necessarily reflect the view of the organizations or agencies that provided support for this project.

Library of Congress Cataloging-in-Publication Data

Institute of Medicine (U.S.). Committee on Cancer Control in Low- and Middle-Income Countries.

Cancer control opportunities in low- and middle-income countries / Committee on Cancer Control in Low- and Middle-Income Countries, Board on Global Health ; Frank A. Sloan and Hellen Gelband, editors.

p. ; cm.

Includes bibliographical references.

ISBN-13: 978-0-309-10384-8 (pbk.)

ISBN-10: 0-309-10384-3 (pbk.)

1. Cancer—Developing countries—Prevention. 2. Cancer—Economic aspects—Developing countries. 3. Cancer—Prevention—International cooperation. I. Sloan, Frank A. II. Gelband, Hellen. III. Title.

[DNLM: 1. Neoplasms—prevention & control. 2. Developing Countries. 3. Health Care Rationing. 4. International Cooperation. 5. Neoplasms—economics. QZ 200 I43845 2006]

RA645.C3I55 2006

362.196'9940091724—dc22

2006100723

Additional copies of this report are available from the National Academies Press, 500 Fifth Street, N.W., Lockbox 285, Washington, DC 20055; (800) 624-6242 or (202) 334-3313 (in the Washington metropolitan area); Internet, http://www.nap.edu.

For more information about the Institute of Medicine, visit the IOM home page at: **www.iom.edu.**

Printed in the United States of America.

The serpent has been a symbol of long life, healing, and knowledge among almost all cultures and religions since the beginning of recorded history. The serpent adopted as a logotype by the Institute of Medicine is a relief carving from ancient Greece, now held by the Staatliche Museen in Berlin.

"Knowing is not enough; we must apply.
Willing is not enough; we must do."

—Goethe

INSTITUTE OF MEDICINE

OF THE NATIONAL ACADEMIES

Advising the Nation. Improving Health.

THE NATIONAL ACADEMIES

Advisers to the Nation on Science, Engineering, and Medicine

The **National Academy of Sciences** is a private, nonprofit, self-perpetuating society of distinguished scholars engaged in scientific and engineering research, dedicated to the furtherance of science and technology and to their use for the general welfare. Upon the authority of the charter granted to it by the Congress in 1863, the Academy has a mandate that requires it to advise the federal government on scientific and technical matters. Dr. Ralph J. Cicerone is president of the National Academy of Sciences.

The **National Academy of Engineering** was established in 1964, under the charter of the National Academy of Sciences, as a parallel organization of outstanding engineers. It is autonomous in its administration and in the selection of its members, sharing with the National Academy of Sciences the responsibility for advising the federal government. The National Academy of Engineering also sponsors engineering programs aimed at meeting national needs, encourages education and research, and recognizes the superior achievements of engineers. Dr. Wm. A. Wulf is president of the National Academy of Engineering.

The **Institute of Medicine** was established in 1970 by the National Academy of Sciences to secure the services of eminent members of appropriate professions in the examination of policy matters pertaining to the health of the public. The Institute acts under the responsibility given to the National Academy of Sciences by its congressional charter to be an adviser to the federal government and, upon its own initiative, to identify issues of medical care, research, and education. Dr. Harvey V. Fineberg is president of the Institute of Medicine.

The **National Research Council** was organized by the National Academy of Sciences in 1916 to associate the broad community of science and technology with the Academy's purposes of furthering knowledge and advising the federal government. Functioning in accordance with general policies determined by the Academy, the Council has become the principal operating agency of both the National Academy of Sciences and the National Academy of Engineering in providing services to the government, the public, and the scientific and engineering communities. The Council is administered jointly by both Academies and the Institute of Medicine. Dr. Ralph J. Cicerone and Dr. Wm. A. Wulf are chair and vice chair, respectively, of the National Research Council.

www.national-academies.org

COMMITTEE ON CANCER CONTROL IN LOW- AND MIDDLE-INCOME COUNTRIES

FRANK A. SLOAN *(Chair)*, Center for Health Policy, Law & Management, Duke University, Durham, NC
DAVID CLARK, International Observatory on End of Life Care, Institute for Health Research, Lancaster University, Lancaster, England
HAILE T. DEBAS, Global Health Sciences, University of California at San Francisco
ELMER E. HUERTA, Cancer Preventorium, Washington Cancer Institute at Washington Hospital Center, Washington, DC
PRABHAT JHA, University of Toronto Centre for Global Health Research, St. Michael's Hospital, Toronto, Canada
DAVID E. JORANSON, Pain and Policy Studies Group, University of Wisconsin Comprehensive Cancer Center, Madison
RANJIT KAUR, Reach to Recovery International and Breast Cancer Welfare Association, Kuala Lumpur, Malaysia
KATHLEEN HARDIN MOONEY, University of Utah College of Nursing, Salt Lake City
TWALIB A. NGOMA, Ocean Road Cancer Institute, Dar es Salaam, Tanzania
D.M. PARKIN, Clinical Trial Service Unit and Epidemiological Studies Unit, Oxford University, England
RICHARD PETO, Clinical Trial Service Unit and Epidemiological Studies Unit, Oxford University, England
YOUCEF M. RUSTUM, Roswell Park Cancer Institute, Buffalo, NY
BHADRASAIN VIKRAM, International Atomic Energy Agency, Vienna, Austria (at IAEA until June 2006)

Consultant

IAN MAGRATH, International Network for Cancer Treatment and Research, Brussels, Belgium

Staff

HELLEN GELBAND, Study Director
PATRICK KELLEY, Director, Board on Global Health
ROGER HERDMAN, Director, National Cancer Policy Forum
PENNY SMITH, Research Associate (until October 2005)
ALLISON BRANTLEY, Project Assistant (since October 2005)

Reviewers

This report has been reviewed in draft form by individuals chosen for their diverse perspectives and technical expertise, in accordance with procedures approved by the NRC's Report Review Committee. The purpose of this independent review is to provide candid and critical comments that will assist the institution in making its published report as sound as possible and to ensure that the report meets institutional standards for objectivity, evidence, and responsiveness to the study charge. The review comments and draft manuscript remain confidential to protect the integrity of the deliberative process. We wish to thank the following individuals for their review of this report:

Eduardo Cazap, Sociedad Latinoamericana y del Caribe de Oncologia Medica, Buenos Aires, Argentina
Susan J. Curry, University of Illinois at Chicago School of Public Health
Silvia Franceschi, International Agency for Research on Cancer, Lyon, France
Robert A. Hiatt, University of California at San Francisco Comprehensive Cancer Center
Edward Katongole-Mbidde, Uganda Virus Research Institute, Entebbe, Uganda
Donald Kenkel, Cornell University, Ithaca, NY
Gerald T. Keusch, Boston University School of Public Health, Boston, MA
Lawrence S. Lewin, Chevy Chase, MD
Shahla Masood, University of Florida, Jacksonville
M.R. Rajagopal, Pallium India,Thiruvananthapuram, India

Raul C. Ribeiro, St. Jude Children's Research Hospital, Memphis, TN
Roberto Rivera-Luna, Instituto Nacional de Pediatria, Mexico City, Mexico
Sylvia C. Robles, The World Bank, Washington, DC

Although the reviewers listed above have provided many constructive comments and suggestions, they were not asked to endorse the conclusions or recommendations nor did they see the final draft of the report before its release. The review of this report was overseen by **David R. Challoner,** University of Florida, Gainesville. Appointed by the National Research Council, he was responsible for making certain that an independent examination of this report was carried out in accordance with institutional procedures and that all review comments were carefully considered. Responsibility for the final content of this report rests entirely with the authoring committee and the institution.

Preface

In high-income countries, cancer has received considerable public attention because it is one of the major causes of mortality, morbidity, and disease burden. In middle- and particularly in low-income countries, cancer has received less public attention because other diseases, especially infectious diseases, have historically been far more pressing. Although less prominent in relative terms, as this report documents, cancer is a major burden in low- and middle-income countries (LMCs) today.

In the future, it is inevitable that cancer will be a more important issue in LMCs. As the competing risk of infectious disease declines, major chronic diseases, including cancer, will move to the forefront as contributors to poor health. Furthermore, to the extent that LMCs adopt the health behaviors of populations in high-income countries, the incidence of chronic diseases such as cancer will increase.

If cancer is to be an even greater health problem in the future, given other pressing social priorities, why should LMCs be concerned about it now? First, it is already a greater burden than is widely appreciated. Second, establishing capacity for cancer prevention, diagnosis, and treatment in a country takes time. Third, some cancers can be prevented, and the latency period from the cause to the development of cancer can be several decades. Tobacco use is a case in point. The vast majority of tobacco use is initiated before age 21. Yet most of the deleterious effects of such use occur after age 50. A message of this report is that countries can implement effective policies for reducing tobacco use in their countries, and they can do this rather inexpensively.

This report is about "opportunities." The committee's concept of opportunity is broad, ranging from data collection and planning to resource-level-appropriate interventions. We did not use cost-effectiveness or cost-benefit analysis to rank individual projects. There is likely to be important variation in benefits relative to costs between low- and middle-income countries, and within countries in each category.

The concept of "resource-level-appropriateness" is central to this report. For the lowest income countries, where most people first present to the health care system with late-stage cancers, cure is usually impossible. Yet much more can be done than at present to promote palliative therapies to improve the quality of life of those who have incurable cancers, particularly near the end of life. At the other end of the spectrum is cancer prevention, which includes educating the public about what they can do to avoid cancer. Some approaches to prevention identified in the report are not costly and are within the ability of lower income countries to finance, sometimes with external assistance.

Investments in cancer diagnosis and treatment should vary depending on resources available in the country. A temptation that high-income countries should resist is focusing on exporting the latest, most expensive technologies that may (or may not!) be appropriate for wealthy countries, but for which alternatives exist that may be preferred in low-, and in some cases, middle-income countries. Partnerships are needed between high-income and other countries in developing resource-appropriate strategies. These partnerships may be government to government, but there is great potential for private partnerships, involving, for example, academic health centers in high-income countries and delivery sites in low- or middle-income countries. The report describes such opportunities. We hope it will prove a valuable resource, not only for the report's sponsors—the National Cancer Institute and the American Cancer Society—for considering how best to use existing knowledge to develop strategies for cancer control that recognize differences among countries in both resources and health care services delivery.

Frank A. Sloan
J. Alexander McMahon Professor of
Health Policy and Management and
Professor of Economics
Duke University

Project Consultants and Commissioned Authors

Benjamin O. Anderson, University of Washington and Fred Hutchinson Cancer Research Center, Seattle
Michael Barton, University of New South Wales, Australia
Vinona Bhatia, University of California at San Francisco Comprehensive Cancer Center
Robert W. Carlson, Stanford University, Stanford, CA
Mariana De Santis, National University of Cordoba, Argentina
Jorge Eisenchlas, Universidad del Salvador, Buenos Aires, Argentina
Alexandru E. Eniu, Cancer Institute I. Chiricuta, Cluj-Napoca, Romania
Michael Frommer, University of Sydney, Australia
Nigel Gray, Victoria, Australia
Ednin Hamzah, Hospis Malaysia, Kuala Lumpur, Malaysia
Diwani Msemo, Ocean Road Cancer Institute, Dar es Salaam, Tanzania
Jesmin Shafiq, University of New South Wales, Australia
Leslie Sullivan, Fred Hutchinson Cancer Research Center, Seattle, WA
Tatiana Vidaurre Rojas, Instituto Especializado de Enfermedades Neoplásicas, Lima, Peru
John Ziegler, University of California at San Francisco Comprehensive Cancer Center

Contents

Summary 1

1 Introduction 17
2 Cancer Causes and Risk Factors and the Elements of Cancer Control 27
3 The Cancer Burden in Low- and Middle-Income Countries and How It Is Measured 69
4 Defining Resource-Level-Appropriate Cancer Control 106
5 Preventing Cancers (and Other Diseases) by Reducing Tobacco Use 138
6 Compelling Opportunities in Global Cancer Control 170
7 Palliative Care 225
8 Cancer Centers in Low- and Middle-Income Countries 253
9 Advocacy for Cancer Control 272
10 Expanding the Role of the Global Community in Cancer Control 285

Appendixes

A Cancer Control in Malaysia and Tanzania 305
B Acronyms and Abbreviations 322

Summary

Cancer is absent or low on the health agendas of low- and middle-income countries (LMCs), and minimally represented in global health efforts in those countries. Even as other chronic diseases—cardiovascular disease and mental disorders, in particular—have gained attention in LMCs, cancer is largely left untouched. Cancer is common everywhere and growing as a share of the burden of disease. Eleven million cases of cancer now occur annually worldwide, six million of them in LMCs. Four million deaths from cancer—one million more than deaths from AIDS—have occurred each recent year in LMCs.

Determining health priorities and allocating resources are national decisions. In LMCs, however, these decisions are deeply influenced by priorities of the "global health community"—the public- and private- (for-profit and not-for-profit) sector agencies and organizations that provide advice, assistance at a variety of levels, products and services, and financial support for health and health care. As the burden of cancer and other chronic diseases increases, LMCs and the global community at large should be increasing resources proportionately, yet this has not happened to any noticeable degree.

The National Cancer Institute and the American Cancer Society—two organizations that have recognized the need to raise awareness about and take action against cancer in LMCs—asked the Institute of Medicine to conduct this study and provided the funding for it. The report calls for governments, health professionals, nongovernmental organizations (NGOs), and others in LMCs, with the help of the global health community, to achieve a better understanding of the current and future burden of cancer in LMCs and to take appropriate and feasible next steps in cancer control. Steps taken now—particularly in prevention—will be rewarded by curbing the growth in cancer rates. Steps taken toward establishing effective cancer diagnosis and treatment (i.e., cancer management), even if modest, can act as a nucleus from which development can grow.

"Low- and middle-income countries" include a wide range of nations vastly different in available resources, in rates of economic growth, in political and social conditions, and in the history and current status of health care services and infrastructure. They range from the low-income countries (defined by the World Bank as having a per capita gross national income—GNI—of less than $825 in 2004) where cancer control activity is minimal or nonexistent, to the upper middle-income countries (defined as having a GNI per capita of $3,256–$10,065) where most of the population may have access to at least some cancer services (Figure S-1).

This report does not suggest a single prescription for these diverse countries, nor does it envision "comprehensive" cancer control being possible without significant improvements in health care systems. Rather, it recognizes certain global priorities and approaches that are feasible at low resource levels, in the context of national cancer control planning. However, without assistance from the broader global health community—the same span of public- and private-sector agencies and organizations involved in traditional developing country health issues such as infant mortality, child and maternal health, tropical infectious diseases, and HIV/AIDS—it is unlikely that countries will be able to make substantial progress in cancer control. Thus, the recommendations in this report are aimed equally at LMCs and the global health and international development communities.

CANCER IN LOW- AND MIDDLE-INCOME COUNTRIES

Cancer is common everywhere. However, the mix of cancers that occurs varies around the world, driven largely by environment, geography, and standard of living. Cancer is also regarded differently in different settings: as a preventable and often curable disease in high-income countries; but as a painful death sentence in many LMCs.

The rise in cigarette smoking has made lung cancer the most common cancer, and cause of death from cancer in LMCs, just as it is in high-income countries in men and overall. Breast cancer is the most common cancer in women in both LMCs and high-income countries. Among men in LMCs, cancers of the stomach and liver are next most common and among women, cancers of the cervix and stomach.

Most cases of stomach and liver cancers, and nearly all cases of cervical cancer are caused by infectious agents: the bacterium *Helicobacter pylori*, hepatitis B and C viruses, and human papillomaviruses, respectively. In

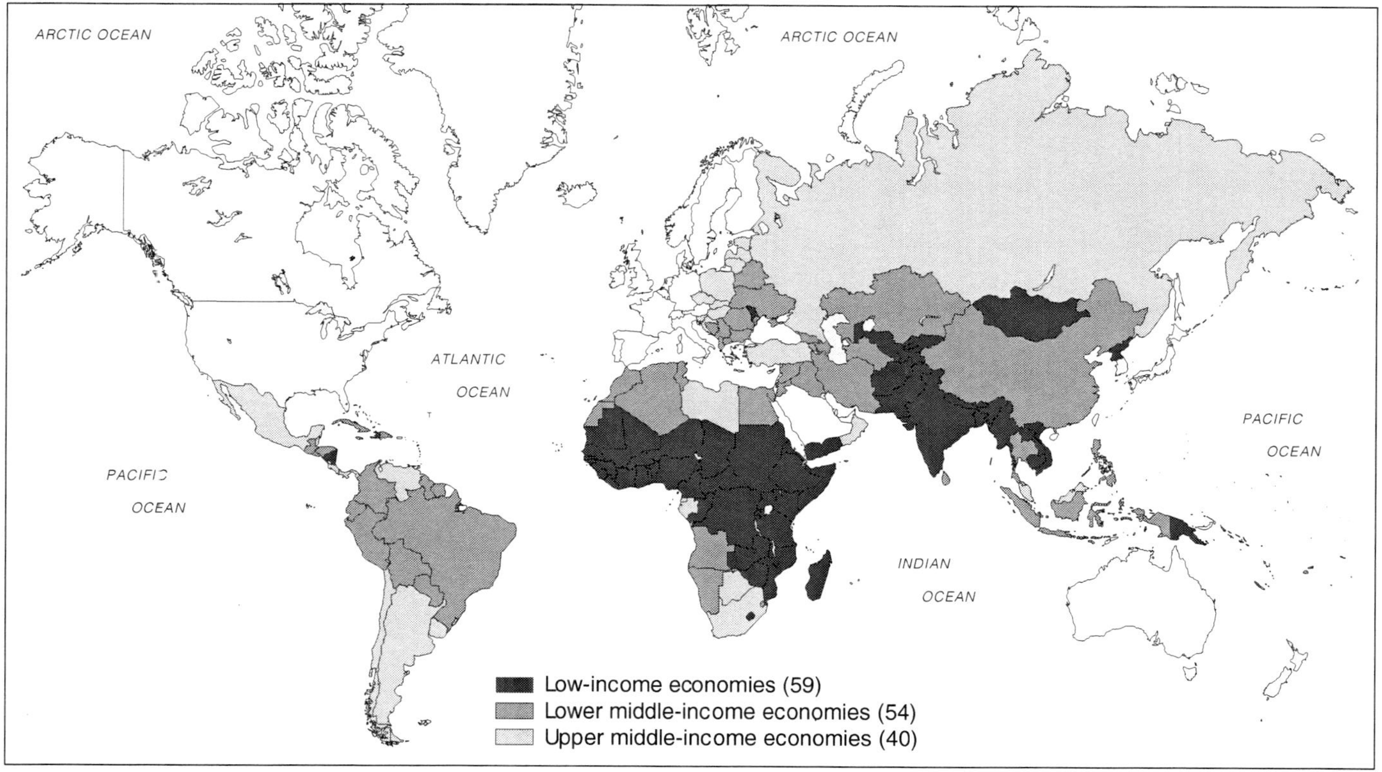

FIGURE S-1 Low- and middle-income countries by World Bank income category, 2004.
SOURCE: Data from World Bank (2005).

developing countries, 26 percent of all cancers are attributable directly to infectious agents; in high-income countries, the corresponding figure is only about 8 percent.

Cancer stage at the time of detection in LMCs is, on average, substantially further advanced than in wealthy countries. In some countries, as much as 80 percent of cancers may already be incurable when first noted (although this figure is impossible to document). Patients in LMCs also tend to have additional health conditions (co-morbidities) that make their recovery from cancer less likely than patients in high-income countries. Wherever they are, whatever their circumstances, these are real people—adults and children—living with and dying from cancer, with all the pain and misery that it brings.

NEXT STEPS IN CANCER CONTROL

"Cancer control" describes the totality of activities and interventions intended to reduce the burden of cancer in a population, either by reducing cancer incidence or mortality, or by alleviating the suffering of people with cancer. Prevention, early detection, diagnosis, treatment, psychosocial support, and palliative care are the components of cancer control that can reduce the cancer burden. Surveillance and monitoring are needed to understand the cancer burden and to track progress. All of these require commitments of financial and human resources, including training and education to build the required human resource base, and information for the public to understand what they can do and the services available to them.

Cancer control activities are not all conducted within the health care system proper, nor do they always involve only health professionals. Many effective tobacco control interventions (e.g., higher taxes, bans on advertising and promotion) are legal and regulatory in nature. Making morphine available for pain control necessarily involves narcotics control authorities as well as the health care system. Other key interventions are allied to parts of the health care system that otherwise are unrelated to cancer. For example, vaccination against hepatitis B virus to prevent liver cancer is conducted by childhood immunization programs. Where cancer shares risk factors with other chronic diseases—tobacco being by far the most important, but also including diet—control measures will produce benefits for a number of diseases. Within the health care system, some aspects of cancer control can be integrated into primary and higher level health care levels (e.g., vaccinations for HBV and human papillomavirus [HPV]), and others require specialized practitioners and equipment (especially aspects of treatment).

From high-income countries, it is obvious that the array of cancer control interventions is huge once basic infrastructure is in place and financing is plentiful. In LMCs, where those conditions do not exist, cancer control must build starting with interventions that are highly effective, cost-effective, and "resource-level appropriate." Additional steps can always be taken for incremental benefits once a cancer control culture exists and resources for cancer control grow.

Cancer Planning

Deciding on national cancer control priorities is best accomplished through a formal process of cancer control planning at the national (or, if appropriate, the subnational) level. Emphasizing the importance of this step, the 58th World Health Assembly (WHA) in May 2005 approved a resolution on cancer prevention and control that calls on all 192 WHO Member States to develop national cancer plans and programs. Although they must eventually be embraced by government to be fully effective, national cancer plans may be developed outside of government, such as those spearheaded by NGOs. Regardless of how the effort is led, the process must involve a broad spectrum of stakeholders and interest groups. Steps in cancer control planning have been well described by WHO and additional guidance is available from the International Union Against Cancer (UICC) (with particular emphasis on the role of NGOs in the development of national cancer plans) and other sources. The plan does not have to cover every aspect of cancer control: e.g., an initial focus on tobacco control and palliative care can lead to success in those areas and open the door to adding further goals later.

> **RECOMMENDATION. Cancer control plans should be developed, or updated, in each country every 3 to 5 years through a process that involves all major stakeholders, public and private sectors, as described by WHO, UICC, and others.** *Cancer control plans should be promoted and supported financially and programmatically through both government action and public advocacy. In both the planning and implementation phases, global partners should provide necessary guidance and financial support.*

OPPORTUNITIES FOR CANCER CONTROL IN LMCs

The following sections identify high-priority opportunities for cancer control in LMCs.

Prevention

Tobacco Control

At a global level, tobacco causes more premature deaths from cancer—and even greater numbers from other causes—than any other single agent. Experience in many high-income countries and a few LMCs has proven that tobacco use and ultimately, its impact, can be reduced substantially through a combination of policy measures. These policy measures include raising prices of tobacco products by increasing taxes on them, banning smoking in public places, banning advertising and promotion of tobacco products, requiring large and dramatic cigarette package warnings, and "counteradvertising" to publicize the adverse health effects of tobacco and the benefits of quitting. The top priority for cancer control is to convince the world's 1.1 billion smokers (80 percent of whom live in LMCs) to quit: Cessation by today's smokers will lead to substantial health gains over the next five decades. Preventing children from starting smoking will have full benefits after 2050. The Framework Convention on Tobacco Control (FCTC), the first and only international public health treaty, includes the measures known—largely from high-income countries—to be effective. As provisions of the FCTC are implemented in LMCs, it will be important to reevaluate their effectiveness under a range of economic and societal conditions.

RECOMMENDATION. Every country should sign and ratify the Framework Convention on Tobacco Control and implement its provisions, most importantly:

- *Substantial increases in taxation to raise the prices of tobacco products (goal is to have taxes at 80 percent or higher of retail price)*
- *Complete advertising and promotion bans on tobacco products*
- *Mandating that public spaces be smoke free*
- *Large, explicit cigarette packet warnings in local languages (which also helps to reduce smuggling)*
- *Support of counteradvertising to publicize the health damage from tobacco and the benefits of stopping tobacco use*

Liver Cancer and Hepatitis B Vaccination

HBV is the cause (often in conjunction with a co-factor) of most cases of liver cancer, taking 500,000 lives each year globally. A safe and highly effective HBV vaccine has been used in most high-income countries and many LMCs since the 1990s, yet vaccination coverage is poor to nonexistent in many countries with the highest rates of liver cancer. In 2001, the latest year for which complete data are available, fewer than 10 percent of babies in Southeast Asia and Africa—among the worst affected areas—were vaccinated against HBV.

A three-dose series of HBV vaccines costs less than $2 through UNICEF, a cost that can be subsidized by the Global Alliance for Vaccines and Immunization (GAVI). The countries where children are not immunized are mainly those with inadequate immunization programs for the more traditional vaccines, thus this is not a problem only for HBV vaccination. The future payoffs for HBV vaccination and other scheduled immunizations are enormous; vaccination should remain as high on the cancer control agenda as it is on the child health agenda.

Vaccination cannot help the 360 million people worldwide who are currently infected with HBV. However, limiting exposure to the most ubiquitous co-factor—aflatoxin—can substantially lower the risk of liver cancer. Contamination of stored grain by aflatoxin—a chemical produced by certain fungi under humid storage conditions—can be reduced by using low technology techniques such as drying crops in the sun, discarding moldy kernels, and storing crops in natural fiber sacks on wooden pallets. Such efforts may be worthwhile, although they are more complex than vaccination. Furthermore, about one-quarter of liver cancer is caused by hepatitis C virus (HCV) for which there is, as yet, no successful vaccine.

RECOMMENDATION. GAVI and other international partners should continue to assist countries to incorporate HBV vaccination into their childhood immunization programs as quickly as possible, with support from the global cancer community.

RECOMMENDATION. Countries with a high liver cancer burden and significant aflatoxin contamination of foodstuffs should examine the options for aflatoxin exposure reduction. *Development partners should help to implement those measures that are feasible and cost-effective.*

Cervical Cancer Screening and Human Papillomavirus Vaccines

Nearly 300,000 women die from cervical cancer each year, 85 percent of them in LMCs. The cause is persistent infection with one of several strains of the human papillomavirus (HPV). A century ago, cervical cancer was as common in the United States and Europe as it is today in LMCs. Improved living standards, effective treatment for early and somewhat advanced cancers, and screening using the Papanicolaou (Pap) smear are responsible for the steep decline in incidence and mortality in high-income countries.

Two developing strategies could transform cervical cancer control in LMCs: (1) vaccines to prevent HPV infection, and (2) screening methods that are more compatible with LMC resources and infrastructure than are Pap smear programs. A vaccine against the two most common carcinogenic strains of HPV entered the market in 2006 and another is expected soon. The initial market is in affluent countries; however, if adopted, the greatest impact of these vaccines will be in LMCs with highest cervical cancer rates. They could prevent of hundreds of thousands of deaths every year, starting several decades after establishment of a vaccination program. Governments and the international health community should take concrete steps now to develop HPV immunization policies and the means to pay for what is currently an expensive vaccine. Operational issues (e.g., developing immunization schedules, including the optimal age for immunization; deciding whether to immunize only girls or both girls and boys) also must be addressed.

For pre-vaccination generations of women, the vaccines cannot help. However, two new approaches to screening and treatment of pre-cancerous lesions are available. Techniques for testing and treatment of precancerous lesions in a single visit, using "direct visualization" (either visualization with coloration with acetic acid [VIA] or with Lugol's iodine [VILI]) have been piloted in trials in LMCs, with positive results. The treatment (for women without advanced disease) is by cryotherapy—freezing of abnormal tissue. Ongoing demonstration projects will provide a firmer information base on which to decide about the suitability and effectiveness of these techniques for broader use. The second technique involves testing for chronic HPV infection. HPV testing currently requires two visits if treatment is needed, but quick-reading tests are being developed that could eliminate the need for a second visit. While these screening methods may be feasible in some settings (mainly middle-income countries), they can only be successful where a reasonable healthcare infrastructure exists and care for detected cancers can be accessed, a requirement that, unfortunately, still excludes many countries. Where they are feasible, the value of such programs can be great: Even one or two appropriately timed screenings in a lifetime could reduce the incidence of invasive cervical cancer by as much as 40 percent.

RECOMMENDATION. Countries should actively plan for the introduction of HPV vaccination as more information becomes available about the vaccines and as they become affordable. The international community should support a global dialogue on HPV vaccine policy and pricing.

RECOMMENDATION. Countries and global partners should follow the evolving information on newer screening approaches and determine the feasibility of adoption, given local resources and infrastructure.

Cancer Management: Diagnosis, Treatment, and Psychosocial Support

In low-income countries, most people with cancer have no access to potentially curative treatment. In middle-income countries, existing services and resources are variable but generally limited. Where few or no services exist, the emphasis should be on establishing a core of expertise and limited cancer management that can be expanded as resources permit. Where some services are available but resources are stretched or inadequate, the emphases should be as follows: (1) ensuring that the most appropriate and most cost-effective measures are provided in well-equipped medical institutions and futile attempts at cure are avoided, and (2) ensuring that the stage is set for services to expand.

Along with clinical medical services, people with cancer and those around them benefit from psychosocial support to deal with the physical, psychological, and social impacts of the disease and improve quality of life. Psychosocial support can commence at diagnosis and continue through treatment and recovery or death. In LMCs, psychosocial support can be offered by a wide range of health care workers and lay people.

Resource-Level-Appropriate Treatment for Curable Cancers

The concept of "resource-level appropriateness" recognizes that effective interventions for the most curable cancers have progressed in high-income countries through more than one generation. The most appropriate choice for an LMC may not be the current choice in New York or Paris. For example, breast-conserving surgery for early-stage breast cancer requires treatment with radiotherapy. If radiotherapy is not available, women's lives can still be saved with more extensive surgery. Comprehensive information on the range of choices is rarely available, however. The major exception is the result of a recent, highly innovative effort, the Breast Health Global Initiative (BHGI).

The BHGI is an international collaboration initiated by an American breast surgeon who eventually attracted a wide range of partners from both high-income and lower income countries. Financial support initially came from a foundation devoted to breast cancer with later support from the National Cancer Institute (NCI) and others. BHGI has produced a comprehensive set of resource-specific, stage-specific evidence-based guidelines, which will be updated biannually, for all aspects of breast cancer management.

The BHGI process involved "summit" meetings with expert researchers, practitioners, and patients from all over the world. A next phase that is under way involves helping centers in LMCs adopt, adapt, and implement the guidelines, and developing procedures for implementation so that the guidelines can be disseminated widely.

The BHGI model could be applied to other cancers for which highly effective treatments are available. The common cancers that fit this description are cancers of the breast, cervix, head and neck, and colon and rectum. A large proportion of cancers affecting children and young adults are also highly curable, in particular, leukemias and lymphomas, retinoblastoma, and testicular cancer. A hurdle in organizing such efforts will be financial support. The BHGI was able to begin and build because of early support from the Susan J. Komen Foundation, the most visible breast cancer advocacy group in the United States. Advocacy does exist for all the cancers in the list above, but they are not as powerful as the forces that have massed against breast cancer. The BHGI example, however, has laid groundwork that should make it easier for public sector sources, professional societies, advocacy organizations, and others to support efforts for other cancers.

> **RECOMMENDATION. Resource-level-appropriate guidelines should be developed for the overall management of major cancers for which treatment can make a substantial difference in a meaningful proportion of patients, and for selected pediatric cancers.** *The BHGI model could be used or others developed. The priority adult cancers for which resource-level-specific guidelines are needed are cervical cancer, colon cancer, and head and neck cancers. Pediatric priority cancers are leukemias and lymphomas. Motivated professionals from high-income countries and LMCs should work together to spearhead these efforts, with financial support from a variety of institutions.*

Cancer "Centers of Excellence"

Providing guidelines for cancer diagnosis and treatment is of no benefit without a medical institution and professionals who can apply them. Countries should consider supporting at least one well-functioning government-supported cancer center where patients can go for diagnosis, treatment, palliation, and vital psychosocial services. The center should also undertake locally relevant research. Even if capacity is limited, such centers can act as focal points for national cancer control and as points of contact for the international cancer control and clinical oncology communities. In the poorest countries, and in small countries that wish to develop this capacity, the center may be a unit in a hospital, focusing only on selected aspects of treatment or on specific types of cancer. In countries that already have one or more cancer centers, it may only require enhancing the functions of one or more center.

Financing to initiate and operate cancer centers in LMCs can come from a variety of public and private sources, including taxes on tobacco products.

Some international support is available for establishing or upgrading cancer centers. A new organizational unit of the International Atomic Energy Agency (IAEA), building on a 25-year history of support for radiotherapy, is the Programme of Action for Cancer Therapy (PACT), which is intended to attract additional funding and collaboration from United Nations Member States and other donors. PACT is likely to be a major source of new and upgraded cancer centers for at least the next decade. Radiotherapy remains a centerpiece, but PACT intends to develop and maintain equivalent capability in medical and surgical oncology.

Institutional "twinning" is an approach that should see expanded use in improving and expanding cancer control in LMCs. Twinning involves long-term pairings of established cancer centers with new or existing centers in LMCs. Hallmarks of successful twinning programs are regular exchanges of information and often personnel, attention to funding (although not necessarily money flowing from the high-income partner), training, and technical issues. The oncology community is well organized in affluent countries and has the capacity to help to organize twinning programs.

A special opportunity and responsibility is the treatment of children and young people with specific highly curable types of cancer. The total numbers are small compared with cancers in adults—approximately 160,000 children and young adults get cancer every year, worldwide. Currently, 80 percent of U.S. children under age 15 with cancer are cured, but 80 percent of the world's children who develop cancer live in countries where most die because of late diagnosis and lack of treatment.

> **RECOMMENDATION. Countries should consider establishing a government-supported cancer "center of excellence" that provides resource-level-appropriate services to the public and acts as a reference point for national cancer control.** *This could be a new center or designation of an existing one.*

> **RECOMMENDATION. International partners should assist in developing and improving cancer centers in LMCs through twinning arrangements and other means.** *The recently formed PACT, established by the IAEA, could—in collaboration with a range of partners—take on this role. Financial contributions from national governments (research funding institutions and bilateral aid agencies) could be channeled into this effort as a means of progressively increasing the global donor community's investments in cancer control in LMCs in ways likely to have the biggest impact.*

> **RECOMMENDATION. Countries should aim to provide access to treatment and psychosocial services for children and young adults**

with highly curable cancers in pediatric cancer units in cancer centers or children's hospitals.

Palliative Care

Late diagnosis of most cancers in LMCs and a lack of treatment options even when diagnosis is early means large numbers of patients who can benefit from palliative care. The cornerstone of palliative care is pain control with oral morphine or other strong opioid analgesics. These medications are largely unavailable in LMCs (and in many high-income countries); in addition to medication, palliative care involves a range of other services to relieve and manage symptoms and to provide psychosocial support to patients and families in the communities where they live. The two major obstacles to palliative care in LMCs are (1) legal, societal, and educational barriers to opioid availability; and (2) lack of programs to deliver palliative care at the community level. Progress in the past 10 years has demonstrated that barriers to opioid availability can be overcome and that palliative care can be delivered effectively and inexpensively, even in LMCs.

A major barrier to making morphine available to cancer patients in severe pain is the irrational fear of opioids that continues to exist among policy makers, regulators, law enforcement, health professionals, and the public. WHO and the International Narcotics Control Board (INCB) play key roles in educating relevant parties and encouraging governments to examine their national policies for unduly strict drug regulations. International collaborations and the provision of funding are vital to continued progress. Because people dying from AIDS require much the same palliative care as do cancer patients, building or adapting organizations to serve both types of patient presents a new set of opportunities.

RECOMMENDATION. Governments should collaborate with national organizations and leaders to identify and remove barriers to ensure that opioid pain medications, as well as other essential palliative care medications, are available under appropriate control. *The INCB and WHO should provide enhanced guidance and support, and assist governments with this task.*

RECOMMENDATION. Palliative care, not limited to pain control, should be provided in the community to the extent possible. *This may require developing new models, including training of personnel and innovations in types of personnel who can deliver both psychosocial services and symptom relief interventions.*

Surveillance and Monitoring

Few LMCs have accurate, recent data about their cancer burden or major risk factors for cancer, consistent with generally poor vital and health statistics. *Estimates* of cancer incidence and mortality by cancer type, age, and gender have been produced for every country by the International Agency for Research on Cancer (IARC). These estimates are useful for setting initial priorities, but cannot be used to track progress or to define priorities.

Major improvements in vital and health statistics are long term goals, but over the short term, modest improvements can be made. In particular, it is relatively inexpensive to gather information on the major risk factors for cancer and other noncommunicable diseases in periodic cross-sectional surveys. WHO has developed standardized survey instruments in "STEPS," a Stepwise Approach to Chronic Disease Risk Factor Surveillance. Questionnaire-based data gathering about tobacco use, alcohol consumption, diet, and physical activity constitute the first "step." Steps 2 and 3 add physical and physiological measurements of risk factors for the other major chronic diseases: weight and blood pressure measurements; and blood glucose and cholesterol, respectively. STEPS has the advantage of producing comparable information across countries as well as over time.

More ambitious is measuring causes of death in a population. In low-income countries in particular, this is difficult because many people die without medical care, or at least without a diagnosis. Systems based on "verbal autopsies" can be developed in place of medical certification, as has been demonstrated in India's "Million Death Study," in areas that constitute a nationally representative sample of deaths.

Longitudinal studies of chronic disease risk factors and causes of death involving in total several million people have been initiated as collaborations between researchers in LMCs and high-income countries. Results have already been produced in a few LMCs such as China, India, and Mexico. In these studies, adults are interviewed briefly about major risk factors (e.g., smoking, diet) and have basic physical measurements taken (and blood, in some cases). Households are revisited periodically to record household members' vital status, and the participants are resurveyed every 3 to 5 years. When cohort members die, the cause of death is ascertained. Such studies are complex, requiring extensive planning and the sustained commitment of human and financial resources. Studies now under way cost on average $1 per person per year to maintain.

Finally, cancer registries that record cancer cases and outcomes over time—in specific hospitals, or more usefully, in defined geographic areas—are important for understanding local cancer patterns of those who come to medical attention. Registries require sustained commitments and trained personnel, which are most feasible in urban areas where diagnosis and treatment are available.

RECOMMENDATION. The following should be considered:

- **Risk factor surveillance** *for chronic diseases should be initiated in many countries using standardized questionnaires (e.g., STEPS).*

- **Collection of cause-specific mortality data should be a long-term goal in every country.** *Where vital statistics systems are weak or nonexistent, initial data collection may be in sentinel sites rather than nationwide. Improved mortality reporting at a level appropriate to the country should be supported as a part of cancer control activities.*

- **Longitudinal studies of chronic disease risk factors and mortality should be initiated in a few additional middle-income countries.**

- **Cancer registries should be developed in conjunction with cancer control activities,** *mainly in urban areas where diagnostic and treatment services exist. Where new or existing cancer centers are developed into centers of excellence, registries in the catchment area should be a part of the development.*

The Global Community

Cancer control will not advance in LMCs without support from the global health and development community for the invariably small constituencies within these countries. Multilateral and bilateral aid agencies, foundations and other philanthropies, professional organizations and the academic community all have roles to play in developing the global cancer control agenda, working with countries to prioritize and plan next steps, and providing resources to carry out plans. With a few exceptions (e.g., tobacco control and to a lesser extent, palliative care), cancer control has had little support while the infectious and nutritional diseases have dominated the efforts of the global health community.

Thus far, it has been cancer-specific organizations or units that have promoted cancer control in LMCs. WHO's small cancer program has continued to provide guidance and other parts of WHO headquarters have taken up specific cancers or types of exposures. IARC has played the leading role in defining the causes of cancer and in surveillance, largely to the benefit of high-income countries, with spillover benefits to LMCs, as well as some efforts, particularly in recent years, more directed to LMC problems (e.g., an emphasis on cervical cancer in LMCs). In the private non-profit sector, the International Union Against Cancer, largely devoted to cancer control and advocacy in resource-rich countries, has become more active in LMCs in recent years. The broader global health community has, by and large, not followed.

Another major untapped resource is the burgeoning interest in global health at universities in the United States and other countries. The recent formation of many global health programs should be seen as an opportunity to expand the topic areas in which these units work. For this to happen, faculty and administrators must become aware of new types of projects, in cancer and other areas, that are possible, in addition to the traditional emphases on infectious and nutritional diseases. Cancer centers in the United States and other wealthy countries also may not be aware of opportunities for twinning and other collaborations with centers in LMCs.

RECOMMENDATION. *International Organizations*
WHO should maintain a strong capacity for cancer control analysis and guidance to assist the many countries that rely on them for health-related information and policy advice. *Capacity is needed both at WHO headquarters and in the regional offices.*

RECOMMENDATION. *Development Assistance*
The bilateral aid agencies, including the U.S. Agency for International Development, should consider adding aspects of cancer control to their discussion agendas with LMCs, *and adding funding for specific projects that fit into national cancer control plans and programs.*

RECOMMENDATION. *Advocacy*
Established cancer advocacy organizations, mainly in high-income countries, should actively support and assist the growth of cancer advocacy in LMCs. *Specific activities would include setting up advocacy networks within countries, within regions and internationally; identifying successful approaches to cancer advocacy and replicating or adapting them for use in other settings; and providing hands-on training and technical assistance.*

RECOMMENDATION. *National Institutions*
The U.S. National Cancer Institute and other established cancer research and funding organizations both in the United States (e.g., the Centers for Disease Control and Prevention) and in other countries should help to establish and facilitate relationships between U.S. cancer centers and centers in LMCs *and encourage U.S. researchers, through grant programs, to undertake collaborative research of relevance to LMCs.*

RECOMMENDATION. ***The Academic Community***
Universities with active global health programs should consider opportunities in cancer control, as well as the more traditional areas of focus. *If a university consortium is developed, one function should be to encourage and facilitate a broader agenda of topics, cancer control among them.*

1

Introduction

You are a 38-year-old woman with abnormal vaginal bleeding because of early-stage cervical cancer. In 4 years, will you be living the rest of your life with little interruption after a lifesaving, low-risk hysterectomy, or dying far from home with advanced and painful cancer, an outcast from friends and family? If you have adequate resources, either because you live in a high-income country or have personal wealth, it is unlikely that you would have found yourself in this situation at all—with early-stage cervical cancer. In the United States, for example, periodic screening with a Pap smear would have detected *precancerous* changes years before, and the abnormal tissue would have been removed in a minimally invasive procedure. But if you are poor and come from a rural village in a low-income country such as Tanzania, the next 4 years will be agonizing physically and psychologically, and crippling financially as you try again and again to get help. You are unlikely to have anything to ease the pain of your final days.

How could this scenario turn out differently, in Tanzania or other resource-limited countries, in the short-to-medium term? Rewinding the story, the 38-year-old woman could have reached the cancer center in the city months sooner, had she not been discouraged by traditional healers, family, and friends. She could have been cared for and lived a full life. Even at a somewhat advanced stage, cervical cancer is curable by radiotherapy, which is practicable and available in many low- and middle-income countries (LMCs) at an affordable cost. If her story could be fast forwarded a decade, she could be screened at age 30 or 35 using one of the single-visit "screen-and-treat" approaches now beginning to gain an evidence base. The slow-progressing lesion on her cervix could have been removed and normal life resumed after possibly a month of some discomfort. In the worst case, if the cervical cancer progressed anyway and eventually led to death, her final days could have been relatively free of pain and her other basic physical, psychological, and emotional needs met by village palliative care workers and family—services already available in some parts of Africa. If the 38-year-old has a daughter entering adolescence, that daughter soon might be able to get a vaccine that will protect her against cervical cancer by preventing its cause, infection with human papillomavirus (HPV). Even in LMCs, these alternate endings are possible, with increased global awareness of the magnitude of the cancer problem, the opportunities that exist already, and those just around the corner.

The long view back over the 20th century in the United States and other wealthy countries, where the picture of cancer incidence and mortality is reasonably clear, gives perspective and reason for optimism that the cancer burden can be lessened in LMCs today.

REASONS FOR OPTIMISM

Over the course of the 20th century, the cancer burden changed dramatically—positively and negatively—in the United States and other wealthy countries. Changing lifestyles, environmental influences, and improved health care all have contributed. In 1900, cancer was eighth in the list of causes of death.[1] By 1950, it was second only to heart disease. Cancer death rates continued to rise through the early 1990s, when overall rates were nearly three times the 1900 rate (National Cancer Institute, 1997). The single greatest cause of the cancer increase was the rise in lung cancer from tobacco use. While lung cancer (and other smoking-related cancers) increased, rates for other cancers were falling. Death rates for stomach cancer—the most frequent cause of cancer deaths early in the 20th century—fell by nearly 90 percent over that period, with the greatest declines occurring in the 1950s. The reasons are thought to be improved living conditions, which reduced chronic infection with the cancer-inducing bacterium *Helicobacter pylori*, and better diet, including more fresh and less preserved food. Treatment of stomach cancer is still relatively ineffective, so medical care contributed little. The story is different for cervical cancer, which claimed more women's lives than any other cancer in the United States in the early 1900s. Declines in death rates began early, again probably due to better living conditions. Death rates decreased quickly and were driven to their current low levels by early detection and curative medical care.

After the earlier continuous increases, by the early 1990s, lung cancer

[1]This statistic is adjusted for the age structure of the population, so it is not simply a reflection of a larger older population.

death rates among U.S. men had declined, following several decades of concerted action against smoking. (The epidemic in women began later and may now be plateauing.) Overall cancer death rates also declined by a few percentage points, reflecting the combined effects of improved environmental conditions, healthier lifestyle choices, and better medical care (Wingo et al., 2003).

The changes that have been seen in wealthy countries during the past century and into this century, and the knowledge gained about the causes of cancer and preventive and other interventions, are evidence that control measures can be effective. These changes and knowledge provide goals for practicable cancer control measures for LMCs that can begin to be established widely over the next few decades, once the opportunities are recognized and pursued. With the growing recognition that chronic, noncommunicable diseases are increasing in importance in LMCs, the time is right to move forward.

The remainder of this chapter introduces the need for greater focus on cancer (and other chronic diseases), defines low- and middle-income countries, and describes the intent and framework of the report.

CANCER AND OTHER CHRONIC DISEASES

> The lives of far too many people in the world are being blighted and cut short by chronic diseases such as heart disease, stroke, cancer, chronic respiratory diseases and diabetes. This is no longer only happening in high income countries. Four out of five chronic disease deaths today are in low and middle income countries.
>
> *J.W. Lee, Director General, World Health Organization*
> *October 2005*

Chronic diseases have recently been called "the neglected epidemic" (Strong et al., 2005). Even the United Nations Millennium Development Goals—the vehicle for improving the health and welfare of the world's poorest starting at the beginning of the 21st century—mention only the major infectious diseases by name. But that has begun to change. The World Health Organization (WHO) has begun a campaign to raise the profile of chronic diseases in LMCs, recognizing that these countries suffer the double burden of the major infectious disease killers and mounting chronic illnesses. WHO dispels the idea that we can wait to conquer infectious diseases before turning to chronic diseases. The two must be addressed simultaneously.

Greater efforts at cancer control in LMCs have long been promoted by those in the cancer community. The WHO cancer program has played its role by providing guidance for governments; the broader cancer interest community, including the International Union Against Cancer and its mem-

TABLE 1-1 World Bank Classification of Countries by Income Level, 2004

Classification	Income Boundaries Gross National Income per Capita
Low income	$825 or less
Lower middle-income	$826–$3,255
Upper middle-income	$3,256–$10,065
High income	$10,066 or more

SOURCE: World Bank (2005).

bers, has reached out to the public and professionals. However, international health efforts historically have been dominated by the immediate problems of infectious diseases that kill infants and children. It is largely the progress made against those diseases that has led to the aging of the global population and the greater impact of chronic diseases.

LOW- AND MIDDLE-INCOME COUNTRIES DEFINED

This report uses the World Bank classification of countries by income level (Table 1-1, Figure 1-1, and Box 1-1). This grouping of LMCs takes in most of the world's population—all but the wealthy countries—and represents a broad spectrum of development. The low-income countries are relatively similar in health profiles and services. This is not so true of the middle-income countries, however. These countries have different levels of infrastructure, different histories, and a much wider range of per-capita health spending. For low-income and some middle-income countries, the challenge is to add services from a very low base. For at least some of the middle-income countries—the emerging economies of Eastern and Central Europe, in particular—the challenge is to upgrade an existing infrastructure that may not provide the most appropriate services and that could become more efficient. In all cases, planners must consider the costs of services and who will pay. Each country must evaluate its own needs and opportunities, regardless of the income rubric in which it falls, and plan accordingly. This report highlights major global opportunities in cancer control that are relevant to most countries regardless of their current situation. It does not prescribe the actions that should be taken by those countries.

INTENT OF THIS REPORT

This report is intended to highlight major opportunities for LMCs toward better cancer control—cancer planning, cancer prevention and early

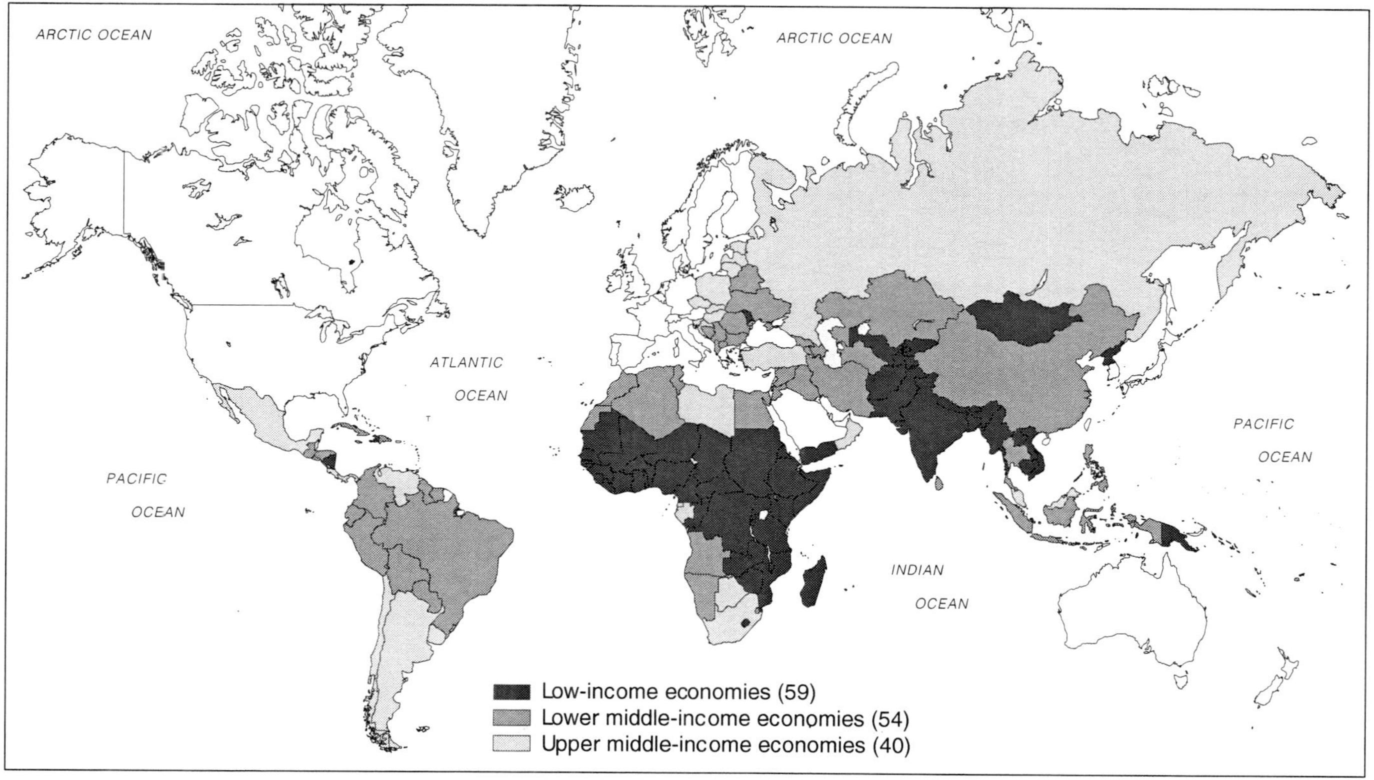

FIGURE 1-1 Low- and middle-income countries by World Bank income category, 2004.
SOURCE: Data from World Bank (2005).

BOX 1-1
Low- and Middle-Income Countries by Category According to 2004 Gross National Income Per Capita

Low-income economies (59): $825 or less

Afghanistan	Haiti	Pakistan
Bangladesh	India	Papua New Guinea
Benin	Kenya	Rwanda
Bhutan	Korea, Dem. Rep.	Sao Tome and Principe
Burkina Faso	Kyrgyz Republic	Senegal
Burundi	Lao PDR	Sierra Leone
Cambodia	Lesotho	Solomon Islands
Cameroon	Liberia	Somalia
Central African Republic	Madagascar	Sudan
Chad	Malawi	Tajikistan
Comoros	Mali	Tanzania
Congo, Dem. Rep.	Mauritania	Timor-Leste
Congo, Rep.	Moldova	Togo
Cote d'Ivoire	Mongolia	Uganda
Eritrea	Mozambique	Uzbekistan
Ethiopia	Myanmar	Vietnam
Gambia, The	Nepal	Yemen, Rep.
Ghana	Nicaragua	Zambia
Guinea	Niger	Zimbabwe
Guinea-Bissau	Nigeria	

Lower middle-income economies (54): $826–$3,255

Albania	El Salvador	Namibia
Algeria	Fiji	Paraguay
Angola	Georgia	Peru
Armenia	Guatemala	Philippines
Azerbaijan	Guyana	Romania
Belarus	Honduras	Samoa

detection (screening), cancer management (diagnosis and treatment, including palliative care) and psychosocial support for patients and families—even where resources are limited. Whatever the status quo, next steps are feasible everywhere. The report is written to bring this message to policy makers in LMCs as well as the many global partners involved in international health, as cancer becomes an ever-widening global health concern. One conclusion of the report—echoing what others have stated—is that cancer is a global disease, and global cooperation and collaboration will allow all countries to move forward. Knowledge sharing among the high-income countries enjoys

BOX 1-1 Continued

Lower middle-income economies continued

Bolivia
Bosnia and Herzegovina
Brazil
Bulgaria
Cape Verde
China
Colombia
Cuba
Djibouti
Dominican Republic
Ecuador
Egypt, Arab Rep.
Indonesia
Iran, Islamic Rep.
Iraq
Jamaica
Jordan
Kazakhstan
Kiribati
Macedonia, FYR
Maldives
Marshall Islands
Micronesia, Fed. Sts.
Morocco
Serbia and Montenegro
Sri Lanka
Suriname
Swaziland
Syrian Arab Republic
Thailand
Tonga
Tunisia
Turkmenistan
Ukraine
Vanuatu
West Bank and Gaza

Upper middle-income economies (40): $3,256–$10,065

American Samoa
Antigua and Barbuda
Argentina
Barbados
Belize
Botswana
Chile
Costa Rica
Croatia
Czech Republic
Dominica
Equatorial Guinea
Estonia
Gabon
Grenada
Hungary
Latvia
Lebanon
Libya
Lithuania
Malaysia
Mauritius
Mayotte
Mexico
Northern Mariana Islands
Oman
Palau
Panama
Poland
Russian Federation
Seychelles
Slovak Republic
South Africa
St. Kitts and Nevis
St. Lucia
St. Vincent and the Grenadines
Trinidad and Tobago
Turkey
Uruguay
Venezuela, RB

a long history among private-sector advocates and cancer control health professionals in and out of government. The sponsors of this report—the U.S. National Cancer Institute (part of the National Institutes of Health) and the American Cancer Society—are among the global leaders in research, training, and advocacy.

The report is not a how-to manual that prescribes specific interventions, a role left best to WHO, the health care professions, and others. Instead, it shines a light on areas of great opportunity that countries should at least be aware of, that could lessen the current and growing burden of cancer.

Reflected in the report framework outlined below, the opportunities include aspects of prevention; services to patients who have cancer, at whatever stage; and building cancer capacity. No report on the global cancer problem could ignore the growth in tobacco use in LMCs, guaranteeing an epidemic of cancer, cardiovascular disease, and respiratory disease, *if* known effective actions are not taken now to curtail tobacco use. Global awareness of the hazards of tobacco has never been higher. Many people in LMCs still have not heard that message, but are beginning to hear messages about the glamor of taking up smoking.

The opportunities that exist for tackling some of the leading causes of death from cancer are less well known. Most liver cancers—among the most numerous and deadly—can be prevented by simple childhood immunization. Future generations can be protected against cancer of the cervix, also caused by a virus, with a new vaccine.

Current generations can be saved with simple, yet highly effective, screening techniques. Treatment for children and young adults with highly curable cancers has been an attractive way to build cancer management infrastructure, guaranteeing success for some significant proportion and demonstrating that cancer does not have to be a death sentence, a message that will be new to many citizens of LMCs. But when death from cancer is inevitable, for adults and children, feasible and inexpensive palliative care to ease symptoms vastly improves the comfort of patients and those around them.

Beyond the specific interventions, a way forward has been demonstrated to tailor cancer control to differing resource levels, maintaining a focus on evidence of effectiveness and appropriateness to the setting. This "resource-level appropriate" approach ties in with recommendations about cancer centers and centers of excellence as focal points for cancer control where none now exists.

All of the opportunities identified are feasible at least in some LMCs. We recognize, however, that undertaking new initiatives and moving existing ones forward requires a long view and a sustained commitment. There are no quick fixes in cancer control, but the payoffs will come for appropriate, effective efforts put in place today in LMCs, with the support of the global health community.

FRAMEWORK OF THE REPORT

The remainder of the report consists of the following chapters:

2. Cancer Causes and Risk Factors and the Elements of Cancer Control
Major and minor causes of and risk factors for cancer in LMCs as a basis for setting the control agenda. The broad elements of cancer control: cancer

planning, cancer prevention and early detection (screening), cancer management—diagnosis and treatment, including palliative care—and psychosocial support for patients and families.

3. **The Cancer Burden in Low- and Middle-Income Countries and How It Is Measured** The best available data on incidence and mortality from cancer in LMCs, trends in the leading types of cancer, the availability of relevant data, and opportunities for improving understanding of the cancer burden.

4. **Defining Resource-Level-Appropriate Cancer Control** "Resource-level appropriateness" introduced, using the example of the Breast Health Global Initiative. An approach to applying this idea to other cancers is presented.

5. **Preventing Cancers (and Other Diseases) by Reducing Tobacco Use** The impact of tobacco use, and the evidence for reducing tobacco use through a series of public policy and personal interventions.

6. **Compelling Opportunities in Global Cancer Control** Opportunities in three areas: (1) furthering the global agenda to eliminate most deaths from liver cancer through universal vaccination against the hepatitis B virus; (2) eliminating most cervical cancers through a combination of new screening techniques and vaccination against HPV, the cause of virtually all cervical cancers; and (3) developing the capacity to treat curable cancers in children and young adults.

7. **Palliative Care** The status of palliative care in LMCs, and feasible and cost-effective measures that can be taken to extend pain control and other measures much more broadly, even in very low-resource environments.

8. **Cancer Centers in Low- and Middle-Income Countries** The role of cancer centers—from modest to sophisticated, as appropriate to available resources—as a path to move forward in cancer control. "Centers of excellence" are proposed as hubs for national cancer control planning and programs, as well as cancer management.

9. **Advocacy for Cancer Control** Needs and opportunities for stepping up advocacy efforts in LMCs. Advocacy from the public and health professionals has played a critical role in advancing cancer control in the United States and other high-income countries, a lesson that should be transferred to LMCs.

10. **Expanding the Role of the Global Community in Global Cancer Control** The "global community"—governments, academia, the private sector—and

their roles in helping LMCs set and carry out their health care agendas, which thus far have lacked a focus on cancer.

Appendix A. Cancer Control in Malaysia and Tanzania Profiles of cancer control in Malaysia (an upper middle-income country) and Tanzania (a low-income country) from papers by cancer professionals in those countries, commissioned by IOM.

Appendix B. Acronyms and Abbreviations.

REFERENCES

National Cancer Institute. 1997. *A New Agenda for Cancer Control Research: Report of the Cancer Control Review Group*. Bethesda, MD: National Cancer Institute.

Strong K, Mathers C, Leeder S, Beaglehole R. 2005. Preventing chronic diseases: How many lives can we save? *Lancet* 366(9496):1578–1582.

Wingo PA, Cardinez CJ, Landis SH, Greenlee RT, Ries LA, Anderson RN, Thun MJ. 2003. Long-term trends in cancer mortality in the United States, 1930–1998 [erratum appears in *Cancer* 103(12):2658]. *Cancer* 97(12 Suppl):3133–3275.

World Bank. 2005. *World Development Indicators 2005*. Washington, DC: World Bank.

2

Cancer Causes and Risk Factors and the Elements of Cancer Control

A logical way to identify cancer control opportunities is to consider what we know about the causes and risk factors for common cancers, and then to consider how easy or difficult it is to eliminate or modify them in ways that would reduce cancer incidence. Where the causes or risk factors are not well understood, are only weak, or cannot readily be changed, the opportunities lie in how easy or difficult it is to "cure" people who get cancer or to care for those with cancer who cannot be cured.

This chapter starts with a review of the causes and known risk factors for the most common cancers in low- and middle-income countries (LMCs), with discussion of the modifiability of these causes and risk factors. The latter part of the chapter is a general review of the approaches to cancer control, beginning with cancer control planning, then prevention and the elements of cancer management (diagnosis and treatment): psychosocial care, radiotherapy, chemotherapy, and surgery. Chapter 7 is devoted entirely to palliative care, the other major pillar of cancer management, so that area is not covered in this chapter.

CAUSES OF AND RISK FACTORS FOR CANCER IN LMCS

Knowing the causes of cancer provides a basis for understanding the potential for preventing cancer. If a cause is known, it is much easier to know whether it can (e.g., tobacco use) or cannot (e.g., ionizing radiation in the atmosphere) be avoided easily. An accounting of the causes also shows up the gaps in knowledge—for example, few specific causes of colon cancer are known. Table 2-1 lists the major risk factors for the top 10 causes

TABLE 2-1 Leading Risk Factors for Cancer Deaths in LMCs (or Developing Countries) and Primary Prevention Strategies

Cancer Type (number of deaths in LMCs in 2002)	Main Risk Factors	Theoretical Minimum Exposure Distribution	Primary Prevention: Currently Available Strategies	PAF %
Lung, trachea, and bronchus (770,938)	Tobacco use	Zero exposure possible	Tobacco control as outlined in Framework Convention on Tobacco Control (FCTC)	60
	Low fruit and vegetable intake	600 grams/day fruit and vegetable intake for adults	Dietary improvements	13
	Urban air pollution	7.5 μg/m^3 for particles with aerodynamic diameters <2.5 microns 15 μg/m^3 for particles with aerodynamic diameters <10 microns	Regulation of automobile exhaust and industrial combustion products	7
	Indoor smoke from cooking and heating	Zero exposure possible	Ventilation and improved low-technology heating and cooking	2
	Radon in buildings (from the earth)	NGE	Building regulations to avoid radon seepage into enclosed buildings, mainly in cold climates	NGE
	Various occupational exposures	NGE	Workplace regulation and controls	9[b]

TABLE 2-1 Continued

Cancer Type (number of deaths in LMCs in 2002)	Main Risk Factors	Theoretical Minimum Exposure Distribution	Primary Prevention: Currently Available Strategies	PAF %
Stomach (695,426)	Chronic infection with *Helicobacter pylori*	Zero exposure possible	Improved living conditions (nonspecific) Future: Vaccine to prevent infection? Future: Drugs to clear infection?	74[a]
	Low fruit and vegetable intake	600 grams/day fruit and vegetable intake for adults	Dietary improvements	19
	Tobacco use	Zero exposure possible	Tobacco control as outlined in FCTC	11
Liver (504,407)	Chronic hepatitis B (HBV), mainly from infection in infancy and childhood; co-factors, such as fungal toxins (e.g., aflatoxin)	Zero exposure possible	Hepatitis B vaccination in infancy Reduced fungal contamination of stored grains Future: Cure of chronic HBV?	59[a]
	Chronic hepatitis C (HCV) from contaminated blood and unsafe injections, and person to person; co-factors such as fungal toxins (e.g., aflatoxin)	Zero exposure possible	Blood supply and injection safety and measures Future: Cure of chronic HCV?	33[a]
	Alcohol use	Zero exposure possible	Reduced alcohol use	23
	Tobacco use	Zero exposure possible	Tobacco control as outlined in FCTC	11

continued

TABLE 2-1 Continued

Cancer Type (number of deaths in LMCs in 2002)	Main Risk Factors	Theoretical Minimum Exposure Distribution	Primary Prevention: Currently Available Strategies	PAF %
Colon and rectum (356,949)	Physical inactivity	At least 2.5 hours/ week of moderate-intensity activity or equivalent (4,000 KJ/week)	Lifestyle changes	15
	Overweight and obesity	BMI (weight/height^2) of 21	Dietary improvements and exercise	9
	Low fruit and vegetable intake	600 grams/day fruit and vegetable intake for adults	Dietary improvements	2
Esophagus (379,760)	Tobacco use	Zero exposure possible	Tobacco control as outlined in FCTC	37
	Alcohol use	Zero exposure possible	Reduced alcohol use	24
	Low fruit and vegetable intake	600 grams/day fruit and vegetable intake for adults	Dietary improvements and exercise	19
Breast (317,195)	Physical inactivity	At least 2.5 hours/ week of moderate-intensity activity or equivalent (4,000 KJ/week)	Exercise	10
	Overweight and obesity	BMI (weight/height^2) of 21	Dietary improvements and exercise	7
	Alcohol use	Zero exposure possible	Reduced alcohol use	4
Mouth and oropharynx (271,074)	Tobacco use	Zero exposure possible	Tobacco control as outlined in FCTC	37
	Alcohol use	Zero exposure possible	Reduced alcohol use	14
Uterine cervix (218,064)	Chronic infection with specific strains of human papillomavirus (HPV)	Zero exposure possible	Screening for precancerous stages Vaccination against HPV in infancy or adolescence	100
	Tobacco use	Zero exposure possible	Tobacco control as outlined in FCTC	2

TABLE 2-1 Continued

Cancer Type (number of deaths in LMCs in 2002)	Main Risk Factors	Theoretical Minimum Exposure Distribution	Primary Prevention: Currently Available Strategies	PAF %
Lymphomas and multiple myeloma[a]	Burkitt's lymphoma (7,800 cases in children in less developed countries): chronic infection with Epstein-Barr virus	Very low exposure possible	None apparent	NGE
Leukemia (190,059)	Ionizing radiation (natural and medical)	Low medical exposure possible; lower radon exposure possible	Improved medical practices Improved building practices to exclude radon	NGE
	Tobacco use	Zero exposure possible	Tobacco control as outlined in FCTC	6
	Various occupational exposures	Lower exposures possible (varying by exposure)	Workplace regulation and controls	2[b]

NOTE: PAFs from the *Global Burden of Disease and Risk Factors* (Lopez et al., 2006) unless otherwise noted. The Institute of Medicine did not independently recalculate these figures. These PAFs refer to fractions of *deaths*, and the denominator is all cancer deaths in LMCs (as defined by the World Bank)—about 5 million deaths. The fractions reported from Parkin (Parkin, 2005) refer to *cases* in developing countries (as defined by the World Health Organization), which total about 6 million. These two types of figures are approximately, but not strictly, comparable. For purposes of this table, however, together they provide a relatively accurate overview of the major risk factors for cancers and cancer deaths.
PAF = Population attributable fraction, which is the proportional reduction in disease that would occur if population exposure to the risk factor were reduced to the theoretical minimum risk level. Many cancers are affected by more than one risk factor (e.g., tobacco and alcohol combining to greatly increase the risk of esophageal cancer); elimination of one or another could prevent a particular cancer from occurring. This means that the PAFs are not mutually exclusive, and added together will generally overestimate the cancer reduction possible by eliminating all identified risk factors.
NGE = No global estimate available.

[a]Data from Parkin (2005).
[b]Data from Rosenstock et al. (2006); refers to worldwide PAF, compared with zero exposure, with no breakdown by country economic level.

SOURCES: Lopez et al. (2006); Parkin (2005); and Institute of Medicine.

of cancer death in LMCs, with their "population attributable fractions" (PAFs). Table 2-2 summarizes the impact of these risk factors for all cancers in LMCs. The PAF represents the proportion of cancer deaths that could be prevented if the risk factor or exposure were reduced to a theoretical minimum. For a number of major risk factors, a zero level of exposure is at least theoretically possible. These include: tobacco use, alcohol use (but see below), indoor smoke from cooking, most carcinogenic infectious agents (if not zero exposure, vastly reduced from current levels). For other factors, zero exposure is not a relevant concept, such as for obesity or for inactivity. The values for those risk factors (from *Global Burden of Disease and Risk Factors*, Lopez et al., 2006) are based on an achievable level that would minimize the risk of all major diseases associated with that risk factor.

Heart disease, stroke, cancer, chronic respiratory diseases, and diabetes—the main chronic diseases—share some common risk factors (Epping-Jordan et al., 2005; WHO, 2005a). Tobacco smoking is overwhelmingly the most significant risk factor for cancer and across the board for chronic diseases. Diet, exercise, and alcohol use also cut across the diseases, and they are significant contributors to cancer, but more significant to other conditions. Of lesser global importance (but in some cases, very important focally), are factors such as occupational exposures to asbestos, coal, and other substances; indoor smoke from cooking and heating; and air pollution, which can cause cancer and a larger burden of chronic respiratory diseases. Beyond these factors, the common cancers in LMCs do not share significant risk factors with other chronic diseases. What stands out is the role of infections in common cancers of LMCs (discussed below). Cancer control will benefit from integrated approaches to chronic disease control, but cancer-specific strategies—which will have little or no impact on other chronic diseases—are also needed.

Table 2-1 describes the risk factors associated with *current* deaths from cancer. Because of the time scale of cancer, the pattern of deaths today reflects the distribution of risk factors some decades ago. For smoking, the peak in smoking-related deaths follows the peak in smoking rates by about 30 years (Figure 2-1). Today's smoking rates will determine the cancer rates 30 years hence. It is important, therefore, to know about levels and trends in risk factors for cancer control planning (see Chapter 3 for a discussion about monitoring risk factors).

Tobacco

Tobacco use is the largest single contributor to cancer mortality: It was a cause of nearly one-fifth of all cancer deaths in LMCs in 2002. It is also the leading cause of death from the totality of major noncommunicable diseases. Chapter 5 goes into considerable detail on the effects of tobacco and its control. What should be noted from Figure 2-1 is where the LMCs are on the epidemic curve. The low-income countries are all in either stage 1 or 2 (tobacco use still low but rising, first among males; tobacco-related deaths low and just beginning to rise), and the middle-income countries in stage 2 or 3 (tobacco use rising steeply or having peaked; mortality following). The challenge to tobacco control is to alter the trajectories in those countries by encouraging adults to quit smoking (benefits that appear in a very short timeframe) and discouraging young people from starting (the long-term solution). They do not have to follow the trajectory we now see in retrospect for the high-income countries. If they do, however, the number of deaths from tobacco will continue to increase steeply. In the year 2000, about 4.9 million deaths from all causes were related to tobacco, about half in developed and half in developing countries. In 2020, *if current trends continue*, 9 million people will die from tobacco-related causes, and 7 million of these will be in developing countries.

Infections

The three leading types of cancer-causing infections—hepatitis B virus (HBV) and hepatitis C virus, human papillomavirus (HPV), and *Helicobacter pylori*—follow tobacco in importance as risk factors for cancer incidence in developing countries. It is clear from their much lesser importance in high-income countries (responsible for an estimated 8 percent of all cancers, compared with 26 percent in developing countries) (Parkin, 2005) that the prevalence of these infections can be greatly reduced, although the means to do so differ. HBV is readily preventable by immunization. Preventing the spread of hepatitis C requires blood bank screening and safe injection practices, which is a more difficult set of interventions to implement. HPV-related cancers have been prevented in high-income countries largely through screening and treatment of precancerous lesions, but infection prevention is newly possible by vaccination as well. HBV- and HPV-related cancers represent immediate opportunities for preventing cancer in current generations.

H. pylori is one major cause of stomach cancer, a cancer that is poorly responsive to treatment. The prevalence of *H. pylori* (and stomach cancer) has declined dramatically without targeted measures in much of the world, suggesting the possibility of developing interventions for places where it is not declining, which includes most LMCs. At present, this is a research question focused on treatment of infected individuals with antibiotics that eradicate the bacteria. Work on vaccines is also reported to be progressing (Parkin, 2005). Progress depends on continued support of promising leads. *H. pylori* research is not pursued further in this report, however.

Other types of infection are locally important and account for about

TABLE 2-2 Summary of Major Risk Factors for All Cancers in LMCs (or Developing Countries)

Cancer Type (number of deaths)	Main Risk Factors	Theoretical Minimum Exposure Distribution
All cancers (~5 million cancer deaths)	Tobacco use	Zero exposure possible
	All carcinogenic infections	
	HBV and HCV	Zero exposure possible
	HPV	Zero exposure possible
	H. pylori	Zero exposure possible
	Low fruit and vegetable intake	600 grams/day fruit and vegetable intake for adults
	Alcohol use	Zero exposure possible
	Physical inactivity	At least 2.5 hours/week of moderate-intensity activity or equivalent (4,000 KJ/week)
	Overweight and obesity	BMI (weight/height^2) of 21
	Urban air pollution	7.5 μg/m^3 for particles with aerodynamic diameters <2.5 microns 15 μg/m^3 for particles with aerodynamic diameters <10 microns
	Indoor smoke from cooking and heating	Zero exposure possible

NOTE: PAFs from the *Global Burden of Disease and Risk Factors* (Lopez et al., 2006) unless otherwise noted. The Institute of Medicine did not independently recalculate these figures. These PAFs refer to fractions of *deaths*, and the denominator is all cancer deaths in LMCs (as defined by the World Bank)—about 5 million deaths. The fractions reported from Parkin (Parkin, 2005) refer to *cases* in developing countries (as defined by the World Health Organization), which total about 6 million. These two types of figures are approximately, but not strictly, comparable. For purposes of this table, however, together they provide a relatively accurate overview of the major risk factors for cancers and cancer deaths.
PAF = Population attributable fraction, which is the proportional reduction in disease that would occur if population exposure to the risk factor were reduced to the theoretical minimum

PAF %	Importance of Risk Factor to Other Serious Health Conditions
18	• Greater burden of cardiovascular disease • Approximately equivalent burden of chronic respiratory disease • Smaller but substantial burdens from other conditions
26[a]	
8.2[a]	Significant burden from other serious liver diseases from HBV and HCV
8[a]	Very small burden from other conditions
6.9[a]	
6	Much greater burden of cardiovascular disease
5	Much greater burden of injuries, neuropsychiatric conditions, cardiovascular conditions, and other causes
2	Much greater burden of cardiovascular and other noncommunicable diseases
1	Much greater burden of cardiovascular and other noncommunicable diseases
1	Greater burden of chronic respiratory disease
<0.5	Much greater burden of cardiovascular and chronic respiratory conditions

risk level. Many cancers are affected by more than one risk factor (e.g., tobacco and alcohol combining to greatly increase the risk of esophageal cancer); elimination of one or another could prevent a particular cancer from occurring. This means that the PAFs are not mutually exclusive, and added together will generally overestimate the cancer reduction possible by eliminating all identified risk factors.
NGE = No global estimate available.

[a]Data from Parkin (2005).

SOURCES: Lopez et al. (2006); Parkin (2005); and Institute of Medicine.

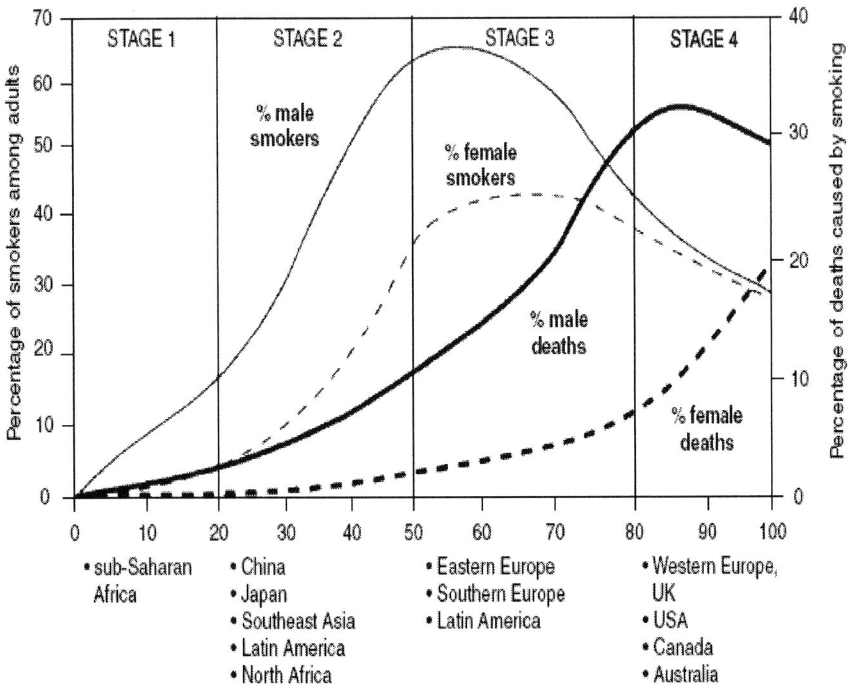

FIGURE 2-1 Four stages of the tobacco epidemic.
SOURCE: Reprinted, with permission, from Lopez et al. (1994). Copyright 1994 by BMJ Publishing Group Ltd.

4 percent of all cancers (Parkin, 2005). The most significant is Epstein-Barr virus, a risk factor for Burkitt's lymphoma and cancers of the nasopharynx, to which 2 percent of cancers in LMCs are attributable. Both of these cancers are much more common in developing than developed countries. Next in importance, the human immunodeficiency virus (HIV) is responsible for an estimated 62,500 cases of Kaposi's sarcoma in developing countries (about 1 percent of all cancers). Somewhat less than 1 percent of cancers are attributable to helminth (worm) infections, including bladder and possibly colorectal cancers ("limited" evidence, according to the International Agency for Research on Cancer, or IARC) (IARC, 1997) caused by schistosomes, and liver cancers caused by liver flukes. Finally, human T-cell lymphotropic virus type 1 (HTLV-1) is the cause of some non-Hodgkin's lymphomas.

It is worth noting that other infectious causes of cancer may be discovered. Current knowledge has been developed largely in the past 30 years. An organism as significant as *H. pylori* was not recognized until the 1980s, originally as the primary cause of gastritis and stomach ulcers, and it was classified as a human carcinogen by IARC only about a decade ago (IARC, 1997).

Diet, Overweight and Obesity, and Physical Inactivity

Diet, body weight, and activity levels are interrelated and seem to act in complex ways to either promote or reduce the risk of cancer. *Global Burden of Disease and Risk Factors* (Lopez et al., 2006) made separate estimates for the three components, based on the best available quantitative evidence and focusing on low fruit and vegetable intake as the best established specific dietary factor. Nine percent of cancer deaths in LMCs are attributable to these three factors, which could be the focus of interventions. As significant as these risk factors are for cancer, they are responsible for considerably greater disability and death from other causes: heart disease, hypertension and stroke, diabetes, and arthritis most important among them. These other conditions are at least five times as important as cancer in terms of disability-adjusted life-years (DALYs) (Lopez et al., 2006).

A high intake of fresh fruits and vegetables (generally excluding root vegetables and pulses (peas and beans), which have a higher carbohydrate content than other types of vegetables), has consistently been found in epidemiologic studies to be associated with lower cancer rates. Fruits and vegetables are generally low in calories (supply less than 5 percent of calories in most countries) and high in fiber, vitamins, minerals, and other active molecules. Studies that have looked at vegetables individually or in classes (categorized several different ways, either botanically or culinarily) have not been able to pinpoint more precisely which vegetables or fruits are more or less beneficial, or which components cause which effects. Eventually, this may be possible, but given the state of the science today, it is best to consider fruits and vegetables collectively (World Cancer Research Fund, 1997).

The evidence is convincing that an adequate intake of fruits and vegetables (for some cancers, mainly vegetables) lowers the risk of the following cancers: colon and rectum, lung, stomach, esophagus, and mouth and pharynx (IOM, 2003; World Cancer Research Fund, 1997). The risk of a number of other cancers also may be lowered, but the evidence is not as strong. Those with the strongest evidence are cancers of the larynx, pancreas, breast, and bladder. The strength of the totality of the research literature underlies the estimate that 6 percent of cancer deaths are attributable to low fruit and vegetable intake (Lopez et al., 2006).

Other estimates of cancers related to "diet and nutrition" are higher. IARC's 2003 *World Cancer Report* (Stewart and Kleihues, 2003) states: "Up to 30 percent of human cancers are probably related to diet and nutrition," using an expansive definition of diet and nutrition. The estimate also refers to the world as a whole, with no separate estimates for countries by income level. In addition to the effects of fruit and vegetable consumption and body weight, salt and salt-preserved food increase the risk of stomach and nasopharyngeal cancers (more important in LMCs than in high-income countries); red meat consumption appears to increase the risk of colorectal cancer (more important in high-income countries than in LMCs); and other factors, such as food additives, have a small overall effect.

Diet and physical activity are clearly very important determinants of cancer (although the specifics of the associations are not clear), and even more so for other major chronic diseases. However, interventions that are known to have a substantial effect on diet and exercise habits are not well established in high-income countries, where virtually all the documented efforts have been made (e.g., changing dietary composition, losing weight, or increasing exercise) (IOM, 2003). In LMCs, food availability, agriculture policies, and the much different lifestyles make this a difficult, though important, area to address in the context of integrated chronic disease control. WHO's "Global Strategy on Diet, Physical Activity and Health," which was endorsed by the May 2004 World Health Assembly, has made a series of recommendations based on the following principles (WHO, 2004):

- Stronger evidence for policy: synthesize existing knowledge, science and interventions on the relationship between diet, physical activity, and chronic disease.
- Advocacy for policy change: inform decision-makers and stakeholders of the problem, determinants, interventions, and policy needs.
- Stakeholder involvement: agree on the roles of stakeholders in implementing the global strategy.
- A strategic framework for action: propose appropriately tailored policies and interventions for countries.

This report concentrates on measures that are mainly or exclusively cancer related, so contains no specific recommendations in this area. Clearly, cancer control authorities in LMCs should join efforts to improve diet and encourage appropriate physical activity in their own countries.

Alcohol Use

Cancers of the oral cavity, pharynx, larynx, esophagus, liver, and breast can be caused by heavy alcohol drinking, with the risk varying by cancer site, but increasing for all sites with greater consumption and resulting in an estimated 5 percent of attributable cancer deaths in LMCs (Lopez et al., 2006). Similar to diet and physical activity, the disease burden from heavy alcohol consumption is several times greater for other conditions—cardiovascular disease, neuropsychiatric illness, and intentional and unintentional injuries—than for cancer in LMCs. What is different is that *moderate* alcohol consumption has the benefit of reducing cardiovascular risks, although this is documented only in high-income countries. The many acute social and psychological problems caused by excessive drinking must be added to the tally of harm from chronic conditions.

Certain interventions to curb heavy drinking have been effective in high-income countries, but have rarely been implemented in LMCs and even more rarely evaluated. Increased excise taxes, reduced access to stores selling alcoholic beverages, advertising bans, random breath testing for motor vehicle drivers, and brief advice to heavy drinkers from physicians are among the effective and cost-effective interventions known (Rehm et al., 2006). Applying these interventions in LMCs, however, will require tailoring to national and local cultural, social, and economic environments.

Occupational Exposures

Workplaces can be hazardous, whether they are factories, family farms, city streets, or any other formal or informal place of work. The International Labor Organization (ILO) estimates that 2 million deaths per year worldwide, among 2.7 billion workers, are attributable to workplace exposures. The burden of disease and disability is enormous, but data to support quantitative estimates are not available for most of the world (Rosenstock et al., 2006).

About 25 chemicals or mixed chemical exposures for which exposures are mostly occupational have been identified by IARC as established human carcinogens, and an equal number are probably carcinogenic (Stewart and Kleihues, 2003). The numbers of workers exposed and exposure levels are largely unknown, however. Certain patterns suggest that at least some hazardous exposures are becoming more frequent in LMCs, and that in general, with industrialization and globalization, occupational health problems are rising in these countries. An example is the relocation of manufacturing involving asbestos from high-income countries to countries such as Brazil, India, Pakistan, and the Republic of Korea, where occupational health control may be less stringent (Stewart and Kleihues, 2003). These operations are also more likely to be on a smaller scale than in high-income countries, often using older machinery and with limited protection for workers.

The World Health Organization (WHO) undertook a thorough assessment of worldwide data for five occupational risk factors, one of which was carcinogens (the others were risks for injuries, airborne particulates, ergonomic risks for back pain, and noise). All five together accounted for about 800,000 annual workplace-related deaths (about 40 percent of the 2 million estimated by ILO). Of these, 100,000 were lung cancers and 2,000 were leukemias, the most prevalent (but not the only) types of occupationally related cancers. By comparison, chronic obstructive pulmonary disease was responsible for about 318,000 deaths per year, behind injuries, the leading cause of occupational death.

The technical means exist to prevent a substantial portion of occupationally related cancers, as has happened in high-income countries. Implementing these preventive measures requires both the knowledge and a regulatory framework to enforce lower exposures. International (e.g., ILO and WHO) and national or state governments, as well as industry, have roles to play in this process. However, many impediments stand in the way of effective protection against workplace exposures to carcinogens and other hazards in LMCs, discussed in detail by Rosenstock and colleagues (Rosenstock et al., 2006). Improvements in occupational health go far beyond cancer control, and the activities necessary for it are largely outside the general health infrastructure.

Pollution

Pollution of the air (indoor and outdoor), water, and soil causes an estimated 1 to 4 percent of all cancers worldwide (Stewart and Kleihues, 2003). Even though the risk levels per person are quite low, the large numbers of people exposed—involuntarily—can mean a substantial population effect. For indoor and outdoor air pollution, lung cancer is the main cancer type implicated. Ambient air pollution is caused mainly by vehicular exhaust, which is a mixture of chemicals. While emission levels in high-income countries have tended to decline over recent decades, they are level or increasing in many LMCs. In poor rural areas of sub-Saharan Africa, and South Asia, East Asia, and the Pacific in particular, indoor air is polluted by heating and cooking fires, and fumes from cooked food. Coal and biomass, the smokiest fuels, are those used most frequently in these places. Much more widespread (but far less hazardous per person exposed) is indoor tobacco smoke. The number of cancer deaths caused by indoor and outdoor air pollution is exceeded by deaths from respiratory and some cardiovascular conditions in adults and deaths from acute respiratory infections in children.

Poor water quality is associated mainly with infectious diseases. Some cancers are probably caused by the by-products of chlorination used to purify water, and by arsenic, which occurs naturally in high concentrations in the soil in certain areas. Focal exposure to a variety of harmful compounds from industrial waste may also cause some cancers in local populations, but these are difficult to sort out and more difficult to quantify.

As with occupational exposures, the main means of reducing exposure to outdoor pollution is through regulation. Reduction of motor vehicle emissions and industrial emissions in air and water have been successful in high-income countries, and have probably produced health benefits, although the cancer prevention benefits have probably been modest. Reducing exposure to indoor air pollution from stoves requires specific policy actions. Those most affected are the poorest and most vulnerable in the population who have no financial means to improve their living conditions, including the use of cleaner fuels and better stoves. In a recent in-depth analysis, Bruce and colleagues (Bruce et al., 2006) reviewed programs over the past few decades aimed at reducing indoor air pollution. Lessons have been learned, but the situation globally has improved little. Various technologies are available, but making them available to those at highest risk, in a sustainable fashion, has proven very difficult.

Other Causes and Risk Factors

Food Contaminants

Apart from the substantial influence of macro- and micronutrients and energy balance in affecting the risk of cancer, food can be contaminated with naturally occurring or manmade carcinogens. The burden of cancer from food contaminants has not been estimated, but it is thought to be quite small globally (Stewart and Kleihues, 2003). The best known (and possibly most important) natural carcinogenic contaminants are mycotoxins produced by fungi, the best characterized of which are aflatoxins. Aflatoxins are produced by fungi of the genus *Aspergillus*, which live on grains and groundnuts (peanuts). Aflatoxins accumulate on these foods particularly if they are stored in hot, moist conditions. Certain aflatoxins and chronic infection with HBV together are the main risk factors for liver cancer in parts of Africa, Asia, and South America. Improved storage conditions can greatly reduce aflatoxin contamination (see Chapter 6).

Food can become contaminated with pesticides and other industrial chemicals either directly or as they move up the food chain. Possibly carcinogenic chemicals are also produced during cooking (e.g., polycyclic aromatic hydrocarbons, N-Nitroso compounds). Any of these could be locally important, but are difficult to detect and quantify, and no broad strategies are available for controlling them.

Medical Drugs

A small number of drugs—often intentionally powerful compounds—have been found to be carcinogenic. The largest group is, ironically, drugs used to treat cancer. Although they increase the risk of a cancer decades later, their immediate benefits outweigh that risk, which may be accepted knowingly. When carcinogenicity has been suspected or proven, other drugs for less serious conditions have been withdrawn (e.g., diethylstilbestrol [DES]) or restricted (e.g., phenacetin). Drugs with hormonal actions may increase some cancer risks (while decreasing others). Drugs with immunosuppressive effects may also increase the risk of certain cancers. The total global cancer burden attributable to medical drugs is thought to be small, and in LMCs, where drug use is limited, probably lower than the global average (Stewart and Kleihues, 2003).

Hormonal and Reproductive Factors

Sex steroid hormones (androgens, estrogens, progestogens) affect the development and growth of certain cancers in women, specifically, cancers of the breast, endometrium, and ovary. While oral contraceptives and hormone replacement therapy contribute to both increased and decreased risks, endogenous hormonal differences related to age at menarche and menopause, and reproductive history also contribute. It is well established that an early age at first birth protects women against cancers of the breast, endometrium, and ovary, and that having no children is associated with higher risks. Even obesity, which alters the circulating levels of various hormones, increases the risk of breast cancer in post-menopausal women, apparently at least in part through this mechanism (Stewart and Kleihues, 2003).

In men, the prostate is responsive to the hormone testosterone, the levels of which may vary and be associated with increased prostate cancer risk. Obesity is also associated with prostate cancer, and at least some of the risk may be mediated by an increase in an insulin-like growth factor (Stewart and Kleihues, 2003).

Risks posed by medical hormones can be reduced, if they are understood. The composition of birth control pills has, in fact, changed markedly both in dosages and combinations of hormones in response to health problems, including cancer, as they were identified. The burden of cancer attributable to these factors must be quite small, however.

Ionizing Radiation from Natural, Industrial, and Medical Sources

Everyone is exposed to ionizing radiation in the form of gamma rays from outer space and from global distribution of manmade gamma and X-radiation from nuclear weapons testing and nuclear reactor accidents (e.g., Chernobyl). Radon gas, which is a natural decay product of uranium from the earth, diffuses through the earth into the atmosphere, where it is ubiquitous. Outdoors, it disperses and is of little consequence. Where radon is concentrated and emerges into buildings that are relatively airtight, the exposure of residents can be substantial. Radon itself is inert, but its decay products include radioactive alpha particles that can lodge in the lung, causing damage near where they are deposited, and resulting in lung cancer in some people. A recent analysis of the available evidence from studies in Europe concluded that 9 percent of all lung cancer deaths—and 2 percent of all deaths from cancer *in Europe*—are attributable to residential radon. Most of these deaths are among smokers, whose risk is about 26 times that of nonsmokers (i.e., most of these deaths would be prevented by elimination of exposure to *either* smoking or radon) (Darby et al., 2005). No estimate of the importance of radon in LMCs has been made. In tropical, lower income countries, where houses are less likely to be tightly enclosed, exposure is likely to be lower than in colder cities. Radon can be largely excluded from buildings by relatively simple measures during construction, and by remedial measures in existing buildings. Most European and other high-income countries have guidelines for doing so (Darby et al., 2001). Although probably not a major problem in most LMCs, it could be locally important in certain areas. It is not a focus of this report, however.

Medical radiation from diagnostic X-rays and radiotherapy represents almost 40 percent of the global human exposure to ionizing radiation worldwide, but is likely to be substantially less in LMCs, where the use of these technologies is far lower.

Ultraviolet (UV) Radiation

Natural UV radiation from sunlight causes most cases of melanoma in the world (about 160,000 per year) (IARC, 2004) about 80 percent of which occur in North America, Europe, Australia, and New Zealand (Stewart and Kleihues, 2003). It is also the cause of most of the more numerous non-melanoma skin cancers, also predominantly in light-skinned populations and generally highly curable by excision. The obvious interventions to prevent UV-related cancer are sun avoidance, protective clothing and sunglasses, and sunscreen, measures that require public awareness and access to the physical items. UV-related cancer is a relatively small problem in most LMCs, and is not considered further in this report. However, some LMCs, e.g., in Eastern and Central Europe, do have significant light-skinned populations and may wish to prioritize UV exposure measures. The U.N. INTERSUN Programme provides comprehensive information and guidance for countries to protect their populations from UV-related cancers (WHO, 2003; 2006b).

Immunosuppression

The body's immune response plays a role in defending the body against cancer, a concept known mainly because certain cancers occur at a greatly increased prevalence among people whose immune systems are suppressed persistently. Medical drugs and certain infections are the most frequent immunosuppressants, with infections being more important in LMCs. The best known is HIV, which is associated with Kaposi's sarcoma, an otherwise rare cancer that is an AIDS-defining condition, and some non-Hodgkin's lymphomas. Immunosuppressive drugs given to organ transplant patients, to prevent rejection of the organ, are also associated with these cancers and some others. Transplant-associated cancers do not constitute a major problem globally, and are not preventable given current transplant standards. Cancers associated with AIDS, however, are largely preventable with standard antiretroviral therapies. In this case, AIDS control can make a significant contribution to cancer control.

Genetic Susceptibility

An increased risk of developing certain cancers can be inherited in the genetic material passed from generation to generation, accounting for up to 4 percent of all cancers worldwide (Stewart and Kleihues, 2003) (there is no separate estimate for LMCs). In some cases, a specific gene mutation can mean an extraordinarily high risk of cancer: women with certain mutations in the BRCA1 gene have a lifetime risk of about 70 percent of developing either breast or ovarian cancer. Fortunately, these and other mutations with such high penetrance are rare in the population as a whole. About 20 cancer syndromes caused by single gene defects are known. Probably more important, however, are susceptibilities—the genetic details of which are largely unknown—that increase cancer risks by much smaller amounts, but occur widely in the population. It is likely that interactions with the environment that cause additional chance mutations are key in whether cancer develops in people with these genetic traits. Strategies to prevent cancer or detect it early in people with genetic susceptibility are limited currently and do not represent major opportunities for cancer control in LMCs.

BASIC ELEMENTS OF CANCER CONTROL

The basic elements of cancer control are the same everywhere in the world: Cancer planning, cancer prevention and early detection (screening), cancer management—diagnosis and treatment, including palliative care delivered by a multidisciplinary team—and psychosocial support for patients and families. Details of what is most important and what is feasible vary according to the cancer burden and the resources available. The opportunities described in the body of this report include elements of each approach. The basic approaches are described briefly here. They are all discussed in the context of breast cancer in Chapter 4. Discussion of cancer control elements is prefaced by a section about national cancer control planning and programs.

National Cancer Control Planning and Programs

For cancer control to advance systematically, it requires priority setting and budgeting, at a minimum, which require an understanding of the cancer problems that exist in a country and the means available to address them. The process by which this logically occurs is cancer control planning. Because of the differences among countries, cancer control planning and programs must be tailored to individual country situations, recognizing the realities of time and place. In the end, an appropriate cancer plan and program may be limited to a single or a few activities, or can be more comprehensive. Plans and programs should be reviewed every few years and should change as needs and resources dictate.

WHO has been the global leader in promoting and providing guidance for cancer control planning and programs. In 2001, fewer than half of 167 WHO Member States responding to a survey reported having a plan to target cancer or other chronic diseases. Eighty percent of the African countries lacked national plans (Alwan et al., 2001). To address this, WHO produced an updated edition of *National Cancer Control Programs: Policy and Managerial Guidelines* (WHO, 2002) in 2002. It provides guidance on planning, implementing, managing, and evaluating cancer programs to help policy makers and program managers make the most efficient use of their available resources. It outlines the scientific basis for cancer prevention, early detection, cure, and care; discusses the appropriateness of particular technologies; and describes how to manage national programs tailored to different resource settings.

Building on the 2002 report, a six-volume "how-to" series, *Cancer Control: Knowledge Into Action. WHO Guide for Effective Programmes* (WHO, forthcoming), will appear in 2006–2007. The impetus for this expanded series is the World Health Assembly resolution on Cancer Prevention and Control. In May 2005, the 192 member countries of the 58th World Health Assembly, the governing body of WHO, approved a resolution that calls on all WHO Member States to develop national cancer programs covering preventive measures, early detection and screening, and improved treatment and palliative care (Box 2-1).

The forthcoming series includes the following modules:

1. Planning: "A practical guide for programme managers on how to plan overall cancer control effectively, according to available resources and integrating cancer control with programmes for other chronic diseases and related problems."
2. Prevention: "A practical guide for programme managers on how to implement effective cancer prevention by controlling major avoidable cancer risk factors."

BOX 2-1
World Health Organization Resolution on Cancer Prevention and Control (Summary)

1. Cancer is one of the most common causes of morbidity and mortality today, with more than 10 million new cases and more than 6 million deaths each year worldwide . . . by 2020 there will be every year 15 million new cancer cases and 10 million cancer deaths.
2. . . . There is now sufficient understanding of the causes to prevent at least one third of all cancers worldwide . . . [and] permit the early detection and effective treatment of a further one third of cases. Effective strategies exist for the relief of pain and the provision of palliative care to all cancer patients in need and of support to their families, even in low-resource settings.
3. . . . Efforts to prevent and control cancer are hampered by the low priority frequently given to the disease by governments and health ministries, excessive reliance and expenditure on treatment, and a considerable imbalance between resources allocated for basic cancer research and those devoted to its prevention and control.
4. The overall goal of cancer prevention and control is to reduce the incidence and mortality of cancer and to improve the quality of life of cancer patients and their families. A well conceived national cancer control programme is the most effective instrument to . . . achieve this goal.
5. Prevention frequently offers the most cost-effective long-term strategy for cancer control . . . [and] can also contribute to preventing other chronic diseases that share the same risk factors. It is estimated that around 43 percent of cancer deaths are due to tobacco use, unhealthy diets, alcohol consumption, inactive lifestyles and infection. Of these, tobacco use is the world's most avoidable cause of cancer.
6. Infectious agents are responsible for almost 25 percent of cancer deaths in the developing world and 6 percent in industrialized countries. In low-resource settings . . . special measures are needed to combat these infections. For example, in areas endemic for liver cancer, hepatitis B virus immunization, integrated with other vaccination programmes, is the principal preventive measure. Vaccines are being developed and tested in human beings that could prove to be effective in preventing cervical cancer in the near future. . . .
7. Early detection, which comprises screening of asymptomatic populations and awareness of early signs and symptoms, increases the probability of cure. . . . Awareness of early signs and symptoms is particularly relevant for cancers of the breast, cervix, mouth, larynx, endometrium, colon and rectum, stomach and skin . . . population screening can currently be advocated only for cancers of the breast, cervix, and colon and rectum, in countries where resources are available for wide coverage of the popula-

tion, appropriate treatment is in place and quality-control standards are implemented . . . studies are under way to evaluate low-cost approaches to screening . . . for low-resource settings.

8. Treatment aims to cure disease, prolong life, and improve the quality of life. The most effective and efficient treatment is linked to early detection programmes and follows evidence-based standards of care . . . .
9. Most cancer patients require palliative care . . . [which] involves not only pain relief, but also spiritual and psychosocial support to patients and their families from diagnosis, throughout the course of the disease, to the end of life and bereavement. . . . These services can be provided simply and inexpensively. . . . Nonetheless, access to pain relief and palliative care services is often limited, even in high-resources settings, because of lack of political will, insufficient information and education of the general public, health care providers and patients, and excessive regulation of opioids.
10. Surveillance and research are crucial for both planning effective and efficient cancer control programmes and monitoring and evaluating their performance. . . . Population-based [cancer] registries provide information on incidence . . . and . . . trends; whereas hospital-based registries provide information regarding diagnosis, stage distribution, treatment methods and survival. . . .
11. Effective partnerships at national, regional and global levels are essential for sustainable prevention and control of cancer. . . . The [World Health Organization (WHO)] network comprises international organizations, agencies of the United Nations system, government bodies, nongovernmental organizations, and private-sector entities, covering such fields of expertise as medicine, nursing, research, public health and communications.
12. IARC [International Agency for Research in Cancer] conducts focused research on cancer etiology and prevention. . . . WHO promotes policy development and programme implementation. The recently published WHO/IARC report [*World Cancer Report*] . . . together with other IARC and WHO monographs, technical reports and scientific publications, provides a sound basis on which to develop effective cancer control strategies.
13. . . . previous resolutions . . . provide the general framework for addressing cancer prevention and control. Resolution WHA51.18 noted that noncommunicable diseases, including cancer, represented a significant and growing burden on public health services; resolution WHA53.17 urged the establishment of comprehensive programmes for the prevention and control of major noncommunicable diseases; resolution WHA55.23 urged the development of a global strategy on diet, physical activity and health; and resolution WHA56.1 adopted the WHO Framework Convention on Tobacco Control.

SOURCE: World Health Assembly (2005).

3. Early detection: "A practical guide for programme managers on how to implement effective early detection of major types of cancer that are amenable to early diagnosis and screening."

4. Diagnosis and treatment: "A practical guide for programme managers on how to implement effective cancer diagnosis and treatment, particularly linked to early detection programmes or curable cancers."

5. Palliative care: "A practical guide for programme managers on how to implement effective palliative care for cancer, with a particular focus on community-based care."

6. Policy and advocacy: "A practical guide for medium level decision-makers and programme managers on how to advocate for policy development and effective programme implementation for cancer control."

This Institute of Medicine report endorses the concept of cancer control planning and programs, and the guidance provided by WHO and others (in particular, the International Union Against Cancer, also known as UICC). We endorse the idea that countries revisit their cancer control plans every few years to reassess and fine tune priorities and programs. As with the operational aspects of cancer control, the role of global partners can be key in helping to organize local stakeholders and providing support to begin the process. An example is the current development of a new cancer control plan in Peru (Box 2-2).

The challenge, of course, lies in moving beyond planning to implementation. The process described by WHO, if followed, would involve a wide range of stakeholders—public and private sectors, including the advocacy community—and forward movement toward action.

Cancer Prevention and Early Detection

Preventing cancer from occurring in the first place—primary prevention—is the most definitive way to lessen the burden of cancer. Developing primary prevention strategies requires knowing something about the causes or risk factors associated with the cancer. If the cause or risk factor can be eliminated or reduced, prevention is possible through behavior modification, modification of the environment, or in the case of infectious agents, vaccination or treatment. Not surprisingly, most of the evidence about cancer prevention and early detection relates to high-income countries. Much of this information may be applicable directly to LMCs, although prevention strategies may have to be modified to fit the conditions in those countries. For a thorough review of the world's literature on cancer prevention and early detection, see the Institute of Medicine report *Fulfilling the Potential of Cancer Prevention and Early Detection* (IOM, 2003).

BOX 2-2
Development of a New National Cancer Control Plan for Peru

A new National Cancer Control Plan and program is under development in Peru, a process initiated in 2002 by the Instituto Nacional de Enfermedades Neoplasicas (National Institute for Neoplastic Illnesses, INEN), the central cancer institute for the country (Coalición Multisectorial Peru Contra el Cáncer, 2006). INEN is collaborating with a large number of Peruvian partners as well as the American Cancer Society, U.S. National Cancer Institute, the Pan American Health Organization, and the International Union Against Cancer (also known as UICC). Support from the American Cancer Society has been made available not only to develop the plan, but to help defray staff costs of the program for the first 2 years of start-up. A major task during the early phase is to secure the future of the program by raising internal funds. This arrangement of support and the centralization of the work in a major cancer center is the first such effort of its kind in Latin America (Personal communication, E. Huerta, Cancer Preventorium, Washington Cancer Institute, 2006).

The one modifiable cause of cancer that dwarfs all others is tobacco use. Fortunately, specific interventions are known to work at reducing tobacco use. Tobacco control is the subject of Chapter 5 of this report. In LMCs, because of the large burden of cancer from infectious agents, prevention through vaccination or treatment is a major focus. When it comes to other preventive measures, much is known about what could be done—eating a healthy diet, maintaining a healthy weight, exercising, not drinking too much alcohol—but how to motivate these changes in people is still a developing field in high-income countries.

Screening for early stages of cancer or precancerous states is the other strategy for reducing the cancer death rate, assuming appropriate management is available when a treatable condition is detected. The cancers for which screening is widely recommended in high-income countries are breast, cervical, and colon. Controversy persists over the value of screening for prostate cancer using the prostate specific antigen (PSA) test. Screening that reaches a substantial proportion of the population requires significant infrastructure for the screening itself as well as the capacity for treatment. Whether or not a country embarks on a screening program will depend on the state of readiness to deal with both aspects—screening and management.

Cancer Management

When cancer is suspected in an individual, either because of a screening test or because of signs and symptoms that lead the person to seek care, a host of services may be needed. Ideally the person would have access to diagnostic services and if a cancer is, in fact, diagnosed, services appropriate to the type and stage of cancer. For some people, this means potentially curative treatment with surgery, radiotherapy, or chemotherapy, or much more frequently, some combination of these modalities, applied by a multidisciplinary medical team working together. Even at early treatable stages, and often as a result of treatment, palliative care for symptom control can be beneficial. For difficult-to-treat cancers, the many cancers of all types not seen until they are advanced beyond probable cure, and other cancers that advance despite treatment, palliative care alone may be most appropriate. Psychosocial services to help deal with the psychological and social impacts of cancer can be appropriate for virtually all people with cancer, and for the survivors of those who die from cancer. These approaches all fall into the "cancer management" category.

Cancer Management: Diagnosis and Staging

An accurate diagnosis is key to receiving appropriate care for cancer. Diagnostic tests include imaging, laboratory, and pathology techniques, in addition to physical examination. The same techniques are applicable to the initial diagnosis and staging and when reassessments are needed to determine a patient's state at later time points. As is the case for other aspects of cancer management, new and more sophisticated (usually more expensive) diagnostic techniques have been added to those available traditionally, requiring choices to be made where resources are limited. A diagnosis may require one or more tests in sequence.

Imaging includes conventional X-rays, as well as ultrasonography, computed tomography (CT) scanning, and magnetic resonance imaging (MRI). These methods are used to visualize the anatomy of tumors. Two types of nuclear imaging techniques have been added more recently to cancer imaging modalities: Positron emission tomography (PET) and single photon emission computed tomography (SPECT). These techniques detect metabolic activity in cells, and can differentiate cancer cells by their different levels of activity.

Laboratory tests include tests on blood, urine, other fluids, and tissues. Specimens are collected by phlebotomy (blood drawing), fine-needle aspiration cytology or fine-needle-biopsy, and surgical procedures. In addition to tests looking directly for cancerous cells, other types of tests, e.g., to assess liver function or look for tumor markers (biological or chemical compounds that may increase when cancer is present) can provide information about the status of the cancer.

Pathologic examination for most solid tumors requires surgically excising a sample of the tumor, a biopsy. Cells found in body fluids are also evaluated by pathologic techniques. Microscopic evaluation of the tissue is carried out to determine the size of the tumor, its growth into other tissues and organs, the type of cancer cells, and the grade of the tumor (how closely the cancer cells resemble normal tissue).

Additional information about cancers is found during surgery. Surgical reports describe the size and appearance of tumors and may include observations about lymph nodes and nearby organs.

Cancer Staging

Once a cancer diagnosis is confirmed, further testing (using the same techniques) may be needed to determine the extent of the cancer. This information is captured in "staging systems," which have developed over time. The principles are common to all cancers, but the details vary depending on the specific cancer. The common elements of staging are:

- location of primary tumor
- tumor size and number (if multiple)
- spread into lymph nodes
- cell type and grade of tumor (i.e., how closely the cancer cells resemble normal tissue)
- spread to distant sites (i.e., metastases)

The "TNM" system is a widely used staging system (although not the only one). The UICC is instrumental in updating and disseminating the TNM system. The initials T, N, and M stand for:

- T, tumor (extent of primary tumor)
- N, nodes (extent of spread to regional lymph nodes)
- M, metastases (presence or absence)

Numbers modify each letter indicating the size or extent of the feature (Table 2-3).

A typical example is a breast cancer classified as T3 N2 M0. This refers to a large tumor that has spread to nearby lymph nodes but has not metastasized to other parts of the body. TNM classifications also correspond to numerical stages 0 through IV (expressed as Roman numerals) (Table 2-4).

Another set of terms is also used to denote cancer stage (National Cancer Institute, 2004):

TABLE 2-3 TNM Staging

T—Primary Tumor	
TX	Primary tumor cannot be evaluated
T0	No evidence of primary tumor
Tis	Carcinoma in situ (early cancer that has not spread to neighboring tissue)
T1, T2, T3, T4	Size and/or extent of the primary tumor (increasing from T1 to T4
N—Regional Lymph Nodes	
NX	Regional lymph nodes cannot be evaluated
N0	No regional lymph node involvement (no cancer found in the lymph nodes)
N1, N2, N3	Involvement of regional lymph nodes (number and/or extent of spread)
M—Distant Metastasis	
MX	Distant metastasis cannot be evaluated
M0	No distant metastasis (cancer has not spread to other parts of the body)
M1	Distant metastasis (cancer has spread to distant parts of the body)

SOURCE: National Cancer Institute (2004).

TABLE 2-4 Cancer Stages

Stage	Definition
0	Carcinoma in situ (early cancer that is present only in the layer of cells in which it began).
I, II, III	Higher numbers indicate more extensive disease: greater tumor size, and/or spread of the cancer to nearby lymph nodes and/or organs adjacent to the primary tumor.
IV	The cancer has spread to another organ.

SOURCE: National Cancer Institute (2004).

- In situ cancer is confined to the layer of cells in which it arose
- Localized cancer is limited to the organ in which it arose
- Regional cancer has spread beyond the primary site to nearly lymph nodes, or organs or tissues
- Distant cancer has spread from the primary site to distant parts of the body

Special classification systems are used for certain types of cancer, including cancers of the brain and spinal cord, leukemias and lymphomas, and other cancers in some circumstances (e.g., childhood cancers).

Cancer Management: Surgery

Surgery was the earliest form of cancer treatment and remains its mainstay where the range of cancer treatment is available. Until the middle of the 20th century, when chemotherapy and radiotherapy were developed as treatment modalities, surgical resection of tumors was the only available approach. For solid tumors today, long-term survival is usually dependent on surgical removal of the primary tumor (and a margin of normal tissue) and regional lymph nodes, often with additional treatment modalities. In the United States, about 90 percent of cures of solid tumors are through surgery alone or with other modalities. Cancers in which surgical resection is a major factor in cure include melanomas and cancers of the breast, colon, rectum, thyroid, stomach, and lung (Fleming et al., 1995). The surgeries involved range from basic to highly complex, which bears on the types of settings in which they can be performed. The trend is toward less radical surgery than previously, using radiotherapy and/or chemotherapy to augment surgery. For example, bone or soft-tissue sarcomas of the extremities used to be treated by surgical amputation of the affected limb. Now, limbs are routinely spared by adding other treatment modalities to more conservative surgery.

Higher technology surgical techniques are common where resources are available. This includes the use of laparoscopic surgery and the extensive use of imaging, such as ultrasound, during surgery.

Not all surgery is done with curative intent (although intent might not be known until surgery is begun). When complete removal of a tumor is not possible, surgery is often still used to reduce (debulk) the tumor, which can prolong life and in some cases reduce symptoms (e.g., if the tumor is interfering with vital functions).

Surgical Settings

Debas and colleagues (Debas et al., 2006) have described a "coordinated model system for surgical care" appropriate for LMCs, consisting of community clinics, district hospitals, and tertiary hospitals. They also analyzed, for the first time, the burden of disease (expressed as disability-adjusted life years) of surgical conditions, defined as conditions requiring surgery for management. The analysis was based on expert opinion of 18 surgeons in different parts of the world. "Surgical DALYs" attributed to cancer are less important as a percentage of total surgical DALYs in LMCs than in high-income countries, but still represent a substantial fraction. In Europe, malignancies are the leading cause of surgical DALYs, at 36 percent, and in the Americas (a mixture of mainly high- and middle-income countries), at 22 percent; in Africa, 8 percent. The level of surgery (i.e., the complexity) is not captured in these estimates. How much could realistically be addressed would have to be critically assessed in each country.

Cancer Management: Radiotherapy

Radiotherapy refers to the application of ionizing radiation (X-rays, γ-rays [gamma rays], or radioactive particles) for treatment. Radiation oncology is the medical discipline of treating malignant disease with radiation. Radiotherapy can be used curatively, as a single modality, or in conjunction with surgery, chemotherapy, or both. It can also relieve symptoms (palliate) in patients with incurable cancer. Radiotherapy has some limited medical uses in noncancerous conditions (e.g., keloid or "heaped-up" scars), but it is overwhelmingly a cancer treatment modality.

How Radiotherapy Works

Different types of cells—normal and malignant—vary in their susceptibility to ionizing radiation. Clinical radiotherapy schedules are designed to exploit the differences between normal tissues and tumors, so that as many malignant cells as possible are killed, while damage to normal tissue is minimized. In radical curative treatments, total radiation doses may be close to the tolerance of normal tissues. In palliative treatments, lower doses are the norm.

Some tumors, such as seminoma of the testis and lymphoma, are very sensitive to radiotherapy and can be cured with relatively low doses. Others, such as glioblastoma multiforme in the brain, are notoriously resistant, even to large doses.

A course of radiotherapy may be spread over days or weeks. This is known as *fractionating*, and the radiation delivered to a patient in a single treatment session is called a *fraction*. Fractionating allows normal tissues to repair much of the radiation damage, while tumor cells, which are less efficient at repair, do not recover. Each fraction of radiotherapy kills a certain proportion of the cancer cells in the irradiated region. A beam of radiation is called a *field*. A fraction consists of one or more fields delivered sequentially.

External-beam radiotherapy can be delivered by cobalt machines or linear accelerators ("linacs"), collectively known as "megavoltage machines." Cobalt machines and linacs deliver very high-energy, highly focused beams that can reach deeper tumor tissues while depositing relatively small doses in the normal tissues through which they pass. Linacs produce the same intensity of radiation throughout operation, but the machines are more complex than cobalt machines and require greater manpower and attention to maintain them. These factors make cobalt machines—with replaceable cobalt sources—more appropriate in many LMCs. As the cobalt source decays, treatment time increases, decreasing the number of patients that can be treated per day. The half-life of cobalt is 5.3 years, so a source that is 5.3 years old will take twice as long to deliver the prescribed dose to a patient as a new source. An 11-year-old source will take *four* times as long as a new source to deliver the same dose.

Side Effects of Radiotherapy

Both early (acute) and late (chronic) side effects can occur after radiotherapy. The occurrence and severity depend on the body site being treated, the volume of normal tissue irradiated (the larger the volume, the higher the risk and severity of side effects), the total dose, and the rate of dose accumulation (the amount per week).

Early side effects result from damage to proliferating tissues (i.e., cells that continually divide and replace old cells with new ones) such as the lining of the gastrointestinal tract, or the skin. For example, radiotherapy to an abdominal tumor may damage the mucosa of the small bowel, causing malabsorption and diarrhea, but most patients recover completely within a few weeks when new cells have replaced the damaged ones.

Late reactions, which are much less common than acute side effects, occur months or years after treatment ends. They may result from damage to nonproliferating differentiated tissues, which cannot compensate for cell death by dividing to replace lost cells. These effects may be difficult to reverse and can be permanent or progressive. Examples include fibrosis of the skin, spinal cord damage, scarring of the lungs, and radiation-induced liver disease.

Side effects can be minimized by meticulous planning and delivery of radiotherapy. Late-reacting tissues are particularly sensitive to the size of each radiation dose, so they can be protected by giving a greater number of smaller fractions of radiation, provided the total dose is not too high.

Second cancers are an even rarer type of late effect. Especially in children, even relatively low doses of radiation increase the risk of developing another malignancy, unrelated to the one that was treated originally. Leukemias appear on average 7 years after exposure and solid tumors after 10 or 20 years.

Curative Radiotherapy

In high-income countries, at least half of all cancer patients treated with radiotherapy—alone or with surgery, chemotherapy, or both—are treated with the goal of achieving a cure. Radiotherapy is used by itself when it has the highest cure rate or because it is likely to have fewer side effects. Examples include treatment of advanced cervical cancer, pituitary tumors, deep-seated gliomas, nasopharyngeal cancer, and early-stage, low-grade lymphomas, including Hodgkin's lymphoma.

Radiotherapy is preferred over surgery when surgery will result in the loss of an organ and the control of the tumor is similar. Examples include laryngeal cancer and prostate cancer. Surgery alone can be effective for small tumors. For large tumors, radiotherapy is often used with surgery to reduce tumor size or reduce the risk of tumor recurrence so that the whole tumor site can be treated with the least effect on the patient's normal functioning. In general, radiotherapy is used along with surgery when:

- Organ preservation is desirable; an example is breast-conserving surgery (lumpectomy);
- The tumor is advanced with a high risk of local recurrence after surgery, such as rectal cancer;
- An inoperable cancer can be rendered operable, such as when advanced rectal cancers that are adhered to other organs, preventing complete excision, can be shrunk by radiation;
- The surgery included too small a margin of normal tissue around the tumor to preclude a high likelihood of local recurrence; radiotherapy reduces that likelihood.

Chemotherapy may improve the results of radiotherapy in the treatment of some cancers (Table 2-5). Radiotherapy can treat large primary tumors, and chemotherapy can work on disseminated micrometastases. The dose-limiting toxicities of radiotherapy and chemotherapy are different, which means that it is possible to deliver a higher overall dose of "treatment" with the two modalities than with one or the other. Other mechanisms are

TABLE 2-5 Beneficial Interactions Between Radiotherapy and Chemotherapy

Mechanism	Benefits	Examples of Cancer
Spatial cooperation	Radiotherapy cures the high-volume local cancer and chemotherapy cures micrometastases	Hodgkin's lymphoma Rectal cancer
Independent toxicity	Because radiotherapy and chemotherapy have different dose-limiting toxicities, it is possible to deliver a higher antitumor dose with fewer side effects than with radiotherapy alone	Cervical cancer Esophageal cancer
Enhanced tumor response	Even if the effects of radiotherapy and chemotherapy are only additive, the steep dose response of tumors means that there can be greater rates of cure than with radiotherapy by itself	Anal cancer
Protection of normal tissues	Some dose-limiting normal tissues can be protected by chemical modifiers such as amifostine, resulting in fewer side effects	Head and neck cancers

SOURCE: Barton et al. (2006).

enhanced tumor response with two modalities, and the use of chemical agents to protect normal tissues from radiation damage, allowing a greater radiation dose.

Palliative Radiotherapy

Growing tumors cause symptoms by their physical presence, e.g., by pressing on adjacent organs or blocking passages or orifices. Radiotherapy can be used to shrink tumors directly causing symptoms. In many cases, it may reduce or eliminate the need for analgesics (including opioids).

Radiotherapy is effective for people with incurable lung cancer, alleviating shortness of breath, cough, and hemoptysis (coughing up blood). For breast cancer, radiotherapy can control fungating masses (large, rapidly growing tissue), and for prostate cancer it can be used to relieve urinary obstruction. Short-course radiotherapy (sometimes just a single treatment, or for more extensive disease, a few treatments) is effective in relieving pain from bone and brain metastases and compression of the spinal cord and various nerves (Roos et al., 2005). Radiotherapy can reverse the effects of spinal cord compression and prevent paraplegia.

With longer courses than those used for symptom relief, radiotherapy can prolong life for patients with some incurable cancers such as high-grade gliomas (Laperriere and Bernstein, 1994).

Infrastructure Needs and Costs of Radiotherapy

Providing a safe and effective radiation oncology service requires an initial capital investment in radiotherapy equipment and specially designed buildings, as well as an ongoing investment in consumable items and maintenance of the equipment; an expert team of doctors, therapists, and physicists; and good access to engineering support. The necessary medical, scientific, and technical expertise is in short supply in many countries and is an even bigger constraint in many LMCs than the shortage of radiotherapy equipment. A shortage of trained staff may limit the number of patients who can be treated, to the point of underutilization of even the existing scarce equipment (Tatsuzaki and Levin, 2001; Radiation Oncology Inquiry, 2002).

The introduction or expansion of radiation oncology services in any health care system inevitably has implications for other services. These include surgical and medical oncology, pathology, imaging, general and specialist medical and surgical services, and nursing and psychosocial support services.

The costs of radiotherapy include the capital costs of the building and equipment, maintenance costs, and staff salaries. Buildings can be relatively expensive, but are durable, so amortized costs are small. Cobalt machines are considerably cheaper than linacs because they are mechanically and electronically simpler. Capital costs also include equipment for planning treatment, including simulators and computers. Staff costs are for radiation oncologists, physicists, and technologists, each of whom is necessary to assess and treat patients.

The cost of establishing a radiotherapy facility in an LMC is about $1 million. If used 12 hours per day, it could deliver half a million doses of radiotherapy over its lifetime, with an amortized cost of about $2 per fraction. Adding the costs of consumables and salaries, each fraction of radiotherapy would cost a few dollars in an LMC. In a study of 11 countries of differing economic status, median costs per treatment dose of radiotherapy were US$11 for linear accelerators and US$4.87 for cobalt machines, with a range from US$1.29 to US$39.59 (Van Der Giessen et al., 2004). One fraction is often enough for producing pain relief for several weeks or months, while 20 to 40 fractions are typically required for curing a cancer such as laryngeal cancer. Radiotherapy is clearly a beneficial technology but is limited in where it can be delivered, in addition to limitations imposed by resources. In general, facilities are limited to urban areas with infrastructure and transportation, and may never be accessible to the largely rural population of much of the developing world.

Cancer Management: Chemotherapy

Chemotherapy refers broadly to the use of drugs to treat cancer with the intention of producing long-term survival (or "cure"), or at least a substantial increase in the length and possibly quality of life. (Drugs that improve the quality of life of cancer patients during their illness and at the end of life by controlling pain and other symptoms are considered separately in the discussion of palliative care in Chapter 8.) Medical oncologists are the medical professionals trained in the use of chemotherapy.

"Cytotoxic" drugs kill cancer cells by several mechanisms. Other drugs—referred to more specifically as hormonal therapy—add, block, or remove hormones to slow or stop the growth of certain cancers (mainly cancers of the breast and prostate). Typically, drugs are used in combinations, not infrequently including three or four drugs, given on a schedule that may be months long. Hormonal therapy with tamoxifen, for breast cancer, may be taken for at least several years. The main classes of cancer chemotherapy drugs are listed in Table 2-6.

WHO Model List of Essential Medicines

The WHO Model List of Essential Medicines was developed and is periodically revised as a guide for the development of national and local essential medicine lists that "satisfy the priority health care needs of the population" (WHO, 2006a), tailored to each specific situation. The list, organized by category of use, includes a core list and a complementary list. The core list includes the "minimum medicine needs for a basic health care system." The most efficacious, safe, and cost-effective medicines for "priority conditions"—selected on the basis of current and estimated future public health relevance, and potential for safe and cost-effective treatment—are included. Cancer chemotherapeutic agents are on a complementary list (Table 2-7), acknowledging that cancer is a priority condition, but that "specialized diagnostic or monitoring facilities, and/or specialist medical care, and/or specialist training" are needed for the appropriate use of the drugs. A full menu of drugs for palliative care, however, is on the core list (see Chapter 7). These are, according to WHO, "intended to be available within the context of functioning health systems at all times in adequate amounts . . . at a price the individual and the community can afford" (WHO, 2006a). Countries, of course, are free to select the drugs that best meet their needs and budgets, and are available to them. What is actually available may differ considerably from the WHO lists.

TABLE 2-6 Major Classes of Chemotherapeutic Drugs for Cancer

Drug Type	Mode of Action and Examples
Alkylating agents	• Kill cells by directly attacking DNA. • Used to treat chronic leukemias, Hodgkin's disease, lymphomas, and certain carcinomas of the lung, breast, prostate, and ovary. • Cyclophosphamide is a commonly used alkylating agent.
Nitrosoureas	• Act similarly to alkylating agents and also inhibit changes necessary for DNA repair. • Cross the blood–brain barrier and are therefore used to treat brain tumors, lymphomas, multiple myeloma, and malignant melanoma. • Carmustine (BCNU) and lomustine (CCNU) are the major nitrosourea drugs.
Antimetabolites	• Block cell growth by interfering with certain activities, usually DNA synthesis, halting normal development and reproduction. • Used to treat acute and chronic leukemias, choriocarcinoma, and some tumors of the gastrointestinal tract, breast, and ovary. • 6-mercaptopurine and 5-fluorouracil (5-FU) are commonly used.
Antitumor antibiotics	• Diverse group of compounds that generally act by binding with DNA and preventing RNA synthesis. • Widely used to treat a variety of cancers. • Doxorubicin, adriamycin, mitomycin-C, and bleomycin are the most common drugs in this category.
Plant (vinca) alkaloids	• Act by blocking cell division during mitosis. • Commonly used to treat acute lymphocytic leukemia (ALL), Hodgkin's and non-Hodgkin's lymphomas, neuroblastomas, Wilms' tumor, and cancers of the lung, breast, and testes. • Vincristine and vinblastine are commonly used agents in this group.
Hormonal agents	• Includes adrenocorticosteroids, estrogens, antiestrogens, progesterones, and androgens that modify the growth of certain hormone-dependent cancers. • Tamoxifen, used for estrogen-dependent breast cancer, is an example.

The Development of Cancer Chemotherapy

Development of chemotherapy began in the 1940s and progressed rapidly through the 1960s. Leukemias and lymphomas were the first major classes of cancer to respond to chemotherapy. Early successes led to extensive screening programs of agents both of biological origin (e.g., plants and sea creatures) and synthesized molecules to find agents with anticancer properties. Early on, it was discovered that cancers easily develop resistance to single agents, leading to the common use of drugs in combination, and a continuing search for more effective combinations. "Responses" to single and multiple agents, leading to a temporary reprieve from the cancer, which may last months or longer, are always more common than long-term free-

TABLE 2-7 WHO Model List of Essential Medicines: Antineoplastic Drugs

Cytotoxic Medicines (complementary list[a])	
Asparaginase	Powder for injection
Bleomycin	Powder for injection
Calcium folinate	Tablet; injectable liquid
Chlorambucil	Tablet
Chlormethine	Powder for injection
Cisplatin	Powder for injection
Cyclophosphamide	Tablet; powder for injection
Cytarabine	Powder for injection
Dacarbazine	Powder for injection
Dactinomycin	Powder for injection
Daunorubicin	Powder for injection
Doxorubicin	Powder for injection
Etoposide	Capsule; injectable liquid
Fluorouracil	Injectable liquid
Levamisole	Tablet
Mercaptopurine	Tablet
Methotrexate	Tablet; powder for injection
Procarbazine	Capsule
Vinblastine	Powder for injection
Vincristine	Powder for injection
Hormones and Antihormones (complementary list[a])	
Dexamethasone	Injectable liquid
Hydrocortisone	Powder for injection
Prednisolone	Tablet
Tamoxifen	Tablet
Medicines Used in Palliative Care[b]	
The WHO Expert Committee on the Selection and Use of Essential Medicines recommended that all the drugs mentioned in the second edition of the WHO publication *Cancer Pain Relief* (WHO, 1996) be considered essential. The drugs are included in the relevant sections of the Model List, according to their therapeutic use, such as analgesics.	

[a]The complementary list includes essential medicines for priority diseases for which specialized diagnostic or monitoring facilities, and/or specialist medical care, and/or specialist training are needed.

[b]See Chapter 7, "Palliative Care."

SOURCE: Reprinted, with permission, from WHO (2005b). Copyright 2005 by WHO.

dom ("cure") from cancer after treatment. A caveat of particular importance in LMCs is that chemotherapy (and other treatments) are more effective in the earlier stages of cancer. Cancers that have spread only locally are often curable; those with distant metastases are much less so (with some exceptions). In this discussion, effective treatment refers mainly to earlier stage cancers. While palliative care and pain control medications can be beneficial to patients with late-stage cancers, even the most effective chemotherapy is unlikely to prolong life significantly.

Through the 1980s, effective drugs for testicular cancer and other malignancies of children and young adults were found. Many of these treatments involve only drugs. Drugs are also used as an "adjuvant" to cancer surgery. Adjuvant chemotherapy is given either before or after surgery (or both) to kill both remaining cancer cells at the primary site and cells that are circulating or lodged at distant sites where, left unchecked, they may proliferate into metastatic lesions. Successful adjuvant treatments that produce long-term survival in a large proportion of patients are available for some cancers, including cancers of the breast and colon, among the common cancers. For other common cancers, including cancers of the liver, pancreas, brain, and melanomas, no currently available drugs produce large benefits for a large proportion of patients. For still others, such as stomach cancer, the diagnosis is most often made (outside of screening programs) at a late stage, when treatment is unlikely to be effective. A new era has begun with the advent of "targeted" agents for cancer chemotherapy (Box 2-3).

Delivery of Chemotherapy

The way chemotherapy is administered has a bearing on the settings in which it can be given. The most common routes of administration are by mouth, intravenously, intramuscularly, and topically. Less commonly, drugs are infused directly into body cavities, such as the abdomen (intraperitoneal), the lung (intrapleural), or the central nervous system (intrathecal). It is not uncommon for more than one route to be used for a chemotherapy regimen that involves several drugs. Depending on the route of administration and other factors (e.g., need for monitoring), treatments can be given in a medical office or clinic, or in a hospital as an inpatient or outpatient. Laboratory tests are usually carried out periodically to monitor the blood and organs for side effects (the specifics depend on the cancer and the treatment).

Treatment regimens not uncommonly stretch over 6 months or more, with treatments occurring in cycles (periods of active treatment and rest). In a cycle, treatment may be daily, weekly, or at some other interval.

Side Effects

The predominant strategy with cytotoxic drugs is to give them at the maximum possible total dosage, but in individual increments and over time. Experience in clinical trials over decades has shown that success rates are best with highest doses. However, dose intensity is limited by side effects that occur because of damage to normal tissues. Certain side effects—such as

BOX 2-3
Targeted Cancer Therapies

Cytotoxic cancer drugs exploit the rapid growth and division of cancer cells compared with normal cells, preferentially killing cancer cells. But cancer cells may not differ so much from normal cells, so significant damage to normal tissue may occur. Newer "targeted" therapies block cancer cells' ability to grow, divide, repair, and/or communicate with other cells by interfering with specific molecules associated with cancer cells, but not found on normal cells (or found in very small numbers). The successful targeted therapy homes in on the cancer-specific target. There are, theoretically, many targets in the pathway of a single cancer cell, involved with the development, growth, and spread of cancer.

Unlike traditional cancer drugs, targeted therapies are taken over a long period of time, possibly for life. In the United States, the dozen or so approved targeted therapies can cost thousands or tens of thousands of dollars per year.

Targeted therapies can be a variety of drug types. Some synthetic small molecule drugs work inside cancer cells to disrupt their function. Monoclonal antibodies target receptors on the cell surface. Antiangiogenesis agents block formation of blood vessels within tumors, causing the cells to die for lack of oxygen. Many of the targeted therapies that have been or are being developed target proteins that are involved in cell signalling, interfering with the molecular signals that instruct cells to grow and divide as cancer cells. These include Herceptin (trastuzumab), a monoclonal antibody; the small molecules Gleevec (imatinib) for some types of myelogenous leukemia (CML) and gastrointestinal stromal tumors; and Iressa (erlotinib), for some cases of lung cancer. Other targeted therapies cause cancer cells to die (undergo apoptosis), including Velcade (bortezomib) to treat multiple myeloma. Avastin (bevacizumab) blocks the formation of blood vessels.

About a dozen targeted therapies have been approved in one or another high-income country, most for limited indications. Many more are in clinical trials. The hope is that eventually, an individual's tumor will be characterized by the particular set of molecular markers present, and treatments will be targeted to interact with them. The specificity of the interactions should mean less damage to normal tissue, hence, fewer side effects.

hair loss—can be distressing, but are usually temporary. More serious are effects on proliferating cells in the digestive tract, bone marrow, or elsewhere, which may result in suppression of blood cell formation, debilitating nausea, and other effects (Stewart and Kleihues, 2003). Little information is available on the impacts of chemotherapy on patients in LMCs, who may have different profiles than those in high-income countries in their co-morbidities and nutritional status, at a minimum.

Implications for LMCs

The facilities and trained personnel for prescribing an appropriate regimen, for administering chemotherapy, for conducting laboratory testing, and for managing side effects are bare necessities where chemotherapy is going to be used. The protracted schedule of chemotherapy regimens means that patients must be able to get to the treatment site and have financial access to treatment. A reliable supply of drugs, which in most LMCs must be imported, is implicit. Based on information assembled for this report, these conditions cannot be met in a large proportion of LMCs. A global view is not available, but in Latin America and the Caribbean, chemotherapy drugs are often not available, out-of-pocket costs for patients are high because few governments cover the costs, and there are few public cancer centers (Eisenchlas, 2006). We know from pediatric cancer treatment experiences in LMCs around the globe that abandonment of treatment—stopping before a long regimen is complete—is among the top problems identified (see Chapter 6).

Cancer Management: Psychosocial Services

People with cancer may experience psychosocial distress at any point from diagnosis through treatment, during advanced illness, and even during long-term survival. Psychosocial distress is defined as an unpleasant emotional experience that may be psychological, social, or spiritual in nature. These feelings may become severe and disabling, and may result eventually in a diagnosis of major depression. Transition points in treatment (time of diagnosis, awaiting treatment, completion of treatment) often trigger worsening distress (IOM, 2004). Psychosocial support enables patients with cancer to cope and deal with the disease, its impact, and with life after cancer. This form of support can be made available at all stages of the cancer experience—at diagnosis, during treatment, and beyond, including during palliative care. Support may also be needed by family members and others close to the patient.

Psychosocial interventions are accepted as an essential component of cancer care, although they are often not well developed. Little information is available about these services in LMCs. At the most basic level, people with cancer need help coping with their illness through personal interaction and empathy from caregivers and other knowledgeable individuals. Social and emotional support focuses on adjusting to the diagnosis, apprehension regarding treatment, and existential concerns (IOM, 2004). In addition to information about the treatment, a wide range of specific interventions have been described, including the following:

1. Psychotherapeutic interventions, including brief crisis counseling, group therapy and counseling, pastoral counseling, family therapy and counseling, grief therapy, and sexual counseling
2. Psychopharmacologic interventions
3. Complementary therapies, such as yoga, massage, exercise, acupuncture, art, music, and dance therapy, and others

A variety of providers can deliver psychosocial services. In many places, nurses are on the front lines of cancer care, and this includes psychosocial support. Physicians, including primary care physicians and specialists, also can provide support, if the patient has access to them. Social workers, psychologists, counselors, and religious workers also can give the needed support. Patient support groups organized by cancer survivors are among the most common sources of support. Community-based traditional resource systems can be tapped to offer psychosocial support to patients and family members.

Reach to Recovery International (RRI) is an example of psychosocial support from breast cancer survivors, under the auspices of the International Union Against Cancer. RRI affiliates have been established in every region of the world, but are all run locally. The program is built on the premise that one woman who has experienced breast cancer herself and received specialized training gives of her time and experience to support another woman facing the same challenges.

The types of services most needed by cancer patients are likely to be similar around the world, but the providers who are available and have sufficient training will vary according to the health care system, as will the resources available, and other social and cultural factors.

SUMMARY AND RECOMMENDATION

The review of causes and risk factors and of cancer control elements sets the stage for the latter chapters of this report, where the greatest opportunities for cancer control are identified. What comes from this review is that a few causes and risk factors are prominent in cancers common in LMCs: tobacco use; infectious agents, particularly hepatitis viruses, HPV, and *H. pylori*; and dietary factors, too little exercise, and too much body mass. A lot of factors have smaller, yet not insignificant, effects. The factors vary with how easily they can be modified. Tobacco smoking is addictive and difficult for people to stop once started, yet certain interventions are effective (more in Chapter 5). We have the tools now to prevent nearly all hepatitis B and most cancer-causing HPV infections. Changing behavior related to diet and exercise has proved exceptionally challenging in the high-income countries where work has been done, and there is little to offer in this regard to LMCs at the moment. In 10 years, new knowledge about behavior change and about the causes of cancer could allow greater scope for direct intervention to prevent cancers.

Cancer management—the mix of treatment and support interventions for people with cancer—has been developed and continues to evolve in high-income countries. While all the elements of cancer management could be applied in LMCs (not only for the rich minorities in LMCs), they may need modification for best effect (as basic as adjusted doses of chemotherapy for populations with different co-morbidities and nutritional status). However, in all cases, they require careful consideration of the circumstances in which they are being used, which may be vastly different from those in high-income countries. The point is made that cancer management often requires multiple interventions, necessitating a mix of medical expertise and support services, and appropriate facilities. The discussion of how this can best be accomplished continues in Chapter 8, which is about cancer centers in LMCs.

Cancer prevention includes an array of activities, some outside the health care system (e.g., increasing tobacco taxes), some in the primary care system (e.g., infant vaccination against HBV), and others under more specialized conditions (e.g., screening for precancerous changes in the cervix). Which prevention activities any country can and will adopt will depend on their specific circumstances.

These decisions and others about cancer control at a national level are best approached through a formal process that weighs the opportunities against the costs within the country context. National cancer control planning and the development of national cancer control programs is the obvious means for making such decisions. In this area, we defer the details to WHO, UICC, and other organizations that provide guidelines and recommendations referenced in this chapter. No other specific recommendations come out of this chapter directly, but the discussion here leads to recommendations in the remainder of the report.

> **RECOMMENDATION 2-1. Cancer control plans should be developed, or updated, in each country every 3 to 5 years through a process that involves all major stakeholders, public and private sectors, as described by WHO, UICC, and others.** *Cancer control plans should be promoted and supported financially and programmatically through both government action and public advocacy.*

In both the planning and implementation phases, global partners should provide necessary guidance and financial support.

REFERENCES

Alwan A, Maclean D, Mandil A. 2001. *Assessment of National Capacity for Noncommunicable Disease Prevention and Control; the Report of a Global Survey.* Geneva, Switzerland: World Health Organization.

Barton MB, Frommer M, Shafiq J. 2006. Role of radiotherapy in cancer control in low-income and middle-income countries. *Lancet Oncology* 7(7):584–595.

Bruce N, Rehfuess E, Mehta S, Hutton G, Smith K. 2006. Indoor air pollution. In: Jamison DT, Breman JG, Measham AR, Alleyne G, Claeson M, Evans DB, Jha P, Mills A, Musgrove P, eds. *Disease Control Priorities in Developing Countries.* 2nd ed. New York: Oxford University Press. Pp. 793–815.

Coalición Multisectorial Peru Contra el Cáncer. 2006. *Documento De Consenso.* Lima, Peru: Ministerio de Salud.

Darby S, Hill D, Auvinen A, Barros-Dios JM, Baysson H, Bochicchio F, Deo H, Falk R, Forastiere F, Hakama M, Heid I, Kreienbrock L, Kreuzer M, Lagarde F, Makelainen I, Muirhead C, Oberaigner W, Pershagen G, Ruano-Ravina A, Ruosteenoja E, Rosario AS, Tirmarche M, Tomasek L, Whitley E, Wichmann HE, Doll R. 2005. Radon in homes and risk of lung cancer: Collaborative analysis of individual data from 13 European case-control studies. *BMJ* 330(7485):223.

Darby S, Hill D, Doll R. 2001. Radon: A likely carcinogen at all exposures. *Annals of Oncology* 12(10):1341–1351.

Debas HT, Gosselin R, McCord C, Thind A. 2006. Surgery. In: Jamison DT, Breman JG, Measham AR, Alleyne G, Claeson M, Evans DB, Jha P, Mills A, Musgrove P, eds. *Disease Control Priorities in Developing Countries.* 2nd ed. New York: Oxford University Press. Pp. 1245–1259.

Eisenchlas J. 2006. *Cancer Prevention and Management in Latin America.* Unpublished paper commissioned by IOM.

Epping-Jordan JE, Galea G, Tukuitonga C, Beaglehole R. 2005. Preventing chronic diseases: Taking stepwise action. *Lancet* 366(9497):1667–1671.

Fleming ID, Brady LW, Mieszkalski GB, Cooper MR.1995. Basis for major current therapies for cancer. In: Murphy GP, Lawrence W, Lenhard RE, eds. *American Cancer Society Textbook of Clinical Oncology.* 2nd ed. Atlanta, GA: American Cancer Society. Pp. 96 ff.

IARC (International Agency for Research on Cancer). 1997. *IARC Monographs on the Evaluation of Carcinogenic Risks to Humans: Schistosomes, Liver Flukes and Helicobacter pylori.* Lyon, France: IARC.

IARC. 2004. *GLOBOCAN 2002.* Lyon, France: IARC.

IOM (Institute of Medicine). 2003. *Fulfilling the Potential of Cancer Prevention and Early Detection.* Curry SJ, Byers T, Hewitt M, eds. Washington, DC: The National Academies Press.

IOM. 2004. *Meeting Psychosocial Needs of Women with Breast Cancer.* Hewitt M, Herdman R, Holland J, eds. Washington, DC: The National Academies Press.

Laperriere NJ, Bernstein M. 1994. Radiotherapy for brain tumors. *CA: A Cancer Journal for Clinicians* 44(2):96–108.

Lopez AD, Collishaw NE, Piha T. 1994. A descriptive model of the cigarette epidemic in developed countries. *Tobacco Control* 1994(3):242–247.

Lopez AD, Mathers CD, Ezzati M, Jamison DT, Murray CJL, eds. 2006. *Global Burden of Disease and Risk Factors.* New York: Oxford University Press.

National Cancer Institute. 2004. *Staging: Questions and Answers.* [Online] Available: http://www.cancer.gov/cancertopics/factsheet/Detection/staging [accessed October 17, 2006].

Parkin DM. 2005. The global health burden of infection-associated cancers in the year 2002. *International Journal of Cancer* 118 (12):3030–3044.

Radiation Oncology Inquiry. 2002. *A Vision for Radiotherapy.* Canberra, Australia: Commonwealth of Australia.

Rehm J, Chisholm D, Room R, Lopez AD. 2006. Alcohol. In: Jamison DT, Breman JG, Measham AR, Alleyne G, Claeson M, Evans DB, Jha P, Mills A, Musgrove P, eds. *Disease Control Priorities in Developing Countries.* 2nd ed. New York: Oxford University Press. Pp. 887–906.

Roos DE, Turner SL, O'Brien PC, Smith JG, Spry NA, Burmeister BH, Hoskin PJ, Ball DL, Trans-Tasman Radiation Oncology Group. 2005. Randomized trial of 8 Gy in 1 versus 20 Gy in 5 fractions of radiotherapy for neuropathic pain due to bone metastases. *Radiotherapy & Oncology* 75(1):54–63.

Rosenstock L, Cullen M, Fingerhut M. 2006. Occupational health. In: Jamison DT, Breman JG, Measham AR, Alleyne G, Claeson M, Evans DB, Jha P, Mills A, Musgrove P, eds. *Disease Control Priorities in Developing Countries.* 2nd ed. New York: Oxford University Press. Pp. 1127–1145.

Stewart BW, Kleihues P. 2003. *World Cancer Report.* Lyon, France: IARC Press.

Tatsuzaki H, Levin CV. 2001. Quantitative status of resources for radiation therapy in Asia and Pacific region. *Radiotherapy & Oncology* 60(1):81–89.

Van Der Giessen PH, Alert J, Badri C, Bistrovic M, Deshpande D, Kardamakis D, Van Der Merwe D, Da Motta N, Pinillos L, Sajjad R, Tian Y, Levin V. 2004. Multinational assessment of some operational costs of teletherapy. *Radiotherapy & Oncology* 71(3):347–355.

World Health Assembly. 2005. Cancer prevention and control. WHA Resolution 58.22. Geneva, Switzerland: WHO.

WHO (World Health Organization). 1996. *Cancer Pain Relief, 2nd edition.* Geneva, Switzerland: WHO.

WHO. 2002. *National Cancer Control Programmes: Policies and Managerial Guidelines, 2nd edition.* Geneva, Switzerland: WHO.

WHO. 2003. *INTERSUN: The Global UV Project, A Guide and Compendium.* Geneva, Switzerland: WHO.

WHO. 2004. *Global Strategy on Diet, Physical Activity and Health.* [Online]. Available: http://www.who.int/dietphysicalactivity/goals/en/ [accessed October 17, 2006].

WHO. 2005a. *Preventing Chronic Diseases: A Vital Investment.* Geneva, Switzerland: WHO.

WHO. 2005b. *Essential Medicines: WHO Model List, 14th edition.* [Online]. Available: http://whqlibdoc.who.int/hq/2005/a87017_eng.pdf [accessed January 28, 2006].

WHO. 2006a. *Essential Medicines.* [Online]. Available: http://www.who.int/medicines/services/essmedicines_def/en/index.html [accessed July 5, 2006].

WHO. 2006b. *Ultraviolet Radiation and the INTERSUN Programme.* [Online]. Available: http://www.who.int/uv/intersunprogramme/en/ [accessed October 16, 2006].

WHO. Forthcoming. *Cancer Control: Knowledge Into Action. WHO Guide for Effective Programmes (Six Volumes).* Geneva, Switzerland: World Health Organization.

World Cancer Research Fund. 1997. *Food, Nutrition, and the Prevention of Cancer: A Global Perspective.* Washington, DC: American Institute for Cancer Research.

3

The Cancer Burden in Low- and Middle-Income Countries and How It Is Measured

Each year, 5 million people in low- and middle-income countries (LMCs) die from cancer, about 10 percent of the 50 million deaths in those countries. This proportion, and the total burden of cancer,[1] will continue to grow as the tobacco-induced cancer epidemic accelerates, and as the world population ages. Looked at another way today, of the 7 million cancer deaths in the world, 5 million are in LMCs. Despite this fact, cancer is not recognized as a high-priority health problem in most of these countries. Where children are dying from malaria and other infectious diseases and suffering the many consequences of malnutrition, where women die in childbirth, and where young adults are dying of AIDS, people with cancer—many dying slowly in their homes—attract less attention. However, the latter half of the 20th century witnessed major reductions in infant and childhood deaths even in the poorest countries, making cancer and the major noncommunicable diseases more prominent in the burden of disease. They now co-exist with the still heavy burden of common infectious diseases and are destined to continue growing in relative importance.

This chapter briefly reviews the major shifts in mortality during the latter half of the 20th century, and then describes what is known of the current cancer burden in LMCs. The final section describes the sources of

[1]The "burden of disease" ideally measures the full impact of a disease on a population. It goes beyond cases and deaths to include functional limitations imposed by the disease and the disability associated with those limitations, and non-health wellbeing (e.g., financial impacts). Quantification of risk factors known to be associated with specific diseases is also part of the measurement of burden of disease (Lopez et al., 2006). The phrase is used in this chapter both specifically and generally to describe how cancer affects populations in LMCs.

data on the global cancer burden and discusses priorities for improving the information base. Cancer mortality, incidence, survival, and risk factor surveillance for cancer and other chronic diseases are highlighted (see Box 3-1 for definitions).

WORLDWIDE CHANGES IN MORTALITY PATTERNS

The decline of childhood mortality in developing countries is one of the most significant public health achievements of the 20th century. In 1950, nearly one-quarter of all children born died before their fifth birthday, most in infancy (Table 3-1). Today, about 8 percent will die before age 5. Much of the improvement is due to vaccinations against childhood infections, antibiotics against a wide range of bacterial infections, oral rehydration therapy for diarrhea, and in some places, generally improved living conditions. The upshot is that many more people are surviving to adulthood and old age—even in developing countries. This means more will eventually die from cancer, cardiovascular disease, chronic respiratory disease, diabetes, or another chronic condition of adulthood.

Today's infants—about 130 million born each year—will experience a much different pattern of deaths than those born in the past century (Table 3-2)—*assuming current patterns in risk factors*. More than half will live to age 70 and older. Nearly one-third (40 million of each year's birth cohort), however, will die in middle age, between ages 35 and 69. Most of these deaths will be from chronic, noncommunicable diseases. As many as half of these "premature" deaths could be prevented if patterns in major risk factors were modified, allowing people to live longer and die in old age. Specifically for cancer, the most practicable measures involve reversing the increases in smoking prevalence; preventing liver cancer through infant vaccination against hepatitis B virus (HBV); and preventing cervical cancer through a combination of vaccination against the cancer-causing human papillomaviruses, or HPVs, (as vaccines become available and affordable) and screening for precancerous or early stages.

The importance of cancer as a cause of illness and death will continue to grow, even with effective preventive measures. Appropriate cancer management—diagnosis and treatment—can extend the lives of many, particularly if diagnosed early. For those eventually dying from cancer (and other causes of death that involve chronic pain and other symptoms), at whatever age, palliative care with good pain control can vastly improve the quality of life of the patient and his or her family.

BOX 3-1
Basic Cancer Population Statistics Defined

Cancer Incidence

Cancer incidence is the number of new cases occurring in a population, expressed either as an absolute number or as a rate. The incidence rate per 100,000 people per year approximates the average risk of developing cancer in a given year and is often used to compare rates over time or across populations. Measurement of incidence rates requires the identification of all new cases of cancer in a defined population, usually in a defined geographic region. The most basic cancer incidence reporting includes information about the person (age, sex, ethnicity) and about the cancer (the date of detection, anatomic site, histology, and the most valid diagnostic method used). The stage of disease at diagnosis (i.e., the extent of disease according to standard definitions) is also a valuable piece of information.

Cancer Mortality

Cancer mortality refers to the number of deaths attributed to cancer in the population, and the cancer mortality rate is the number of deaths per 100,000 people per year. These statistics are usually reported as rates, relating the number of deaths to the underlying population (i.e., the census population). As with incidence, reports can be more and less detailed, but information about the person (age, sex, ethnicity) and the cancer (anatomic site) is very useful.

Mortality is the product of the incidence and fatality from cancer. Fatality is the proportion of people with cancer who die in a given time period, usually a year. It conveys the risk that an individual with cancer will die, while the mortality rate describes the average risk of dying from cancer in the population.

Mortality rates are often used as proxies for cancer incidence, especially where incidence data are not available. For cancers with a poor prognosis everywhere, mortality may, indeed, mirror incidence, and comparisons made across time and place may be valid. In places where people are unlikely to receive curative treatment, even for cancers otherwise considered "curable," mortality may also be a surrogate for incidence, but comparing across areas may not be straightforward.

A statistic derived from cancer mortality is person-years of life lost (PYLL), which weights deaths at different ages: Death at a young age results in more PYLLs than death in old age. PYLL can be modified further by adding aspects of quality of life, such as a year spent in extreme pain would result in loss at a fraction of a "quality-adjusted life-year" or QALY.

continued

BOX 3-1 Continued

Cancer Survival

Cancer survival describes the proportion of individuals with cancer who are still living for defined periods after diagnosis, often aggregated by type of cancer, age group, sex, and place of residence. This statistic is often referred to as the "survival rate," although it actually describes an individual's probability of being alive, and not actually a rate. Cancer survival statistics are derived by calculating the proportion of people originally diagnosed with a type of cancer who are still alive at specified points after diagnosis, such as 1-year survival. For many cancers, 5-year survival is synonymous with "cure," because relatively few of those surviving 5 years go on to die from the cancer (breast cancer is the most important exception). Survival is influenced strongly by the stage of disease at diagnosis and the availability of effective treatment. If no adjustment for stage at diagnosis is made in calculating survival, people diagnosed at earlier stages will appear to have better survival than those diagnosed with later stage disease, regardless of treatment, but this is simply a statistical artifact. But for cancers for which effective treatments exist, early detection and treatment means a real survival advantage. If existing treatments are not very effective (e.g., for pancreatic cancer, lung cancer, and stomach cancer) or if the person does not have access to medical services, the stage of disease makes little difference in survival. Survival is, therefore, a crude measure of the effectiveness and/or availability of cancer treatment.

Cancer Prevalence

Cancer prevalence indicates the number of people alive with cancer in a population. Unlike incidence and mortality, there is no standard definition of a prevalent cancer case. The most appropriate definition may depend on how the information is going to be used. One approach is to count people with cancer who are in active treatment or follow-up, which has strong economic effects. As a practical matter, this has been interpreted by some as cases within 5 years of diagnosis. However, many cancer survivors live with long-term effects of the disease itself and the treatments, some of which require further management, so an argument could also be made for a more inclusive definition. Cancer prevalence can be calculated from cancer registries with good long-term follow-up, or the more usual, estimated from incidence and survival data.

TABLE 3-1 Worldwide Childhood Mortality, 1950–2000

Year of Birth	Percentage Dying Before Age 5
1950–1954	23
1970–1974	14
1990–1994	9
2000–2004	8 (about 10 million of 130 million born each year)

TABLE 3-2 Approximate Distribution of Deaths by Age Group of Those *Dying* in the Early 21st Century and Anticipated for Those *Born* in the Early 21st Century

Age Range	Deaths Each Year in Early 21st Century	Future Deaths of Those *Born* in Early 21st Century
0–34 (children and young adults)	20 million[a] (33%)	20 million (15%)
35–69 (middle age)	20 million (33%)	40 million[b] (30%)
70+ (old age)	20 million (33%)	70 million (54%)
TOTAL	60 million	130 million

[a]In 2001, there were 7 million deaths (out of 56 million), but this number is increasing because of deaths from AIDS.

[b]Deaths at ages 35–69 (in 2035–2069) will be mainly from noncommunicable disease: cardiovascular diseases, cancer, chronic respiratory diseases, etc.

SOURCE: Personal Communication, R. Peto, University of Oxford, June 2006.

BASIC CANCER STATISTICS

In 2002, about 11 million new cases of cancer occurred and about 7 million people died of cancer worldwide. LMCs account for more than 80 percent of the world's population, 72 percent of the world's cancer deaths, 78 percent of years of life lost (YLL), and 77 percent of disability-adjusted life-years (DALYs) (Table 3-3).

Cancer becomes relatively more important as other causes of premature death decline. This leads to substantial variation in the *proportion of deaths* attributable to cancer in different parts of the world and at different income levels. In 2002, cancer accounted for 12.5 percent of deaths worldwide, but just over 25 percent of all deaths in the low-mortality countries of Europe. In contrast, among the highest mortality countries of Africa, 3.6 percent of deaths were from cancer, and in the highest mortality countries of South-east Asia, 7.1 percent (World Health Organization, 2003). Deaths from

TABLE 3-3 Deaths, Years of Life Lost (YLL), and Disability-Adjusted Life Years (DALYs), All Causes and Cancers by Country Income Level, 2002 (all figures in millions)

	All Causes of Death			Cancer			
	Deaths	YLL[a]	DALYs[b]	Deaths	YLL[a]	DALYs[b]	Population
Country Income Level							
Low	28.5	606.4	877.7	1.8	20.8	21.4	2,560,762
Lower middle	17.2	221.0	402.6	2.7	29.4	30.3	2,214,697
Upper middle	3.4	42.2	90.4	0.6	5.9	6.3	513,406
High	7.9	52.4	118.7	2.1	15.4	17.4	933,917
All LMCs	***49.1***	***869.6***	***1,370.7***	***5.1***	***56.1***	***58.0***	5,288,865
World	**57**	**922.5**	**1,490.1**	**7.1**	**71.6**	**75.5**	**6,224,985**
LMC share of global burden	86%	94%	92%	72%	78%	77%	85%

[a]The component of the DALY that measures years of life lost by a population due to premature mortality.

[b] A measure of the gap in healthy years of life lived by a population as compared with a normative standard.

SOURCE: Data from World Health Organization (2006).

communicable diseases, maternal and perinatal conditions, and nutritional deficiencies are of greater importance as the income level is lower, but cancer still occupies a prominent place in the overall statistics (Table 3-4).

Clearly, cancer is not rare anywhere, even where other health problems are more pressing, but significant variations exist (Figure 3-1). For men, cancer *incidence* is highest in North America, with an age-standardized rate of about 400 per 100,000, or an 18 percent risk of developing cancer by age 65. The risk of *dying* from cancer is highest for men in Eastern Europe, at about 200 per 100,000, and the cumulative risk of dying before age 65 is about 10 percent. For women, *incidence* is also highest in North America, at about 300 per 100,000, while cancer *mortality* is highest in East Africa, at about 120 per 100,000. As with all age-standardized international comparisons, the data are adjusted for differences in population age distribution—which is heavily influenced by birth rates and mortality from other diseases—by applying age-specific rates from the country in question to a "standard" population in order to focus on comparable cancer risks and rates for *individuals* within a population.

Patterns of Cancer in LMCs

Knowing approximately how many cancers are occurring in a population, the distribution of types, and who is being affected are essential for

TABLE 3-4 Deaths by Cause, Sex, and Age, 2001 (thousands)

	Low- and Middle-Income Countries					World				
	Males		Females		M + F	M + F	Males		Females	
Cause	0–29	30–69	0–29	30–69	**Total**	**Total**	0–29	30–69	0–29	30–69
All causes	7,975	10,853	7,437	7,312	48,351	56,242	8,117	12,263	7,515	8,088
Communicable, maternal, perinatal, and nutritional conditions	5,797	2,532	5,956	1,829	17,613	18,166	5,822	2,598	5,977	1,862
Noncommunicable diseases	871	6,699	827	4,810	26,023	32,891	915	7,871	859	5,495
Malignant neoplasms	**111**	**1,691**	**95**	**1,255**	**4,955**	**7,021**	**121**	**2,186**	**101**	**1,597**
Injuries	1,307	1,623	654	673	4,715	5,186	1,379	1,792	678	730
Percentage of deaths from cancer	**1.4**	**15.6**	**1.3**	**17.2**	**10.2**	**12.5**	**1.5**	**17.8**	**1.3**	**19.7**

SOURCE: Lopez et al. (2006).

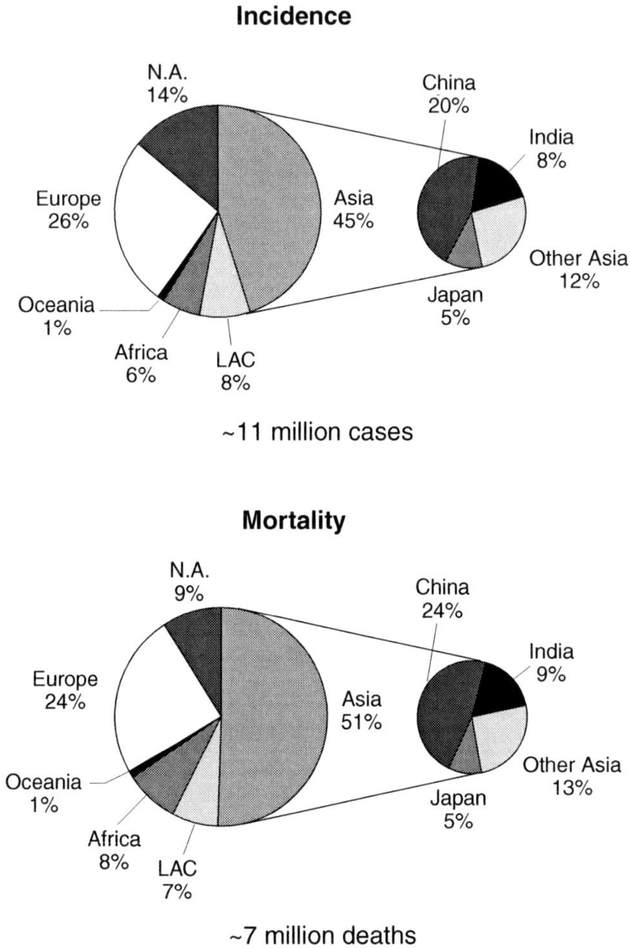

FIGURE 3-1 Cancer incidence and mortality by geographic area, 2002.
LAC = Latin America and the Caribbean.
SOURCE: Reprinted, with permission, from Parkin et al. (2005). Copyright 2005 by Lippincott Williams & Wilkins.

understanding the burden that cancer imposes on society. Any attempt to assess needs and priorities in health logically starts with an examination of the extent of the problem, and cancer is no exception. How important is cancer? Who in the population is most affected? Is the burden of disease from cancer increasing or decreasing? How does it compare with other health problems along these dimensions? Unfortunately, health statistics are poor where health problems are most severe.

More so than for other health conditions, however, enormous effort goes into constructing best estimates for cancer incidence and mortality for every country on the globe. The International Agency for Research on Cancer (IARC, an agency of the World Health Organization, or WHO) is the source of the most widely respected global cancer database, GLOBOCAN. WHO compiles vital and health statistics for all countries and all causes of death. The statistics presented in this chapter come from these two sources. They are considered broadly accurate and indicate the magnitude of the cancer burden in LMCs, though they are mainly estimates, made in the absence of directly collected data, particularly in the lowest income countries. The status of direct data collection in LMCs is reviewed later in this chapter.

The mix of common cancers varies between high-income and low- and middle-income countries (Figure 3-2 and Tables 3-5 and 3-6), and among LMCs in different parts of the world. The patterns vary by geography and economic status, which correlate roughly with the causes of cancer in the "environment" in its broadest sense. Genetic variation plays a lesser role overall. The majority of cancers in more developed countries are those associated with more affluent lifestyles—cancers of the lung, colon and rectum, breast, and prostate. All except lung cancer have a reasonably good prognosis where comprehensive cancer management is available. In contrast, cancers of the liver, stomach, esophagus, and cervix—all related to infectious agents—are relatively more common in developing countries. Where treatment is largely unavailable, all cancers have a poor prognosis, but in this group, all but cervical cancer have poor outcomes everywhere (Parkin et al., 2005).

Differences in rankings between developed and developing countries in both incidence and mortality are broadly explicable by differences in exposures, both to infectious and environmental agents, and the availability of medical care.

Stage Distribution of Cancers at Diagnosis

Most cancers in LMCs are detected at later stages than in high-income countries. Although this is the common wisdom and too logical to dispute, the actual evidence on which to judge this is sparse. Population-based data are not available, but a number of hospital-based studies have been published that report the cancer stage distribution of patients at those hospitals. Table 3-7 is a compilation of these studies for breast cancer. The percentage of advanced cancers ranges from 30 to 98 percent.

CANCER TRENDS AND CURRENT STATUS OF COMMON CANCERS

Over time—mostly over fairly long periods of years and decades—certain cancers become more or less common. This is known largely from

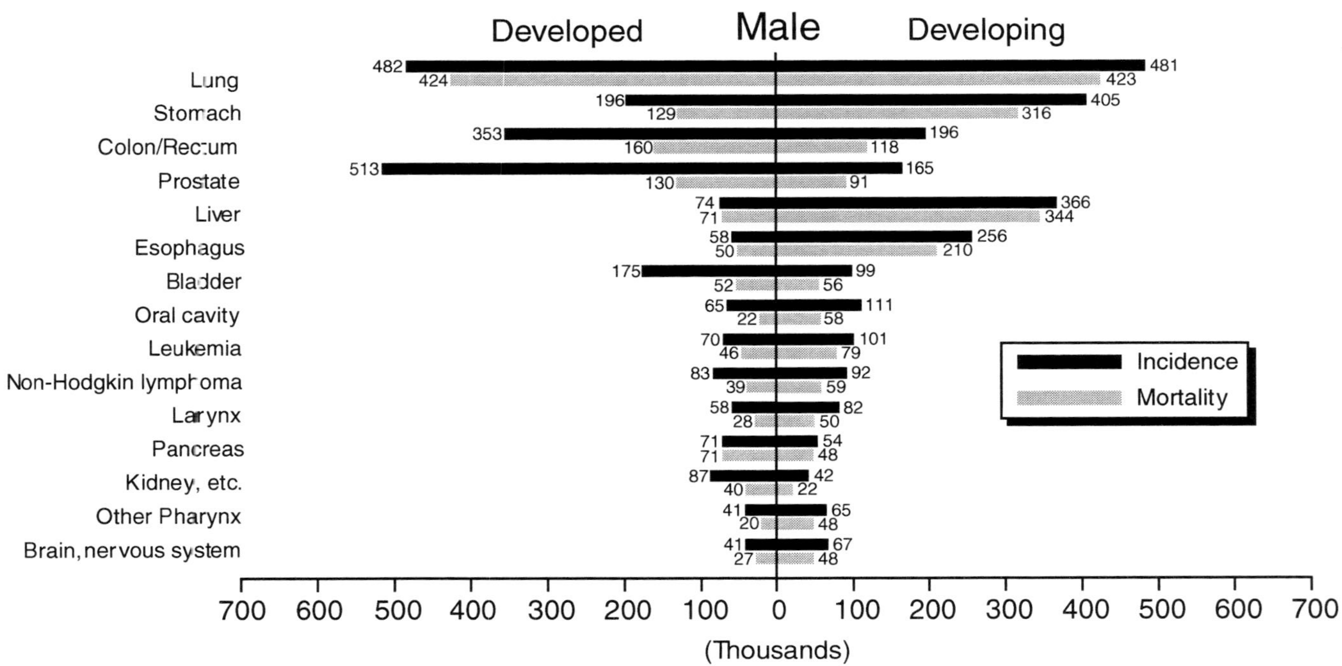

FIGURE 3-2 Continues

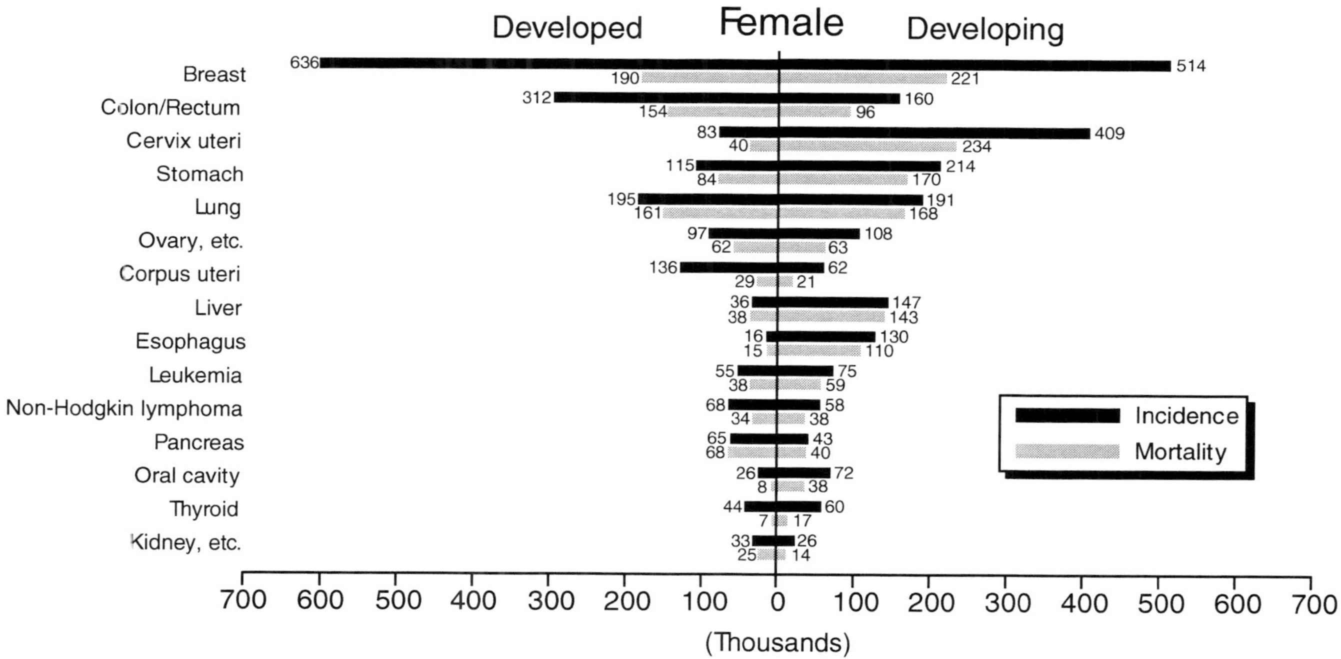

FIGURE 3-2 Estimated global cancer incidence and mortality, 2002.
SOURCE: Reprinted, with permission, from Parkin et al. (2005). Copyright 2005 by Lippincott Williams & Wilkins.

TABLE 3-5 Leading Cancers (Incidence) in Developing and Developed Countries, Males and Females, 2002 (thousands of cases)

	Males		Females	
Rank	Developing	Developed	Developing	Developed
1	Lung (481)	Prostate (513)	Breast (514)	Breast (636)
2	Stomach (405)	Lung (482)	Uterine cervix (409)	Colon/rectum (312)
3	Liver (366)	Colon/rectum (353)	Stomach (214)	Lung (195)
4	Esophagus (256)	Stomach (196)	Lung (191)	Uterine corpus (136)
5	Colon/rectum (196)	Bladder (175)	Colon/rectum (160)	Stomach (115)

SOURCE: Parkin et al. (2005).

TABLE 3-6 Leading Cancers (Mortality) in Developing and Developed Countries, Males and Females, 2002 (thousands of deaths)

	Males		Females	
Rank	Developing	Developed	Developing	Developed
1	Lung (423)	Lung (424)	Cervix uteri (234)	Breast (190)
2	Liver (344)	Colon/rectum (160)	Breast (221)	Lung (161)
3	Stomach (316)	Prostate (130)	Stomach (170)	Colon/rectum (154)
4	Esophagus (210)	Stomach (129)	Lung (168)	Stomach (84)
5	Colon/rectum (118)	Liver (71)	Liver (143)	Pancreas (68)

SOURCE: Parkin et al. (2005).

high-income countries and inferred for low- and middle-income countries. An exception is the relatively rapid rise in the incidence of Kaposi's sarcoma associated with AIDS, most notably in Africa. Over longer periods, the most obvious trend is the steep climb in lung cancers that, with a decade or more delay, parallels the increases in manufactured cigarette smoking. The incidence of stomach cancer, on the other hand, has declined over at least the past 50 years in most high-income countries for reasons that are only partially understood. The current global toll in incidence and mortality for the common cancers is depicted in Figure 3-2. The recent global patterns of the common cancers (arranged by numbers of deaths in developing countries)[2] are described below (based on Parkin et al., 2005).

[2]Parkin and colleagues follow the United Nations convention, which defines "developed" countries as all of North America, Japan, all of Europe, and Australia and New Zealand. All other countries are defined as "developing."

TABLE 3-7 Proportion of Breast Cancer by Stage at Diagnosis in Selected LMCs

Region	Country	Number of Cases	Stages Reported	Stage I %	Stage II %	Stage III %	Stage IV %	Reference
Asia	Mumbai–India		I–IV	8	57	29	6	(Chopra, 2001)
	Trivandrum–India		I–IV	4	42	41	13	(Chopra, 2001)
	Pakistan	566	I–IV	17	33	33	17	(Malik, 2002)
	Hospital Kuala Lumpur–Malaysia	774	I & II, III & IV combined	40–50		50–60		(Hisham and Yip, 2004)
	University Malaya Medical Centre–Malaysia	752	I & II, III & IV combined	60–70		30–40		(Hisham and Yip, 2004)
Africa	South Africa–Black	2,194	I–IV	5	17	42	36	(Vorobiof et al., 2001)
	Tanzania	50		0	2	88	10	(Amir et al., 1997)
	Nigeria	124	I & II, III & IV combined	44		56		(Anyanwu, 2000)
	Egypt	400	I–III	4	26	70		(Omar et al., 2003)
Latin America	Sao Paolo–Brazil	1,796	I–IV	10	22	53	14	(Schwartsmann, 2001)
	Porto Alegre–Brazil	1,783	I–IV	16	54	19	11	(Schwartsmann, 2001)
	Lima–Peru	9,003	I–IV	9	42	33	16	(Schwartsmann, 2001)
	Range (%)				2–70%		30–98%	

SOURCE: Barton et al. (2005).

Lung Cancer

Lung cancer tops the list for cancer incidence and mortality in the world population and among men. It has been the most common cancer since 1985, with 1.35 million cases in 2002, representing 12.4 percent of all new cancers. The 1.18 million lung cancer deaths comprise 17.6 percent of all cancer deaths in that year. Lung cancer is about three times more common among men than women (35.5/100,000 versus 12.2/100,000, age-standardized rates). Half (49.9 percent) of the cases now occur in developing countries; just 20 years ago, the corresponding figure was 31 percent. The explanation for the current distribution of lung cancer around the world and the differences between men and women is no mystery. Nearly all cases are caused by cigarettes and other tobacco smoking although there are localized exceptions, such as smoke from indoor cooking fires as a significant risk for lung cancer among women in parts of China.

The 44 percent increase in lung cancer *cases* among men is due to population growth and aging. The *age-standardized incidence rate* has actually declined slightly since 1985. The 76 percent increase in *cases* among women, however, is due to those factors and to higher smoking rates, leading to a 22 percent increase in the age-standardized rate.

Lung cancer is at once one of the most deadly common cancers—average 5-year survival in Europe is 10 percent, barely better than the 8 to 9 percent in developing countries—and the most preventable.

Stomach Cancer

Stomach cancer ranks fourth in incidence worldwide, but because of its lethality, second among causes of cancer death. The distribution is highly specific geographically. China has the highest rates and 42 percent of worldwide cases. Other high-risk areas are East Asia (including Japan and Korea), Eastern Europe, parts of Central and South America, and Central Africa. Rates are low in South Asia, North and East Africa, North America, and Australia and New Zealand.

Survival from stomach cancer is very low in developing countries (6 percent 5-year survival in sub-Saharan Africa). Japan has the highest survival rate by a wide margin, at 52 percent, a result of mass screening and early detection since the 1960s. The most significant risk factor for stomach cancer is infection with the bacterium *Helicobacter pylori* (which is the cause of most duodenal ulcers). Co-factors, probably diet related, must also be important, however. Some salt-preserved and pickled traditional foods and low intake of fresh fruits and vegetables, seem to be important. Tobacco smoking also increases the risk of stomach cancer.

For reasons that are poorly understood, stomach cancer rates have been declining steadily for more than 50 years in the United States and other high-income countries. Worldwide, incidence rates have declined by about 15 percent since 1985 and continue downward, at least in higher income countries. Possible reasons are lower rates of *H. pylori* infection over time (possibly a result of better living conditions), better food storage and preservation, and greater availability of fresh fruits and vegetables. Even if the current secular trends continue, however, there will be more than 1 million cases of stomach cancer in 2010.

Breast Cancer

Nearly one-quarter (23 percent) of all cancers among women are breast cancers, with an estimated 1.15 million cases in 2002, making it by far the most common cancer among women, and the second most common cancer in the overall population. Incidence is much higher in industrialized countries, where more than half of all cases are diagnosed. Some fraction of the difference is due to widespread breast cancer screening in industrialized countries, which identifies cancers that would never become clinically apparent. The exception is Japan, where, despite screening, the incidence of breast cancer is about one-third that in North America. Although the rates are much lower in most of Africa, Western Asia, South America, and Eastern Europe, breast cancer is still the most common cancer among women. Among regions, the age-standardized incidence rate is lowest in Central Africa (16.5/100,000) and highest in North America (99.4/100,000).

Survival from breast cancer is better than for many cancers. The 5-year survival is about 73 percent in industrialized countries, and 57 percent overall in developing countries. In the poorest countries, however, the prognosis is much worse. Of the estimated 411,000 women who died of breast cancer worldwide in 2002, 221,000 were in developing countries and 190,000 were in industrialized countries. Worldwide, there are more survivors of breast cancer than of any other cancer type (excluding the common and relatively harmless skin cancers).

Breast cancer is increasing in incidence everywhere, but more so where rates historically have been low. Between 1990 and 2002, the global increase was about 0.5 percent per year. In China, annual increases of 3 to 4 percent are reported. If these rates are representative, 1.5 million cases of breast cancer are expected in 2010.

The large differentials in breast cancer incidence around the world and many epidemiologic studies over the past decades implicte the environment in its broadest meaning (including patterns of childbearing and obesity) in breast cancer causation. The evidence has not, however, led to strategies for breast cancer prevention.

Liver Cancer

Liver cancer is among the most lethal cancers. Although it is sixth in incidence worldwide, it is third in mortality, after lung and stomach cancers. With 5-year survival at 5 percent or less even in developed countries, the yearly death toll (598,000) and number of new cases (626,000) are not far apart. More than 80 percent of liver cancers occur in developing countries, and the incidence is substantially higher among men than women (overall, a ratio of 2.4). High-risk areas include East and Southeast Asia, sub-Saharan Africa, and Melanesia. Risk is low in most developed countries, Latin America, and South Central Asia.

Chronic infection with hepatitis B virus (HBV) is the main risk factor for liver cancer worldwide, and hepatitis C virus is also a factor. The best known co-factor is aflatoxin, a food contaminant produced by a common fungus of grains.

Most liver cancers—those caused by HBV—are preventable by childhood vaccination. This is discussed in detail in Chapter 5.

Cervical Cancer

After breast cancer, cervical cancer is the next most common cancer among women worldwide. It is much more important in developing countries. There cervical cancer accounts for some 15 percent of cancers among women, compared with less than 4 percent in developed countries. A large proportion of these cancers and deaths appear in younger women, well before age 65. The highest incidence rates are in sub-Saharan Africa, Latin America and the Caribbean, Melanesia, and South Central and Southeast Asia. Rates are low in China and Western Asia.

Nearly every case of cervical cancer is now known to be caused by one of a few strains of oncogenic HPV. This knowledge has opened a new avenue for prevention through vaccines. But even before the discoveries that contributed to that understanding, a dramatic decline in rates of cervical cancer incidence and death in developed countries was under way, representing one of the greatest successes of public health in the 20th century. Although rates already had begun falling in developed countries, it was the widespread adoption of the Pap smear to screen for precancerous lesions that brought levels down to their current lows. This and other developments are discussed in more detail in Chapter 6.

Treatment for cervical cancer can be very effective, even at somewhat advanced stages. As a result, survival rates are higher than for most other cancers, even in developing countries, where 5-year survival is estimated at about 40 percent.

Esophageal Cancer

Cancer of the esophagus is another cancer that is more common in developing countries, but extremely variable even among those countries. Rates are 20 times higher in China than in West Africa. Survival from esophageal cancer is poor, so it ranks higher in the frequency of cancer deaths (sixth) than in incidence (eighth).

The specific causes of esophageal cancer are not all known, but a large proportion of cases can be attributed (at least in part) to direct exposure of the esophageal surface to various ingested items. In the United States and Europe, most cases are attributable to a combination of tobacco smoking and alcohol. In the Indian subcontinent, chewing tobacco and betel nuts are important. In the Middle East and parts of South America, drinking very hot beverages poses a risk. Certain foods, in particular pickled and moldy foods common in Asia, are thought to play a role, and some micronutrient deficiencies have also been implicated. In some developed countries, a recent increase in certain types of esophageal cancer suggests increasing obesity as a factor, which is associated with esophageal reflux, another known risk factor.

Colon and Rectal Cancer

About 1 million new cases of cancer of the colon and rectum occurred in 2002, with 529,000 deaths. Unlike most cancers, these cancers occur with similar frequency in men and women (although with a slightly higher incidence in men). Survival at 5 years is much better in North America (65 percent) and Western Europe (54 percent) than in LMCs where data are available: 34 percent in Eastern Europe and 30 percent in India.

The incidence of colon and rectal cancers varies about 25-fold from the high-income and high incidence areas (North America, Australia and New Zealand, Western Europe, and Japan) to Africa and Asia, where incidence is lowest. Although detailed explanations are elusive, the variation is assumed to be environmental, with the leading factors related to major dietary components. International correlations (i.e., "ecologic correlations") with the level of animal fat intake (positive correlation) and fiber (negative correlation) and the risk of large bowel cancer are well accepted, as are findings from epidemiologic studies implicating obesity and a lack of physical activity. In countries where rates are already high, incidence rates are more or less stable, but mortality rates are falling. Where rates historically have been low (particularly in Asia), they seem to be rising.

Prostate Cancer

Prostate cancer is relatively common, more so in developed than developing countries (19 versus 5.3 percent). Three-quarters of all cases are in men age 65 and older. Recorded incidence rates are influenced strongly in developed countries by widespread screening, which not only detects earlier stage disease, in general, but cases that would never progress to clinical attention at all. As a result of screening and better treatment, the reported 5-year relative survival in the United States is 99 percent. The picture is somewhat different for mortality, which may be a better indicator of the risk of invasive or metastatic prostate cancer. Rates are high not only in North America, Northern and Western Europe, and Australia/New Zealand, but also in the Caribbean, Southern and Central Africa, and South America. Rates are low in Asia and North Africa. The U.S. prostate cancer mortality rate is 16 times higher than China's.

The impact of screening on prostate cancer statistics makes it difficult to interpret trends, but incidence and mortality appear to be increasing worldwide. The exception is the developed countries with high initial rates, where mortality has been decreasing, attributed mainly to early detection through screening. The causes of prostate cancer are not well understood. Geographic differences are mirrored by racial and ethnic differences documented not only in the United States, but in Brazil, where black populations have higher rates than whites, and whites have higher rates than those of Asian origin.

HOW THE CANCER BURDEN IN LMCS IS ESTIMATED

The most basic cancer statistics in populations are incidence, mortality, and survival. Incidence and survival data are collected in cancer-specific registries, while mortality from cancer is derived from national mortality statistics. Together, these can tell us about the magnitude of the current cancer burden in terms of the need (and unmet need) for medical care, the loss of life (in life-years), the DALYs lived while people are surviving with cancer, and something about the quality of cancer care (from survival, assuming a usable benchmark). Over time, trends emerge that reflect changes in the population, the environment, health, or other risk conditions (e.g., the appearance and increase in Kaposi's sarcoma in conjunction with the AIDS epidemic). More recently data are being collected on major risk factors for cancer and other chronic diseases through population surveys; concentrating on smoking habits, diet, and physical activity; and physiological and biochemical measurements (e.g., blood pressure and cholesterol).

These statistics are important for two reasons. The first is understanding the burden of cancer and thus, the most important opportunities for cancer control in a given population. Comparison to other populations can also be very useful. Second, the statistics are important for tracking progress, to determine whether control measures are having the intended effect. Therefore, consideration of the available data and the need for additional efforts should be part of national cancer control efforts. At the same time, it is unrealistic to propose that comprehensive data collection systems be established where, in fact, very little exists today in LMCs. The current status of relevant cancer data collection is reviewed next, ending with GLOBOCAN, the main international cancer data resource. The final part of this chapter discusses approaches to data collection useful for cancer control that are appropriate in resource-constrained countries.

Cancer Data Collection in LMCs

The amount and quality of vital and health statistics correlate generally with the economic status of countries. About 18 percent of low-income countries have recorded mortality data any time since 1950, and about 35 percent have published some population-based incidence data, although fewer than half of them are represented in the most recent edition of IARC's *Cancer Incidence in Five Continents*. Population-based cancer registries that are IARC members cover about 21 percent of the world population, with large disparities among areas (Figure 3-3).

Most (77 percent) lower middle-income countries do record mortality, and about 65 percent have reported some population-based incidence data, but again, far fewer are currently active (Table 3-8). Upper middle-income countries have a similar level of mortality reporting (72 percent) and about 60 percent have reported some population-based incidence data, but again, with fewer currently active. The quality of mortality data (as rated by WHO, discussed below) also improves with economic status. Of countries that collect mortality data, the data of 7 of 26 upper middle-income countries were rated as high quality, as were 2 of 40 lower middle-income countries, and none of 12 low-income countries.

Cancer Mortality Data

Most countries have established legal requirements for vital registration systems to count births and deaths, and censuses to enumerate the population. In reality, these systems are fully operational in a minority of countries. The countries with the least resources also tend to have the poorest vital information. Mortality—how many people are dying, at what ages, and from what underlying causes—is the most important information for cancer control planning. The population at risk, by age and gender (from census information), is also essential for calculating age- and sex-specific mortality rates by cause. Vital statistics have broad value, not limited to cancer or any

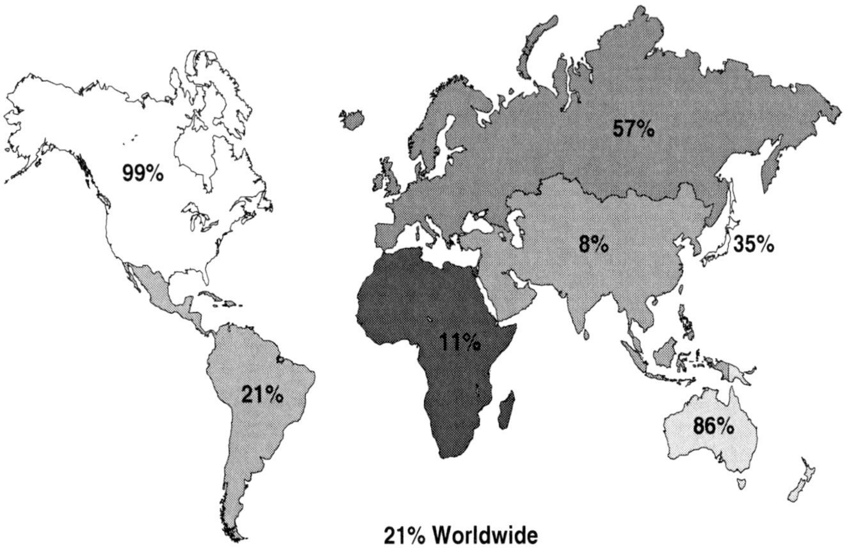

FIGURE 3-3 Population coverage by membership of the International Association of Cancer Registries, 2006.
SOURCE: Reprinted, with permission, from Parkin (2006). Copyright 2006 by Macmillan Publishers Ltd.

other single disease. Accordingly, decisions to invest in new or upgraded vital statistics systems, which entail long-term, sustained support, will not be made on the narrow basis of benefits to cancer control alone. The status of national mortality data globally is reviewed here.

All countries report their death registration data to WHO, which encourages and supports better reporting. A recent assessment of global cause of death reporting provides the first detailed examination of coverage (Mathers et al., 2005). In 1970, about 65 countries reported data; in 1990, 90 countries; and in 2003, 115 countries were reporting some usable cause of death data. Progress has not been uniform, however: For 75 countries, either no cause of death data are available at all or the latest information is from before 1990. Coverage by region ranges from nearly 100 percent of the countries in Europe reporting usable, recent information, to less than 10 percent in Africa.

Of the 115 countries reporting, coverage is considered to be essentially complete in 64. China and India do not have complete registration, but each has a defined sample registration system that provides reasonably represen-

TABLE 3-8 Mortality and Incidence Data Collected in Low- and Middle-Income Countries

World Bank Economic Level	Number of Countries	Some Mortality Any Time Since 1950	Quality of Mortality Data	Incidence in CA5C, Vol. 8: Number of Countries (%)	Any Incidence Data Since 1950
Low	66	12 (18%)	L: 3 M: 6 Representative but <50% coverage: 1 Not rated: 2 (<50% coverage, not representative)	6 (9%)	23 (35)
Lower middle	52	40 (77%)	L: 14 M: 13 H: 2 Representative but <50% coverage: 1 Not rated (various reasons): 10	9 (17%)	34 (65)
Upper middle	36	26 (72%)	L: 2 M: 17 H: 7	13 (36%)	22 (60)

CA5C = *Cancer Incidence in Five Continents;* L = low quality; M = medium quality; H = high quality.

SOURCES: Parkin et al. (2002); Mathers et al. (2005).

tative information on the whole population (Mathers et al., 2005). Coverage in many countries is incomplete either by design or because of difficulties in collecting the data. In some countries, only the urban areas or certain provinces or states are part of the system. Registration can be less complete in rural areas and areas with poor living conditions and is often worse for infants and children than for adults. Some residents (e.g., guest workers or refugees) may not be registered at all (Lopez et al., 2002). Including the sample systems in China and India, mortality data are available for about 72 percent of the world's population.

The quality of reported data is not uniform and is rated using generally accepted criteria (e.g., proportion of deaths of unknown cause). For countries that have supplied cause of death information to WHO for 1990 or later (until 2003), 23 are in the "high-quality" category, 55 are in the "medium-quality" category, and 28 are rated "low-quality." Most, but not all, of the countries with low-quality data are LMCs; those with medium-quality data are a mixture of countries, including a dozen or so in the high-income category. Data of low quality are unlikely to produce an unbiased picture of the distribution of causes of death (Mathers et al., 2005).

Strategies to Improve Cause of Death Reporting

Complete and ongoing reporting of vital events and periodic censuses are the ideal for all countries, but are unrealistic immediate goals for countries with minimally functioning systems. The sample systems already mentioned (India, China) are models for what has been described as a more cost-effective way to gather useful data on the levels, patterns, and causes of mortality in large populations. If resources become available, such systems can be expanded.

Cancer Incidence Data

Cancer incidence data are collected by specialized cancer registries. Cancer is not the only disease for which such surveillance exists, but it is the most prominent and best organized internationally. Two main types of cancer registries exist: hospital based and population based. Hospitals keep track of the patients with cancer diagnosed and/or treated, with at least some pertinent patient demographic and disease information. A hospital will generally know how many cases of various cancers are seen each year. This is useful information for the hospital and somewhat indicative of the types of cancer occurring in the community, but for a number of reasons may indicate substantially different patterns than are occurring in the population as a whole.

Not everyone has access to hospital care. Many simply die at home with or without a diagnosis, others may travel to another place (e.g., an ancestral area) when they are sick, and a host of other reasons may keep people from being treated at a hospital. Population-based registries, in which attempts are made to determine every case of cancer occurring in a population (e.g., a major metropolitan area, a state, or a country), are the gold standard for cancer incidence reporting. Unlike a hospital-based registry, they involve data collection through outreach to all possible places a patient might go or to which specimens might be sent for diagnosis, such as physicians' offices, clinics, and laboratories. Obviously, people who die without receiving a diagnosis will not be captured in such a system, but even in very poor countries, in or around major cities, most people come to some attention. From this information and census data on the demographic makeup of the population, age- and sex-specific incidence rates are calculated. Survival data also come from such systems. Attempts are made to track those in the system to find out whether they are still alive at defined points after diagnosis, and if they have died, to find out the cause.

The world's population-based cancer incidence has been gathered together by IARC in *Cancer Incidence in Five Continents*, published in 2002 for the eighth time (Parkin et al., 2002). The aim of this volume is "to present data on cancer incidence for all the populations of the world for which good quality data are available." Repeating words from the first volume, published in 1966, "The most valuable data are, undoubtedly, the rates obtained by recording the occurrence of every case of cancer over a specified period" in a specified population.

Worldwide, cancer incidence reporting has increased over time. In the early 1960s, 32 registries in 29 countries representing 35 populations were included in Volume 1 of *Cancer Incidence in Five Continents*. Volume 8, in 2002, included 186 registries in 57 countries representing 214 populations, representing data collected in the mid-1990s. However, only 29 LMCs are included in Volume 8 (Table 3-9). A number of the smaller, mostly upper middle-income, countries collect nationwide incidence data, and most of the rest represent urban areas only.

Cancer Survival

How long an individual survives once cancer develops, and whether death is ultimately related to the cancer or to some other cause, depends on many things. Factors related to the cancer itself—the site, histologic type, and stage at which it is diagnosed—the effectiveness of any treatment, and factors related to that person all affect survival. Across populations, cancer survival assumes specific patterns, and these are of interest mainly for purposes of comparison: How does survival—generally cancer-specific survival—compare across countries and populations, and how has it changed over time?

Population-based cancer survival has been reported for decades from registries in the United States, Europe, and other more developed areas. The first and only comparative analysis of cancer survival from other parts of the world waited until 1998, when IARC published *Cancer Survival in Developing Countries* (Sankaranarayanan et al., 1998). That report includes data from nine population-based cancer registries in five countries in Asia, and from the National Cancer Registry of Cuba. Countries of Africa and South America have yet to be represented in such a compilation. Had there been any with adequate data, they would have been included (but see Box 3-2, which discusses cancer survival in Kampala, Uganda). The reasons for the lack of data are not hard to fathom: Few cancer registries exist in developing countries and of those operating, some are relatively new. Most effort, with limited resources, is spent on improving the identification of new cases, and

TABLE 3-9 Low- and Middle-Income Countries Represented in Volume 8, *Cancer Incidence in Five Continents*

Continent/Income Level/Country	Area of Country Covered by Registry
Africa	
Low Income	
The Gambia	Nationwide
Mali	Bamako
Uganda	Kayadondo County (Kampala)
Zimbabwe	Harare
Lower Middle Income	
Algeria	Algiers
Asia	
Low Income	
India	Ahmedabad; Bangalore; Chennai; Delhi; Karunagappally; Mumbai; Nagpur; Poona; Trivandrum
Pakistan	South Karachi
Vietnam	Hanoi; Ho Chi Minh City
Lower Middle Income	
China	Beijing; Changle; Cixian; Jiashan; Qidong County; Shanghai; Tianjin; Wuhan
Philippines	Manila; Rizal
Thailand	Bangkok; Chiang Mai; Khon Kaen; Lampang; Songkla
Upper Middle Income	
Oman	Omani
Europe	
Lower Middle Income	
Belarus	Nationwide
Yugoslavia (Serbia and Montenegro)	Vojvodina
Upper Middle Income	
Croatia	Nationwide
Czech Republic	Nationwide
Estonia	Nationwide
Latvia	Nationwide
Lithuania	Nationwide
Malta	Nationwide
Poland	Cracow; Kielce; Lower Silesia; Warsaw City
Slovak Republic	Nationwide
South and Central America/Caribbean	
Lower Middle Income	
Colombia	Cali
Cuba	Villa Clara
Ecuador	Quito
Upper Middle Income	
Argentina	Bahia Blanca; Concordia
Brazil	Campinas; Goiania
Costa Rica	Nationwide
Uruguay	Montevideo

SOURCE: Parkin et al. (2002).

BOX 3-2
Cancer Survival in Kampala, Uganda

The Kampala Cancer Registry has demonstrated the potential to collect informative cancer incidence data in a low-income country at very low cost. Most recently, data from the registry were used to describe cancer survival in the mid-1990s (Gondos et al., 2005). These data provide a much clearer picture than is possible from the estimates of incidence and mortality that are used as surrogates for most of sub-Saharan Africa. The only other set of information on cancer survival in Africa comes from a registry in Harare, Zimbabwe (Gondos et al., 2004).

The Kampala Cancer Registry was established in 1951, making it one of the longest running registries in Africa. The registry ceased functioning entirely during the most severe political upheavals in the country, from 1980 until 1989, but since resuming, it has operated continuously. The area covered includes Kampala, the Ugandan capital, and neighboring urban and semiurban areas with a total estimated population of 1.2 million.

Changes in cancer incidence from the 1960s through the 1990s have been tracked, documenting, for example, the appearance and rise in AIDS-related cancers in the 1990s. These include large increases in Kaposi's sarcoma, squamous cell carcinoma of the conjunctiva (part of the eye), and non-Hodgkin's lymphoma.

Case Finding

Even in the poorest countries, most people with cancer contact the health care system sometime before they die. Where people have access to urban hospitals, they may be even more likely to seek treatment. Cancer cases are identified for the Kampala registry by actively searching the patient records of six hospitals, three pathology laboratories, and Hospice Uganda, which provides palliative care for people dying from cancer and AIDS. Registration of cancer cases is about 90 percent complete, according to an evaluation carried out in the mid-1990s (Parkin et al., 2001).

Survival

In the United States and most countries with adequate vital statistics systems, we expect accurate data on the numbers and causes of death. We also expect that, given cancer registries, we can track people until their deaths (or link to death records) and thereby calculate survival rates from different types of cancer, and more narrowly, using data in the patient records on, for example, stage and co-morbidities. This capability is not built into systems in poor countries, where mortality data are not

continued

BOX 3-2 Continued

complete and may be unreliable. This is the case in Uganda, where a survival analysis was undertaken recently.

The study reports survival from the 13 most common types of cancer reported between 1993 and 1997 in the Kampala registry. Vital status was recorded up to the end of 1999. If records of the institution that reported on the patient could provide information, it was used. In all other cases, verification of vital status had to be sought through visits to patients' homes. With few street addresses, and often just the name of the village or area, even after intense efforts, just under three-quarters of the patients could be traced. In the analyses, the data for untraceable patients were included appropriately (recorded as "alive" the last time they were seen, and "censored" thereafter). It is unlikely that the patients lost to follow-up fared better than those with complete information. Study personnel often found out something about these people, including many who neighbors said had gone to their ancestral homes, most likely to die. With no cancer services anywhere outside of Kampala, they would have little chance of further treatment.

During the target years, 2,337 patients were reported to the Kampala registry. Of these, 506 did not have sufficient information recorded about their cancers to include them further. Of the 1,831 remaining, 1,205 had complete follow-up data. Histological verification of the tumor was available for just over 60 percent of all those included in the analysis (1,831). Except for those with cancers of the thyroid and prostate, the Ugandan patients were younger than African Americans in the United States with the same cancers (this was taken into account in the analysis).

For each type of cancer, both absolute and relative survival were calculated. Absolute survival is simply the proportion of all patients still alive, over time. Relative survival takes into account the probability of dying from other causes during the period of survival, applying estimates of survival for the entire Ugandan population. The relative survival rates were also compared with the corresponding rates for African Americans, using data from the U.S. Surveillance, Epidemiology and End Results (SEER) Program.

Results

The survival of the Ugandan patients was uniformly poor (Table 1). In comparison with African Americans, survival was similar only for those cancers that were rarely treated successfully anywhere, including esophageal, stomach, liver, and lung cancers. The biggest differences between the two populations were recorded for cancers for which there were effective treatments. The most dramatic difference was for thyroid cancer, which is highly curable. Among African Americans, 95 percent

TABLE 1 Five-Year Relative Survival (in %) of Ugandan Patients with Cancer, Kampala, Uganda, 1993–1997

Cancer Site	5-Year Relative Survival (%)	Number of Patients Contributing to Analysis[a]
Nasopharynx	0.0	50
Esophagus	4.5±2.3	182
Stomach	0.0	91
Colon/rectum	8.3±3.9	104
Liver	3.2±2.2	117
Lung	0.0	50
Breast	45.4±7.1	174
Cervix	18.2±4.8	285
Ovary	16.2±8.1	69
Prostate	46.9±7.7	161
Eye	34.2±9.8	88
Thyroid	13.4±11.4	41
Lymphomas	35.4±5.8	199
Kaposi's sarcoma, HIV positive	9.1±3.6	188
Kaposi's sarcoma, HIV negative	65.7±14.2	32

[a]This includes patients with complete and incomplete follow-up; overall, 27 percent were lost to follow-up before 5 years.

SOURCE: Gondos et al. (2005).

survived 5 years, compared with only 12 percent of the Ugandans. Large gaps between the two populations also were apparent for nasopharyngeal, colorectal, cervical, ovarian, and prostate cancers.

Discussion

Cancer patients in Uganda have very poor survival odds—lower than the few other developing countries where survival has been documented (Sankaranarayanan et al., 1998). This is the outcome that must be expected where annual per capita incomes are less than $300 (World Bank, 2003) and health care spending is less than $50 per capita. An estimated 5 percent of the population has access to the meager cancer treatment facilities, all of which are centered in Kampala. Data on cancer stage at presentation are lacking, but the evidence points to the majority being in late stages. Sixty percent of the deaths occurred in the first year after diagnosis, and 80 percent by the end of 2 years. Those presenting at earlier stages would have a better chance of finding life-saving treatment, but with treatment so scarce, earlier diagnosis may make little difference.

only once that area is sufficiently developed will the task of following up on registered cases commence.

The 10 registries included in *Cancer Survival in Developing Countries* are likely to include what are among the best survival experiences in the developing world. These countries were among those developing rapidly, with better cancer services than other countries. The existence of the registries also signals an urban catchment area with above-average cancer services.

Findings from *Cancer Survival in Developing Countries*

The 10 registries and the time periods represented in the volume are listed in Table 3-10. To the extent possible, the data were made comparable (Sankaranarayanan et al., 1998). Even among these developing countries, wide variations in survival from some cancers was reported. The analysis also includes comparisons with registries in the United States (white population) and Europe, so differences were also noted between the higher- and lower income areas. Figure 3-4 broadly summarizes the relationships found. These are not surprising and are, in fact, intuitive, but it is useful to see them drawn on the basis of evidence. Three major patterns are apparent:

1. **Cancers with poor prognosis:** These cancers have the smallest survival differential between low- and high-income countries, and include cancers of the esophagus, liver, lung, and pancreas. They are often detected at advanced stages in both low- and high-income countries, because no

TABLE 3-10 Registries Included in *Cancer Survival in Developing Countries*

Registry Area	Cancer Registration Period (diagnosis)	Closing Date of Follow-Up
China		
Qidong	1982–1991	31 Dec 94
Shanghai	1988–1991	31 Dec 94
Cuba	1988–1989	31 Dec 94
India		
Bangalore	1982–1989	31 Dec 93
Barshi	1988–1992	31 Dec 95
Bombay	1982–1986	31 Dec 93
Madras	1984–1989	31 Dec 93
Philippines: Rizal	1987	31 Dec 93
Thailand		
Chiang Mai	1983–1992	30 Jun 94
Khon Kaen	1985–1992	31 Dec 95

SOURCE: Sankaranarayanan et al. (1998).

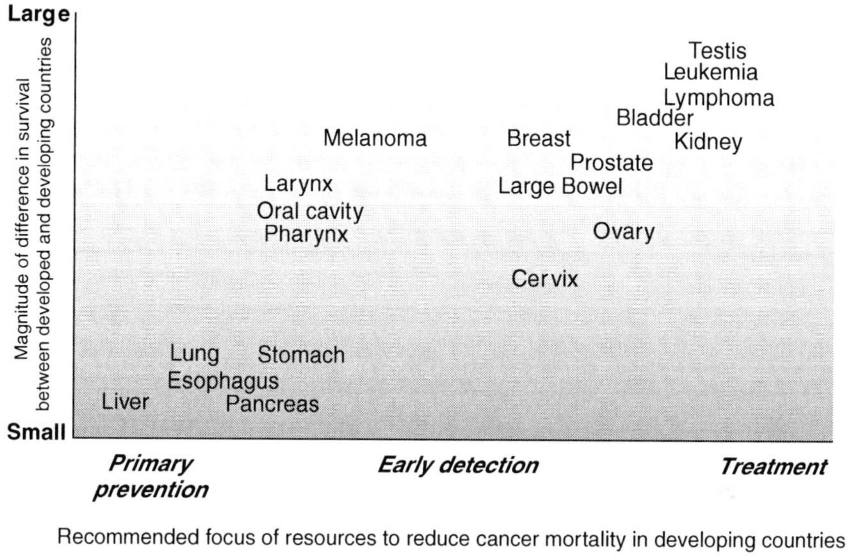

FIGURE 3-4 Cancer survival differences between developed and developing countries and implications for control measures.
SOURCE: Reprinted, with permission, from Sanakaranarayanan et al. (1998). Copyright 2006 by the International Agency for Research on Cancer.

effective screening or early diagnosis techniques are available. Even with the best available treatment, most people who develop these cancers anywhere in the world do not survive for an extended period of time.

2. **Cancers with early detection, diagnosis, and treatment options that are relatively easy to implement:** For a second group of cancers, including melanoma and cancers of the head and neck, large bowel, breast, cervix, ovary, urinary bladder, and thyroid, there is greater variation in survival between developing and developed countries, and probably between low-income and middle-income countries, at least in some cases. For these cancers, early detection, diagnosis, and treatment that, in principle, can be delivered through basic health care facilities is effective and improves survival. To the extent they are implemented in low-resource settings, survival will be improved.

3. **Cancers with effective diagnostic and treatment interventions that require improved logistics:** A third group of cancers, including leukemia, lymphoma, and testicular cancer, are marked by an even greater variability in survival between developing and developed countries. Effective treatments are available for these cancers, but they are multimodal treatments requir-

ing a greater degree of medical resources, a good health care infrastructure, and sophisticated knowledge. The cancers in this group are relatively less common in developing countries.

GLOBOCAN: Cancer Incidence, Mortality, and Survival for All Countries

Given that neither mortality nor cancer incidence data are recorded directly in most LMCs, how are we able to include numbers representing global cancer mortality and incidence, such as those at the beginning of this chapter? How do we know there were 11 million cases and 7 million deaths from cancer in 2002? As referenced earlier, these are estimates from GLOBOCAN, a database created by IARC, part of WHO, that includes estimates of the incidence and prevalence of, and mortality from, 27 cancers for all countries in the world, most recently for 2002.

GLOBOCAN data reflect all reliable information from cancer registries and mortality reporting, and where these sources of information are missing or incomplete, estimates of incidence, mortality, population, and prevalence made following explicit rules (see http://www-dep.iarc.fr/). GLOBOCAN is accessible through the IARC Cancer*Mondial* webpage (see http://www-dep.iarc.fr/) and on CD-ROM, and is widely cited in the global cancer literature.

Surveillance of Risk Factors

In addition to knowing how many cancers are occurring and how many people are dying from cancer, knowing the distribution of risk factors—in particular, those that are modifiable—can be extremely useful. As noted in a WHO report, "the risk factors of today are the diseases of tomorrow" (Bonita et al., 2001). Cancer shares risk factors with other major causes of death from noncommunicable diseases, and it is surveillance of these major, shared risk factors that are the basis of two approaches described in the next sections. The first is WHO's approach, cross-sectional sample surveys that can be adapted for use in every country, even in low-resource areas. The second is longitudinal studies that involve following large cohorts of people over decades; these studies are generally more appropriate for middle-income countries.

WHO "STEPwise" Approach

WHO has developed an initial three-step approach to population surveys for surveillance of risk factors in response to a resolution on the prevention and control of noncommunicable diseases, passed by the World Health

Assembly in 2000. The steps provide flexibility in the level of effort that can be made initially, while allowing for expansion when resources permit. The use of standard survey instruments across time and countries allows for more valid comparisons on those dimensions. Countries may also choose to add more detailed questions or tests, depending on their situation. As with all surveys, the sampling frames must be carefully defined and the numbers surveyed sufficient to provide reliable estimates of the actual population rates. (WHO provides step-by-step guidance for all aspects of the survey through a series of documents available at http://www.who.int/chp/steps/en/, and carries out training programs all over the world.)

The major noncommunicable diseases are cardiovascular diseases, cancers, diabetes, and chronic respiratory diseases. The most important common risk factors that are amenable to intervention are identified as smoking, unhealthy alcohol consumption, unhealthy diet (specifically, low intake of fruits and vegetables), physical inactivity, overweight and obesity, raised blood pressure, raised blood glucose, and raised blood lipids. Of these, smoking has the greatest impact on cancer, but all except raised blood pressure are considered by WHO to have some relevance to cancer (Bonita et al., 2001).

The steps are the following:

1. **Questionnaire-based assessment:** Reports from respondents on socio-economic data, data on tobacco and alcohol use, and some measurements of nutrient status and physical inactivity.
2. **Step 1 plus physical measurements:** Simple physical measurements are added to step 1, including at least blood pressure, height, weight, and waist circumference.
3. **Step 2 plus biochemical measurements:** Measurements on blood samples, including at least fasting blood sugar and total cholesterol.

At each step, a "core" set of data is defined, and an "expanded core" and optional items are suggested. The exact measures should be tailored to specific country needs. Steps 1 and 2 are considered "desirable and appropriate for most countries," while step 3 is not recommended by WHO in "less well-resourced settings unless low-cost technology is used" (Bonita et al., 2001).

The STEPwise approach is meeting with success in terms of training and initial surveys. WHO has provided training to 82 countries, including every country in Africa, and 23 countries have completed initial reports (Personal communication, J. Lippe, WHO, May 2006). It will be at least a few years before sufficient data are built up from different countries to appreciate the full value, but this tool appears to be a good choice for most countries, regardless of other data collection efforts.

Large Prospective Studies of Risk Factors and Deaths

Surveying for well-known risk factors for cancer and other noncommunicable diseases is of clear benefit for disease control planning and monitoring. In order to extend our understanding of these risk factors in populations not yet studied, and identify and characterize risk factors not yet well studied, a different approach is needed. Large prospective (longitudinal) studies serve this function, as well as providing surveillance for *known* risk factors. In each such study, hundreds of thousands of adults are interviewed briefly about major risk factors (e.g., smoking, diet) and have basic physical measurements taken (and blood samples stored, in some cases). Households are revisited periodically to record household members' vital status, and the participants are resurveyed periodically (e.g., every 3 to 5 years) for changes in risk factors. When cohort members die, the cause of death is ascertained. Such studies, involving more than 2 million people, are under way in a handful of countries. A modest number of additional studies should be started periodically to capture unstudied populations, expand the information base on known risk factors, add measures based on new science, and exploit new technologies (e.g., genetic and information) to gather information on large cohorts economically. This is already the case in the current studies, which have an estimated cost of follow-up of $1 per person per year (Personal communication, R. Peto, University of Oxford, June 2006).

A leader in large prospective studies to date has been the Clinical Trial Service Unit and Epidemiological Studies Unit (CTSU) at the University of Oxford, England (Clinical Trial Service Unit, 2006), in collaboration with researchers and governmental and academic organizations in the survey areas. The most mature of the CTSU collaborative studies is a nationally representative study of men only, in China. In 1991, information was recorded on smoking, drinking, weight, height, blood pressure, lung function, medical history, and various social factors in about 225,000 adult men throughout China. Reliable systems of follow-up were put into place, and by 1996 the dates and causes of 12,000 deaths had been recorded. Of these deaths, vascular, neoplastic, respiratory, and all other causes each accounted for about one-quarter. Preliminary analyses were consistent with the conclusion from other studies that, during the 1990s, at least 0.6 million deaths each year in China were directly attributable to smoking (Niu et al., 1998).

Long-term follow-up of the initial Chinese study is continuing, with periodic resurveys of all middle-aged adults living in the study areas. In addition, it is proposed that blood samples be collected at the next resurvey so that nested case-control analyses can be conducted subsequently, as is being done already in some other sites, which include women as well as men. This will allow the age-specific relevance of established risk factors and of newer risk factors (e.g., various details of the lipid profile, coagulation factors, antioxidants, micronutrients, antibodies, genetic variants, etc.) for vascular and other diseases to be studied reliably in "nested" case-control studies. Additional studies are under way in Mexico City (200,000 adults over age 40); Russia (four regions: 100,000 adults); Egypt (150–200,000 adults); Trivandrum, south India (200,000 adults); Bombay, west India (200,000 adults); Madras, east India (300,000 adults); and Cuba (200,000 adults).

Many of CTSU's prospective studies have been paired with large retrospective studies that can provide a reliable snapshot of tobacco-attributable deaths at about the time the prospective studies begin. This was done in southern India, where the smoking habits of 43,000 men who had died of various diseases in the late 1990s were compared with the habits of 35,000 living men (the study was restricted to men because few women smoked). About one-quarter of the smokers studied died at ages 25–69, with those dying at these ages losing, on average, 20 years of life. The expected results for cancer and vascular diseases were confirmed, but an unexpected finding also emerged: about half of the deaths from tuberculosis, which causes more than 10 percent of deaths in this population, were attributable to smoking (Gajalakshmi et al., 2003). Had these people not smoked, they would not have died of tuberculosis. This is not a finding about cancer, but it demonstrates that even in a study of smoking—about which quite a lot is known, mainly from wealthy countries—new and surprising (and potentially life saving) information can come to light.

There may be a misperception that little more can be learned from further studies of this kind, particularly for established risk factors (such as smoking and blood lipids). But the effects of such factors can vary enormously from one population to another, and there is still substantial uncertainty as to how important they are in different settings and how their importance is changing with time. CTSU's studies, for example, have defined the outlines of the future epidemic of deaths due to tobacco in developing countries: If current smoking patterns persist, worldwide deaths from tobacco will increase from about 3 million a year now to about 10 million a year by 2025.

SUMMARY AND RECOMMENDATIONS

There should be no doubt that cancer imposes a substantial burden on all countries, even though the *proportion* of mortality (and other burden measures) is less in LMCs than in high-income countries. Infectious diseases are still the biggest killers, particularly in low-income countries and some middle-income countries. What lies behind the cancer burden figures, however, is a very thin veneer of data and a great deal of estimation, mainly of cancer incidence and mortality. A small amount of data on survival also exists. Conceptually, burden would also include disability, loss of productivity, caregiving burden, out-of-pocket expenditures, etc., but such information is largely unavailable for these countries.

Few LMCs have accurate recent data about their cancer burden or major risk factors for cancer (or other chronic diseases). The lack of health status information extends well beyond cancer to the entire range of vital and health statistics. The estimates produced by IARC for each country are useful for setting initial priorities, but cannot be used to track progress—positive or negative—or to define more precisely what priorities should be in the medium to long term.

Major improvements in overall vital and health statistics will take time. Over the short term, it is feasible to propose modest improvements in the information base, however. In particular, it is relatively inexpensive to gather information on the major risk factors for cancer and other noncommunicable diseases in periodic cross-sectional surveys. WHO's STEPwise Approach to Chronic Disease Risk Factor Surveillance is well developed, and training and other assistance is available from WHO. The standardized STEPwise Approach has the advantage of producing comparable information across countries as well as over time.

Measuring causes of death in a population is more ambitious, but nevertheless highly worthwhile. In low-income countries in particular, this is difficult because many people die without medical care, or at least without a diagnosis before death. Systems based on "verbal autopsies" (determinations based on interviews of family members, health care workers, and others with information about the circumstances of a person's death) can be developed in place of medical certification, as demonstrated in India's "Million Death Study" in a network of sample registration areas that constitute a nationally representative sample of deaths (Jha et al., 2006).

Prospective (longitudinal) studies of chronic disease risk factors and causes of death involving several million people have been initiated as collaborations between researchers in LMCs and high-income countries. Results are already available from a few LMCs, such as China, India (including the "Million Death Study"), and Mexico. These studies have documented the unique patterns of diseases and their risk factors, such as the strong link between smoking and tuberculosis deaths in India or smoking and lung cancer and chronic lung disease in China. Cohort studies such as these are complex, requiring extensive planning as well as the sustained commitment of human and financial resources for data collection, processing, and analysis. The investment is a significant one on all counts, but the cost need not be prohibitive. Studies now under way cost on average $1 per person/per year to maintain (Personal communication, R. Peto, University of Oxford, April 2006).

Finally, cancer registries that record cancer cases and the outcomes of those cases—at least in specific hospitals, and more usefully, in defined geographic areas—are important for understanding local conditions, at least for those who come to medical attention. Registries require sustained commitments and trained personnel, which are most feasible in urban areas where diagnosis and treatment are available.

International assistance and collaboration should be available for all of these monitoring and surveillance activities, to take advantage of existing knowledge and experience.

The recommendations from this chapter focus on better characterizing the cancer burden (along with other diseases) in LMCs to support cancer control planning and monitoring. They are based on the usefulness and feasibility (including cost, although we were not able to make specific cost estimates) following from the discussion in the chapter.

RECOMMENDATION 3-1. The following should be considered:

Risk factor surveillance *for chronic diseases should be initiated in many countries using standardized questionnaires (e.g., STEPS).*

Collection of cause-specific mortality data should be a long-term goal in every country. *Where vital statistics systems are weak or nonexistent, initial data collection may be sentinel sites rather than nationwide. Improved mortality reporting at a level appropriate to the country should be supported as a part of cancer control activities.*

Longitudinal studies of chronic disease risk factors and mortality should be initiated in a few additional middle-income countries.

Cancer registries should be developed in conjunction with cancer control activities, *mainly in urban areas where diagnostic and treatment services exist. Where new or existing cancer centers are developed into centers of excellence, registries in the catchment area should be a part of the development.*

REFERENCES

Amir H, Azizi MR, Makwaya CK, Jessani S. 1997. TNM classification and breast cancer in an African population: A descriptive study. *Central African Journal of Medicine* 43(12):357–359.

Anyanwu SN. 2000. Survival following treatment of primary breast cancer in eastern Nigeria. *East African Medical Journal* 77(10):539–543.

Barton M, Frommer M, Shafiq J. 2005. *The Role of Radiotherapy in Cancer Control in Low- and Middle-Income Countries.* Commissioned by the Institute of Medicine. Typescript.

Bonita R, de Courten M, Dwyer T, Jamrozik K, Winkelmann R. 2001. *Surveillance of Risk Factors for Noncommunicable Diseases: The WHO STEPwise Approach. Summary.* Geneva, Switzerland: World Health Organization.

Bray F, Sankila R, Ferlay J, Parkin DM. 2002. Estimates of cancer incidence and mortality in Europe in 1995. *European Journal of Cancer* 38(1):99–166.

Chopra R. 2001. The Indian scene. *Journal of Clinical Oncology* 19(18 Suppl):106S–111S.

Clinical Trial Service Unit, University of Oxford. 2006. *Need for Large-Scale Observational Epidemiology.* [Online]. Available: http://www.ctsu.ox.ac.uk/projects/observational.shtml#rp [accessed May 31, 2006].

Gajalakshmi V, Peto R, Kanaka TS, Jha P. 2003. Smoking and mortality from tuberculosis and other diseases in India: Retrospective study of 43,000 adult male deaths and 35,000 controls. *Lancet* 362(9383):507–515.

Gondos A, Brenner H, Wabinga H, Parkin DM. 2005. Cancer survival in Kampala, Uganda. *British Journal of Cancer* 92(9):1808–1812.

Gondos A, Chokunonga E, Brenner H, Parkin DM, Sankila R, Borok MZ, Chirenje ZM, Nyakabau AM, Bassett MT. 2004. Cancer survival in a southern African urban population. *International Journal of Cancer* 112(5):860–864.

Jha P, Gajalakshmi V, Gupta PC, Kumar R, Mony P, Dhingra1 N, Peto R, RGI-CGHR Prospective Study Collaborators. 2006. Prospective study of one million deaths in India: Rationale, design and validation results. *PLoS* 3(2):e18.

Lopez AD, Ahmad O, Guillot M, Ferguson B, Salomon J, Murray CJL, et al. 2002. *World Mortality in 2000: Life Tables for 191 Countries.* Geneva, Switzerland: World Health Organization.

Lopez AD, Mathers CD, Ezzati M, Jamison DT, Murray CJL. 2006. *Global Burden of Disease and Risk Factors.* New York: Oxford University Press.

Malik IA. 2002. Clinico-pathological features of breast cancer in Pakistan. *Journal of the Pakistan Medical Association* 52(3):100–104.

Mathers CD, Ma Fat D, Inoue M, Rao C, Lopez AD. 2005. Counting the dead and what they died from: An assessment of the global status of cause of death data. *Bulletin of the World Health Organization* 83(3):171–177.

Niu SR, Yang GH, Chen ZM, Wang JL, Wang GH, He XZ, Schoepff H, Boreham J, Pan HC, Peto R. 1998. Emerging tobacco hazards in China: Early mortality results from a prospective study. *BMJ* 317(7170):1423–1424.

Omar S, Khaled H, Gaafar R, Zekry AR, Eissa S, el-Khatib O. 2003. Breast cancer in Egypt: A review of disease presentation and detection strategies. *Eastern Mediterranean Health Journal* 9(3):448–463.

Parkin DM. 2006. The evolution of the population-based cancer registry. *Nature Reviews Cancer* 6:603–612.

Parkin DM, Bray F, Ferlay J, Pisani P. 2005. Global cancer statistics, 2002. *Ca: A Cancer Journal for Clinicians* 55(2):74–108.

Parkin DM, Wabinga H, Nambooze S. 2001. Completeness in an African cancer registry. *Cancer Causes & Control* 12(2):147–152.

Parkin DM, Whelan SL, Ferlay J, Teppo L, Thomas DB. 2002. *Cancer Incidence in Five Continents, Volume VIII.* Lyon, France: International Agency for Research on Cancer.

Sankaranarayanan R, Black RJ, Parkin DM. 1998. *Cancer Survival in Developing Countries.* Lyon, France: International Agency for Research on Cancer. IARC Scientific Publications No. 145.

Schwartsmann G. 2001. Breast cancer in South America: Challenges to improve early detection and medical management of a public health problem. *Journal of Clinical Oncology* 19(18 Suppl):118S–124S.

Vorobiof DA, Sitas F, Vorobiof G. 2001. Breast cancer incidence in South Africa. *Journal of Clinical Oncology* 19(18 Suppl):125S–127S.

World Bank. *2003 World Development Indicators.* Washington, DC: World Bank.

World Health Organization. 2003. *The World Health Report 2003: Shaping the Future*. Geneva: World Health Organization.

World Health Organization. 2006. *Revised Global Burden of Disease (GBD) 2002 Estimates*. [Online]. Available: http://www.who.int/healthinfo/bodgbd2002revised/en/index.html [accessed January 4, 2006].

World Health Organization. 2006. *Core Health Indicators*. [Online] Available: http://www3.who.int/whosis/core/core_select.cfm?strISO3_select=MYS&strIndicator_select=MortInfantBoth&intYear_select=latest&language=english [accessed 7/10/06].

4

Defining Resource-Level-Appropriate Cancer Control

Interventions for cancer, from prevention through palliative care, have been developed largely in high-income countries. In these countries, where cancer is often referred to as "the most feared disease," the emphasis has always been on maximizing effectiveness and safety. Cost—in terms of money and of other inputs—has been a secondary concern, and other factors that would affect the appropriateness or feasibility of applying an intervention in resource-constrained settings have been considered very little. Specifically, a health care infrastructure sufficient to cover the population, from primary through tertiary care, is assumed. An educated public, reached by at least some basic information about cancer, and access to health care and good nutrition, is taken for granted. Finally, in most high-income countries health care is free or affordable for all or most. Developing cancer control in places where conditions are much different means that all these factors, as well as societal factors, must be considered in deciding on the best approaches. Explicit analysis of effectiveness and costs of alternative approaches and interventions may also help to counter the natural attraction of the medical community and politicians, in low- and middle-income countries (LMCs), as well as in high-income countries, to the newest, high-technology (and expensive) interventions. This is the basic idea behind "resource-level-appropriate" cancer control.

The World Health Organization (WHO), in its 1992 report on guidelines and policies for National Cancer Control Programmes, gave prominence to the idea of tailoring interventions to three scenarios: low, medium, and high resource levels, in a very general sense (WHO, 2002) (Table 4-1). The underlying concepts were enunciated, but not the "how to." The idea

TABLE 4-1 Priority Actions for National Cancer Control Programs, According to Level of Resources

Aspect	All Countries	Scenario A: Low Level of Resources	Scenario B: Medium Level of Resources	Scenario C: High Level of Resources
National cancer control program	• Develop a national cancer control program to ensure effective, efficient, and equitable use of existing resources • Establish a core surveillance mechanism to monitor and evaluate outcomes as well as processes • Develop education and continuous training for health care workers	• Consider the implementation of one or two key priorities in a demonstration area with a stepwise approach • Consider palliative care as an entry point to a more comprehensive approach • Use appropriate technologies that are effective and sustainable in this type of setting	• When initiating or formulating a cancer control program, consider implementation of a comprehensive approach in a demonstration area using a stepwise methodology • Use appropriate technologies that are effective and sustainable in this type of setting	• Full, nationwide implementation of evidence-based strategies guaranteeing effectiveness, efficiency, and accessibility • Implement a comprehensive surveillance system, tracking all program components and results • Provide support for less affluent countries

continued

TABLE 4-1 Continued

Aspect	All Countries	Scenario A: Low Level of Resources	Scenario B: Medium Level of Resources	Scenario C: High Level of Resources
Prevention	• Implement integrated health promotion and prevention strategies for noncommunicable diseases that include legislative/regulatory and environmental measures as well as education for the general public, targeted communities, and individuals • Control tobacco use, and address alcohol use, unhealthy diet, physical activity, and sexual and reproductive factors • Promote policy to minimize occupational-related cancers and known environmental carcinogens • Promote avoidance of unnecessary exposure to sunlight in high-risk populations	• Focus on areas where there are great needs and potential for success • Ensure that priority prevention strategies are targeted to those groups that are influential and can spearhead the process (e.g., policy makers and teachers) • In areas endemic for liver cancer, integrate hepatitis B virus vaccine with other vaccination programs	• Develop integrated clinical preventive services for counseling on risk factors in primary health care settings, schools, and workplaces • Develop model community programs for an integrated approach to prevention of noncommunicable diseases	• Strengthen comprehensive evidence-based health promotion and prevention programs and ensure nationwide implementation in collaboration with other sectors • Establish routine monitoring of ultraviolet radiation levels if the risk of skin cancer is high

Early diagnosis	• Promote early diagnosis through awareness of early signs and symptoms of detectable and curable tumors that have high prevalence in the community, such as breast and cervical cancer • Ensure proper diagnostic and treatment services are available for the detected cases • Provide education and continuous training to target populations and health care providers	• Use low-cost and effective community approaches to promote, in a first phase, early diagnosis of one or two priority detectable tumors in pilot areas with relatively good access to diagnosis and treatment	• Use low-cost and effective community approaches to promote early diagnosis of all priority detectable tumors	• Use comprehensive nationwide promotion strategies for early diagnosis of all highly prevalent detectable tumors
Screening	• Implement screening for cancers of the breast and cervix where incidence justifies such action and the necessary resources are available	• If there is already infrastructure for cervical cytology screening, provide high coverage of effective and efficient cytology screening for women aged 35 to 40 years once in their lifetimes or, if more resources are available, every 10 years for women aged 30 to 60 years	• Provide national coverage cytology screening for cervical cancer at 5-year intervals to women aged 30 to 60 years	• Effective and efficient national screening for cervical cancer (cytology) of women over age 30 years and breast cancer screening (mammography) of women over age 50 years

continued

TABLE 4-1 Continued

Aspect	All Countries	Scenario A: Low Level of Resources	Scenario B: Medium Level of Resources	Scenario C: High Level of Resources
Curative therapy	• Ensure accessibility of effective diagnostic and treatment services • Promote national minimum essential standards for disease staging and treatment • Establish management guidelines for treatment services, essential drugs list, and continuous training • Avoid performing curative therapy when cancer is incurable and patients should be offered palliative care instead	• Organize diagnosis and treatment services, giving priority to early detectable tumors	• Organize diagnosis and treatment services, giving priority to early detectable tumors or to those with high potential of curability	• Reinforce the network of comprehensive cancer treatment centers that are active for clinical training and research and give special support for the ones acting as national and international reference centers
Pain relief and palliative care	• Implement comprehensive palliative care that provides pain relief, other symptom control, and psychosocial and spiritual support • Promote national minimum standards for management of pain and palliative care • Ensure availability and accessibility of opioids, especially oral morphine • Provide education and training for caregivers and public	• Ensure that minimum standards for pain relief and palliative care are progressively adopted by all levels of care in targeted areas and that there is high coverage of patients through services provided mainly by home-based care	• Ensure that minimum standards for pain relief and palliative care are progressively adopted by all levels of care and nationwide there is rising coverage of patients through services provided by primary health care clinics and home-based care	• Ensure that national pain relief and palliative care guidelines are adopted by all levels of care and nationwide there is high coverage of patients through a variety of options, including home-based care

SOURCE: Reprinted, with permission, from WHO (2002). Copyright 2002 by WHO.

of resource-level-appropriate thinking is intuitively simple, but filling in the details requires systematic analyses of varying complexity. How do policy makers know what specific approach or intervention is likely to succeed under their own circumstances? What is a "comprehensive approach"? What are "necessary resources"? What level of incidence justifies a prevention or early detection program? What WHO laid out was actually an agenda for operations research to develop the information needed to guide complex decisions at the national and local levels in low- and middle-income countries (LMCs), but not the information itself. This agenda is now beginning to be addressed, but it requires significantly more effort.

This chapter discusses the means of generating the resource-level-specific information and guidance needed to put this notion into practice. This is not to suggest that decisions and policy cannot be made and actions taken today. Although the concept of resource appropriateness applies to the entire spectrum of cancer control interventions (as well as to research toward defining and testing resource-level-appropriate interventions), some measures may be appropriate and effective everywhere, regardless of national economic status, and may not require a great deal of resource-level analysis. Taxes on cigarettes and other tobacco products have worked to reduce tobacco use in a wide range of countries, including some LMCs, and every country has the ability to levy taxes. Specific tax laws will vary as will the level of tobacco sales and the types of tobacco smoked or consumed in other ways, which may dictate the details of tax programs, but these must be worked out at the country level. For the types of interventions where this may not be the case, however, there exists a need to develop an evidence-based consensus on resource-level-appropriate interventions and make it readily available to decision makers at all levels in LMCs.

The aim is for countries and individual institutions to make the best decisions for their individual patients and for the populations they serve, to maximize the value of existing inputs, and to create a context for incremental investment. The example of how this objective may begin to be achieved (described in detail in this chapter) is the Breast Health Global Initiative (BHGI), an ongoing international collaboration that has taken the first steps to produce detailed, resource-level-specific guidelines for all relevant aspects of breast cancer, from early detection through palliative care. The next phase of the BHGI, working with LMC partners to develop experience in adapting and applying the guidelines, is just beginning. This involves several layers of decision making, from policy and programmatic decisions that could be taken at the national or subnational level, to the level of the institution determining the mix of services it should offer. Still farther down the line is the challenge of persuading physicians and other health care workers to follow guidelines that have been adopted, and to develop systems that encourage this and that monitor their use and patient outcomes. The guidelines themselves are a necessary tool in the process, although not an end in themselves.

CONSIDERATIONS FOR RESOURCE-LEVEL APPROPRIATENESS

A number of factors may contribute to defining which interventions are most appropriate in different settings, with cost being important, but not the only consideration. The point should also be made that what is most appropriate is likely to vary within countries and among countries of similar economic status. In particular, the same services may not be available in major urban areas and in rural areas. In some cases, a single option could be best for every low- or middle-income country, but this cannot be assumed. Even where there are choices to be made, however, the number of options in most cases is likely to be limited, making decisions manageable.

Basic factors that may affect decisions about appropriate services include:

- The monetary cost of the intervention
  - –To patients
  - –To governments or other payers
- Characteristics of patients and their cancers presenting for treatment
  - –Prevalent cancer types
  - –Stage distribution of cancers
  - –Common co-morbidities and nutritional status
  - –Availability of social support for patients during and following treatment
- Characteristics of effective interventions
  - –Time course, including total inpatient and outpatient requirements, and follow-up
  - –Acute toxicity
  - –Long-term effects, including permanent disability, disfigurement, and effect on quality of life
  - –Need for and availability of rehabilitation
- Institutional requirements
  - –General infrastructure
  - –Specific equipment and drugs
  - –Infection control measures, including isolation facilities
  - –Medical, nursing, technician, and psychosocial personnel needs

This chapter draws on the BHGI experience specifically related to guideline development which, at this writing, remains the only available model. However, practitioners in LMCs and those who work with them do implicitly or explicitly weigh alternatives and make "resource-based" decisions in their daily practices. The idea surfaces as well in particular projects and reports. *Comprehensive Cervical Cancer Control: A Guide to Essential Practice* (WHO, 2006), developed by WHO, is a current example. It is presented as a "how-to" manual for cervical cancer, aimed at LMCs in terms of the range of technologies addressed. It does not simply present the best practices of high-income countries as the only effective approaches, and it recognizes that all possible resources are not available everywhere.

That said, very little of the published evidence base is derived from LMCs. Few clinical trials of cancer interventions have taken place in these countries. The point has been made already that conditions regarding the patient and the environment may be significantly different in LMCs. Thus there is also a need for resource-level-appropriate research on questions of particular importance in LMCs. These could be trials of treatments already in use, to confirm their effectiveness and safety in different populations and under different conditions; questions that are largely relevant only to LMCs (e.g., treatment of Burkitt's lymphoma or advanced retinoblastoma, both in children); or modified treatment protocols (e.g., "resource-sparing" protocols for radiotherapy) for common cancers.

THE BREAST HEALTH GLOBAL INITIATIVE: A BLUEPRINT FOR DEVELOPING RESOURCE-LEVEL-APPROPRIATE INTERVENTIONS

The BHGI has developed evidence-based, culturally appropriate sets of guidelines that can be used in countries with limited resources—low- and middle-income countries—to improve breast health outcomes. The program is ongoing, co-sponsored by the Fred Hutchinson Cancer Research Center and the Susan G. Komen Breast Cancer Foundation, in collaboration with a number of national and international health organizations, breast health and cancer societies, and nongovernmental organizations (NGOs) (Box 4-1). The BHGI is the brainchild of Dr. Benjamin Anderson, a breast surgeon at the Fred Hutchinson Cancer Center in Seattle, who has led the effort since the beginning.

The first BHGI Global Summit Consensus Conference on International Breast Health Care was held in October 2002 in Seattle (the conference is hereafter referred to as the 2002 Global Summit). The aim of the 2002 Global Summit was to establish breast health guidelines for countries where health care resources are significantly limited (Anderson, 2003). The guidelines were developed using a panel consensus approach with analysis of evidence-based breast cancer research. The panel consisted of breast cancer experts, scientists, and patient advocates from 17 countries and 9 world regions. They were provided with materials prior to the meeting describing the goals of the project as well as literature related to guideline development. Selected panelists prepared presentations relevant to breast

BOX 4-1
BHGI Collaborating Organizations

American Society for Breast Disease
Breast Surgery International
Centers for Disease Control and Prevention
International Atomic Energy Agency of the United Nations
International Network for Cancer Treatment and Research
International Society for Nurses in Cancer Care
International Society of Breast Pathology
International Union Against Cancer
Middle East Cancer Consortium
National Cancer Institute, Office of International Affairs
Pan American Health Organization
WHO Programs:

- Alliance for Health Policy and Systems Research
- Cancer Control Programme
- Health System Policies and Operations

World Society for Breast Health

SOURCE: Anderson et al. (2005).

cancer care in countries with limited health care resources. At the meeting, three panels were formed, on Early Detection, Diagnosis, and Treatment. Each panel was asked to define guidelines for care in their assigned area, using WHO defined criteria for "low-level" and "medium-level" resource countries (WHO, 2002). The resulting BHGI guidelines were published and have been made available in an unrestricted fashion on the Internet for worldwide access (Anderson et al., 2003a; Anderson et al., 2003b; Carlson et al., 2003; Vargas et al., 2003).

The first summit and development of guidelines was a learning process. The next sections of this chapter discuss issues that were important in creating an appropriate context for the guideline effort, and then describe the refined and improved procedures, used in the second summit and to revise the guidelines.

GUIDELINE DEVELOPMENT FOR LIMITED-RESOURCE SETTINGS: SPECIAL CONSIDERATIONS REGARDING BREAST CANCER

To be applicable and effective, practice guidelines must go beyond summarizing the available evidence and prescribing interventions using strictly quantitative criteria. Social norms and values cannot be ignored in the way practice questions are framed and outcomes chosen, and these may differ among health care systems (Redman, 1996). In the case of breast cancer, gender inequalities that exist between men and women in many societies carry over into health care disparities. Particularly where resources are limited, women may bear more than their share of deprivation in the extent and quality of health services available to them (Gijsbers van Wijk et al., 1996). At the 2002 Global Summit, two axioms were adopted as principles for guideline development:

1. All women have the right to access health care, but considerable challenges exist in implementing breast health care programs when resources are limited.
2. All women have the right to education about breast cancer, but it must be culturally appropriate, and targeted and tailored to the specific population.

In countries with limited resources, most women have advanced or metastatic breast cancer at the time of diagnosis (Pal and Mittal, 2004). Based on evidence-based review and consensus discussion, four observations were made:

1. The more advanced breast cancer is at diagnosis, the poorer the survival and the more resource intensive it is to treat. Efforts to increase early detection can reduce the stage at diagnosis, potentially improving the odds of survival and cure, and enabling simpler and more effective (and more cost-effective) treatment. These efforts are likely to have the greatest overall benefit in terms of both survival and efficient utilization of available resources.
2. Each country must build programs that fit its unique situation.
3. In the low-income countries where it is not yet possible to deliver breast cancer care to women nationwide, the development of cancer centers can be a stepping stone to providing high-quality care to at least some women.
4. Collecting data on breast cancer is imperative for deciding how best to apply resources and for measuring improvements in outcome following programmatic changes.

These observations from the first Global Summit served as the basis of the 2005 BHGI Global Summit Consensus Conference on International Breast Health Care (hereafter referred to as the 2005 Global Summit), where specific recommendations were addressed.

The 2005 Global Summit

The BHGI guidelines were reexamined, revised, and extended at the second Global Summit, held January 12–15, 2005, hosted by the National Cancer Institute in Bethesda, Maryland. Twelve national and international groups and three WHO programs collaborated (Box 4-1). More than 60 experts from 33 countries participated. They represented expertise in screening, pathology and cytology, surgery, medical oncology, radiation oncology, health economics, surveillance, medical ethics, sociology, and advocacy. Participants were organized into four panels:

1. Early Detection and Access to Care
2. Diagnosis and Pathology
3. Cancer Treatment and Allocation of Resources
4. Health Care Systems and Public Policy

Each panel drafted a consensus manuscript summarizing their deliberations and decisions (Anderson et al., 2006a; Eniu et al., 2006; Shyyan et al., 2006; Smith et al., 2006).

Panel Organization and Conference Preparation

Panel co-chairs organized speakers to cover their panels' topics and drafted the consensus manuscript. Each panel held one full-day meeting for all summit participants, split between plenary sessions and discussion and debate to achieve consensus. Each day began with a presentation by a breast cancer advocate from a limited-resource country sharing the personal experience of facing breast cancer in that country.

Consensus Process

Each panel was asked to stratify the health care interventions relevant to their areas into four levels:

1. **"Basic" level**—Core resources absolutely necessary for any breast health care system to function. Basic-level resources are typically applied in a single clinical interaction.
2. **"Limited" level**—Second-tier resources that produce major improvements in outcome. Limited-level resources may involve single or multiple clinical interactions.
3. **"Enhanced" level**—Third-tier resources that are optional, but important. Enhanced-level resources may produce minor improvements in outcome, but increase the number of therapeutic options and patient choices.

4. **"Maximal" level**—Resources applied in a modern breast health care practice in countries or settings with high-level resources.

This stratification scheme assumes incremental resource allocation; for example, the limited level assumes that a setting already has all of the resources recommended for the basic level. All interventions available in the basic level are assumed still to be available for use as appropriate at higher levels, and this pattern of building up continues up through the maximal level. Using this scheme, the short-term goal is to move to the next level, and the long-term goal is to move to the enhanced or maximal levels. Of note, multiple resource levels generally co-exist within a country, a region, or even an individual health care facility. For example, a country may have community clinics that provide care at the basic level, regional hospitals that provide care at the limited level, and a national cancer center that provides care at the enhanced or maximal level. Because circumstances vary so widely around the world, decisions about how to plan the overall structure of a national breast program must be made on a country-by-country, region-by-region, and facility-by-facility basis.

Panels were also asked to develop checklists organized by country resource level, with the intention of creating a series of checklists or tables. These checklists describe the strengths, limitations, and necessary resources to apply a given approach in the areas of early detection, diagnosis, treatment, or health care systems and policies. Finally, the panels were asked to identify areas where evidence is lacking and research is needed to better inform future versions of the guidelines.

Manuscript Preparation and Review

Much of the discussion within panels involved creating the tables (Tables 4-2 through 4-8) that stratify interventions according to the four levels. The consensus draft manuscripts were compared centrally for internal consistency in stratification of interventions by a subpanel of co-authors. Differences among recommendations from the panels were reviewed with panel co-chairs and adapted to minimize inconsistencies, when this was possible. However, there were cases of irreconcilable differences, where interventions were definitively stratified in different ways by different panels. In these cases, the panel recommendations were maintained in the tables and the nature of the disagreements was summarized, explained, and discussed in an overview manuscript (Anderson et al., 2006a).

In addition to panel consensus papers, plenary speakers were invited to submit individual manuscripts for publication together with the consensus manuscripts. These papers are more detailed, and on more focused topics, than could be included in the consensus manuscripts, but were vital to an

TABLE 4-2 Early Detection and Access to Care Guidelines

Level of Resources	Detection Method(s)	Evaluation Goal
Basic	Breast health awareness (education ± self-examination) Clinical breast examination (CBE) (clinician education)	Baseline assessment and repeated resurvey
Limited	Targeted outreach/education encouraging CBE for at-risk groups Diagnostic ultrasound ± diagnostic mammography	Downstaging of symptomatic disease
Enhanced	Diagnostic mammography Opportunistic mammographic screening	Opportunistic screening of asymptomatic women
Maximal	Population-based mammographic screening Other imaging technologies as appropriate: High-risk groups, unique imaging challenges	Population-based screening of asymptomatic women

SOURCE: Reprinted, by permission, from Anderson et al. (2006a). Copyright 2006 by the Breast Health Global Initiative, Fred Hutchinson Cancer Research Center.

overall understanding of the guideline recommendations. In the end, some manuscripts on topics of more general interest were referred for journal submission outside the BHGI process. Some were incorporated into guideline consensus articles. Manuscripts with specific merit in support of the guidelines were accepted for publication along with the consensus documents. The combination of consensus and individual manuscripts represents the complete BHGI guideline compendium, which is the final work product of the 2005 Global Summit. It was published in its entirety as a supplement to the January/February 2006 edition of *The Breast Journal.*

2005 Global Summit Guideline Outcome Summary

The cumulative work of the four panels results in a matrix guideline spanning the spectrum of breast health care from early detection to treatment and palliation of advanced disease, and considers the full spectrum of available resources (Tables 4-3–4-7). A matrix for health care systems and public policy was also developed (Table 4-8).

In most areas, there was good alignment and agreement between consensus panels in the assigned stratification levels. Furthermore, the stratification from basic to maximal levels generally mirrors the evolution of breast cancer diagnosis and treatment that has developed in high-income countries, with a few exceptions, which are described below.

TABLE 4-3 Diagnosis and Pathology Guidelines

Level of Resources	Clinical	Pathology	Imaging and Lab Tests
Basic	History Physical examination Clinical breast examination Surgical biopsy Fine-needle aspiration biopsy	Interpretation of biopsies Cytology or pathology report describing tumor size, lymph node status, histologic type, tumor grade	
Limited	Core needle biopsy Image-guided sampling (ultrasonographic ± mammographic)	Determination and reporting of ER and PR status	Diagnostic breast ultrasound ± diagnostic mammography Plain chest radiography Liver ultrasound Blood chemistry profile/CBC
Enhanced	Preoperative needle localization under mammographic or ultrasound guidance	Onsite cytopathologist	Diagnostic mammography Bone scan
Maximal	Stereotactic biopsy Sentinel node biopsy	HER-2/*neu* status IHC staining of sentinel nodes for cytokeratin to detect micrometastases	CT scan, PET scan, MIBI scan, breast MRI

CBC = complete blood count; CT = computed tomography; ER = estrogen receptor; IHC = immunohistochemistry; MIBI = 99mTc-sestamibi; MRI = magnetic resonance imaging; PET = positron emission tomography; PR = progesterone receptor.
SOURCE: Reprinted, by permission, from Anderson et al. (2006a). Copyright 2006 by the Breast Health Global Initiative, Fred Hutchinson Cancer Research Center.

Introduction of Breast Ultrasound and Diagnostic Mammography in Low-Income Countries

Ideally, diagnostic mammography is a core resource for work-up for all types of breast lesions (NCCN, 2005), and ultrasound is used to examine localized findings from the diagnostic mammogram or clinical breast examination (CBE). Screening breast ultrasound (general survey of the whole breast in clinically asymptomatic women) is generally discouraged because it has a high false-positive rate if strict criteria are followed (Stavros et al., 1995).

In low-resource settings, however, diagnostic ultrasound usually becomes available before diagnostic mammography, for understandable reasons. First, mammography is a highly specialized imaging tool that is con-

TABLE 4-4 Treatment and Allocation of Resources: Stage I Breast Cancer Guidelines

Level of Resources	Local-Regional Treatment		Systemic Treatment (Adjuvant)	
	Surgery	Radiation Therapy	Chemotherapy	Endocrine Therapy
Basic	Modified radical mastectomy			Ovarian ablation
Limited	Breast-conserving therapy[a]	Breast-conserving whole-breast irradiation as part of breast-conserving therapy Postmastectomy irradiation of the chest wall and regional nodes for high-risk cases	Classical CMF[b] AC, EC, or FAC[b]	
Enhanced			Taxanes	Aromatase inhibitors LH-RH agonists
Maximal	Sentinel node biopsy Reconstructive surgery		Growth factors Dose-dense chemotherapy	

CMF = cyclophosphamide, methotrexate, and 5-fluorouracil; AC = doxorubicin and cyclophosphamide; EC = epirubicin and cyclophosphamide; FAC = 5-fluorouracil, doxorubicin, and cyclophosphamide; LH-RH = luteinizing hormone-releasing hormone.

[a]Breast-conserving therapy requires mammography and reporting of margin status.
[b]Requires blood chemistry profile and complete blood count testing.

SOURCE: Reprinted, by permission, from Anderson et al. (2006a). Copyright 2006 by the Breast Health Global Initiative, Fred Hutchinson Cancer Research Center.

siderably more expensive than ultrasound. Until the recent advent of digital technology—which itself is very expensive—all mammography required the use of X-ray film, which can be a critical barrier in a low-income country (Zotov et al., 2003). Second, many health facilities will not purchase mammography equipment because it is dedicated to the single use of breast imaging. In contrast, ultrasound is commonly available in a wide span of resource settings. It can be used for imaging many parts of the body and it requires no film unless records are needed. Thus, breast ultrasound may be used in settings where mammography is unavailable, simply because the tool exists.

Furthermore, breast ultrasound as an initial diagnostic test may have more utility in low-income countries than it does in high-income countries

TABLE 4-5 Treatment and Allocation of Resources: Stage II Breast Cancer Guidelines

Level of Resources	Local-Regional Treatment		Systemic Treatment (Adjuvant)	
	Surgery	Radiation Therapy	Chemotherapy	Endocrine Therapy
Basic	Modified radical mastectomy	Chest wall and regional lymph node irradiation, if available	Classical CMF[a] AC, EC, or FAC[a]	Ovarian ablation Tamoxifen
Limited	Breast-conserving therapy[b]	Breast-conserving whole-breast irradiation as part of breast-conserving therapy Postmastectomy irradiation of the chest wall and regional nodes for high-risk cases		
Enhanced			Taxanes	Aromatase inhibitors LH-RH agonists
Maximal	Sentinel node biopsy Reconstructive surgery		Growth factors Dose-dense chemotherapy	

CMF = cyclophosphamide, methotrexate, and 5-fluorouracil; AC = doxorubicin and cyclophosphamide; EC = epirubicin and cyclophosphamide; FAC = 5-fluorouracil, doxorubicin, and cyclophosphamide; LH-RH = luteinizing hormone-releasing hormone.

[a]Requires blood chemistry profile and complete blood count testing.
[b]Breast-conserving therapy requires mammography and reporting of margin status.

SOURCE: Reprinted, by permission, from Anderson et al. (2006a). Copyright 2006 by the Breast Health Global Initiative, Fred Hutchinson Cancer Research Center.

for two reasons. First, patients in these settings commonly present with locally advanced, palpable disease, where breast ultrasound becomes a useful adjunct to CBE to evaluate the extent of disease (Vargas et al., 2003). Second, premenopausal breast cancer is more commonly diagnosed in low-income than high-income countries (Chow and Ho, 2000). The usually dense breast tissue of younger women makes cancers more difficult to image by mammography. For these reasons, the guidelines support the introduction of breast ultrasound before mammography in low-income countries (Table 4-2), which reverses the order generally accepted in high-income countries.

TABLE 4-6 Treatment and Allocation of Resources: Locally Advanced Breast Cancer Guidelines

Level of Resources	Local-Regional Treatment		Systemic Treatment (Adjuvant)	
	Surgery	Radiation Therapy	Chemotherapy	Endocrine Therapy
Basic	Modified radical mastectomy		Neoadjuvant AC, FAC, or classical CMF[a]	Ovarian ablation Tamoxifen
Limited		Postmastectomy irradiation of the chest wall and regional nodes		
Enhanced	Breast-conserving therapy[b]	Breast-conserving whole-breast irradiation	Taxanes	Aromatase inhibitors LH-RH agonists
Maximal	Reconstructive surgery		Growth factors Dose-dense chemotherapy	

AC = doxorubicin and cyclophosphamide; FAC = 5-fluorouracil, doxorubicin, and cyclophosphamide; CMF = cyclophosphamide, methotrexate, and 5-fluorouracil; EC = epirubicin and cyclophosphamide; LH-RH = luteinizing hormone-releasing hormone.

[a]Requires blood chemistry profile and complete blood count testing.

[b]Breast-conserving therapy requires mammography and reporting of margin status.

SOURCE: Reprinted, by permission, from Anderson et al. (2006a). Copyright 2006 by the Breast Health Global Initiative, Fred Hutchinson Cancer Research Center.

While breast ultrasound is useful for determining the extent of the invasive component of a breast cancer, it will predictably underestimate the extent of some cancers, particularly when they have a large noninvasive component. For example, ductal carcinoma in situ (DCIS, or stage 0 breast cancer) is not seen on breast ultrasound, but can be seen on mammography because it is associated with the deposition of microcalcifications. For this reason, diagnostic mammography (along with good pathology examination) is considered mandatory for breast conservation therapy (Tables 4-4, 4-5, and 4-6) because negative margins are needed with a partial mastectomy, whether it is for invasive or noninvasive disease (Carlson et al., 2000).

Endocrine Therapy and Hormone Receptor Testing

Oral endocrine therapy is among the simplest therapies for breast cancer in women with high tumor estrogen receptor (ER) levels and is recommended at every level, from basic to maximal. If tamoxifen, the standard drug,

TABLE 4-7 Treatment and Allocation of Resources: Metastatic (Stage IV) and Recurrent Breast Cancer Guidelines

	Local-Regional Treatment		Systemic Treatment (Adjuvant)		
Level of Resources	Surgery	Radiation Therapy	Chemotherapy	Endocrine Therapy	Supportive and Palliative Therapy
Basic	Total mastectomy for ipsilateral breast tumor recurrence[a]			Ovarian ablation Tamoxifen	Nonopioid and opioid analgesics
Limited		Palliative radiation therapy	Classical CMF[b] Anthracycline monotherapy or in combination[b]		
Enhanced			Taxanes Capecitabine Trastuzumab	Aromatase inhibitors	Bisphosphonates
Maximal			Growth factors Vinorelbine Gemcitabine Carboplatin	Fulvestrant	

CMF = cyclophosphamide, methotrexate, and 5-fluorouracil.

[a]Required resources are the same as those for modified radical mastectomy.
[b]Requires blood chemistry profile and complete blood count testing.

SOURCE: Reprinted, by permission, from Anderson et al. (2006a). Copyright 2006 by the Breast Health Global Initiative, Fred Hutchinson Cancer Research Center.

is too expensive, surgical or radiation-induced oophorectomy—ovarian ablation—is also effective for premenopausal women. For this reason, the Cancer Treatment and Allocation of Resources panel categorized ovarian ablation and tamoxifen as basic-level resources for all stages of invasive cancer. However, the Diagnosis and Pathology panel designated ER testing as a limited-level resource, reasoning that even in the absence of testing, all patients can be given tamoxifen and/or oophorectomy. With this rationale, ER testing does not meet the formal definition of basic-level resource. This discrepancy between panels was not fully resolved during the 2005 Global Summit.

Treating all patients with endocrine therapy without ER testing means that a large fraction of patients—those without elevated ER levels—will get no benefit. In terms of costs and benefits, limiting hormonal treatments

TABLE 4-8 Health Care Systems and Public Policy Guidelines

Level of Resources	Services	Facilities	Recordkeeping
Basic	Primary care Surgical Oncology Nursing Palliative care	Health care Surgical Pathology laboratory Pharmacy Outpatient care	Individual medical records and service-based patient registration
Limited	Imaging Radiation oncology Peer support Early detection	Imaging Radiation therapy Clinical information system Health system network	Facility-based medical records and centralized patient registration Local cancer registry
Enhanced	Opportunistic screening Cancer follow-up Rehabilitation Group support	Centralized referral cancer center(s)	Facility-based follow-up systems
Maximal	Population-based screening Individual psychosocial care	Satellite (noncentralized or regional) cancer centers	National cancer registry

SOURCE: Reprinted, by permission, from Anderson et al. (2006a). Copyright 2006 by the Breast Health Global Initiative, Fred Hutchinson Cancer Research Center.

to women likely to benefit will save enough to offset, in part, the cost of hormone receptor testing. Thus, regardless of the designation as basic or limited, hormone receptor testing has obvious utility, making it a high-priority test at all levels.

Cytotoxic Chemotherapy and Related Infrastructure

In high-income countries, systemic therapy is usually recommended for all cancers larger than 1 cm, regardless of whether lymph nodes are positive or negative (Carlson et al., 2000). For ER-negative cancers, cytotoxic chemotherapy is needed to reduce the risk of disease recurrence. Chemotherapy is a mainstay of treatment for more advanced cancers. However, because the prognosis for stage I cancer following local therapy (surgery with or without radiotherapy) is already good, chemotherapy increases survival only marginally (Eniu et al., 2006). Thus, the relative utility of cytotoxic chemotherapy, given its cost, can be debated for early-stage, node-negative cancer. To properly reflect this difference in the utility of chemotherapy between early and later stage disease, the Cancer Treatment and Allocation of Resources

TABLE 4-9 Therapy Overview: Modified Radical Mastectomy and Breast-Conserving Therapy

Therapy	Strengths	Weaknesses	Required Resources
Modified radical mastectomy	Effective local treatment Uses surgical techniques widely available Rapid treatment Short posttreatment convalescence Limited long-term complications Radiation therapy can be avoided in some cases	Loss of body image (mutilation) Negative psychosocial impact Radiation therapy is often still necessary	Core surgical resources • Trained surgeon • General anesthesia • Operating room • Postoperative care facility • Pathology Postmastectomy irradiation of the chest wall and regional lymph nodes
Breast-conserving therapy	Equivalent survival to modified radical mastectomy Preservation of body image for the woman Improved quality of life	Slight increase in the rate of recurrence (in breast) compared with modified radical mastectomy Lower acceptance among less educated people Prolonged treatment course Requires access to a radiation therapy facility	High-quality breast imaging (mammography and, if available, ultrasound) Core surgical resources (same as for modified radical mastectomy) Pathology for margin assessment Surgical services experienced in the procedure Breast-conserving whole-breast irradiation Geographic accessibility Support systems that allow receipt of radiation therapy over a period of weeks

SOURCE: Reprinted, by permission, from Eniu et al. (2006). Copyright 2006 by the Breast Health Global Initiative, Fred Hutchinson Cancer Research Center.

panel determined that cytotoxic chemotherapy is a limited-resource therapy for stage I cancer and for metastatic cancer, but is a basic-level resource for patients with stage II or locally advanced cancer.

In a health care system that lacks the infrastructure for providing systemic chemotherapy, stage I, ER positive cancers can be effectively treated and stage IV ER positive cancers can be palliated, but stage II and locally advanced disease can only be palliated at best regardless of ER status. Unfortunately, these more advanced but treatable cancers are the most common presentations in low-income countries. The conclusion, then, is that to provide a reasonable level of breast cancer treatment, the infrastructure for cytotoxic chemotherapy must be there from the beginning, even though this is considered higher than a basic-level resource for some stages of breast cancer.

THE GLOBAL PARTNERSHIP UNDERLYING THE BHGI

Improving breast health care in a low-resource setting is bound to be complex, requiring the collaboration of multiple sectors, including health care ministries and governmental agencies, NGOs, and public and patient groups (Glassman et al., 1999; Lim, 2002; Mathew et al., 2003; McCabe et al., 1995). The relative contribution of each sector will depend on the country's governmental structure, the extent of focus on health care and breast cancer, available resources, the strength of the NGO sector, and the ability of patients, survivors, and advocates to act collaboratively.

A strength of the BHGI guideline development process is its collaborative nature, creating partnerships to improve health care in limited-resource countries (Figure 4-1). The guidelines serve as a framework for these organizations to interact and create projects of common interest. The challenges extend beyond the capacity of any one partner or sector to address effectively. This is especially true in a global world where traditional boundaries between what are "public" and "private" responsibilities have become blurred, where civil society organizations have taken on important new roles, and where technology enables the creation of effective networks

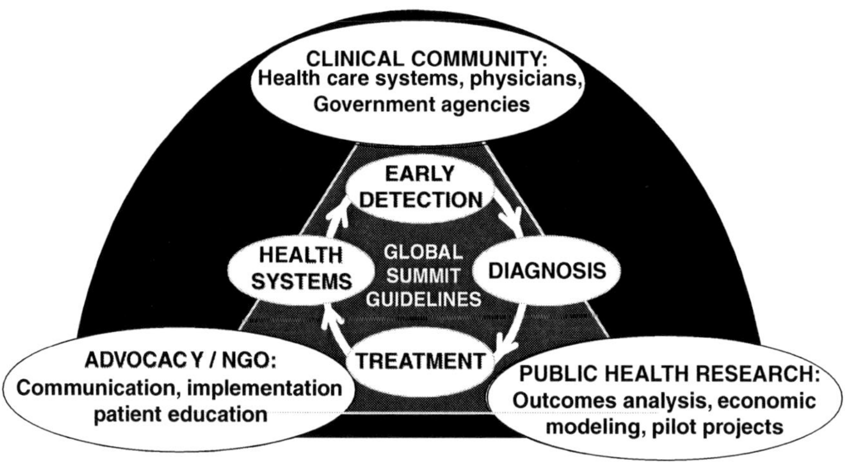

FIGURE 4-1 Linkages among the clinical community, advocacy groups and nongovernmental organizations (NGOs), and the public health research community.

with lowered cost. A next step is to transform the guideline alliance into operational alliances that take the guidelines into practice in low-resource settings.

LESSONS FROM THE BHGI MODEL FOR OTHER CANCERS

The guidelines development process for countries with limited resources tries to offer a practical solution to the implausibility of applying guidelines developed for high-resource countries. In a limited-resource country, many barriers stand between the average patient and the level of care dictated by guidelines applicable to high-resource settings. These include inadequate numbers of trained health care providers; inadequate diagnostic and treatment infrastructure such as pathology, pharmacy, infusion centers, and microbiology laboratories; lack of drugs; lack of radiographic film; and inadequate transportation and communications systems.

Physicians working in a limited-resources environment may be forced to make decisions at odds with their medical knowledge. Despite knowing the optimal management for a patient, less-than-optimal solutions are offered to patients because diagnostic and/or treatment resources are simply lacking. Lack of mammography and radiotherapy facilities, for example, precludes the use of breast-conserving therapy, and unavailability of chemotherapy agents and infrastructure may make it impossible or unsafe to deliver cytotoxic chemotherapy in the adjuvant setting.

Resource limitations frustrate clinicians who are unable to offer "gold standard" treatment to any or only to some patients. This tension is often amplified by the clinicians' added responsibility for managing inadequate resources from an insufficient cancer program budget. Does a clinician decide to treat 10 patients with an older, less expensive chemotherapy regimen, or to treat 2 patients with a newer, more efficacious, but also more expensive regimen?

To establish a cancer treatment program in a limited-resource setting, key treatment alternatives should be considered, weighing costs, efficacy differences, and the expected availability of resources and personnel to implement the program. Flexibility must be built into recommendations because heterogeneous social, economic, and health system development among countries and often among regions of the same country, make uniform recommendations impractical.

The expert panels asked to develop meaningful, justifiable, and scientifically rigorous guidelines for LMCs requires the same type of multidisciplinary expertise as needed to develop guidelines for resource-rich areas. They must also be willing and competent to estimate the magnitude of relative benefit from the available therapies and to prioritize these therapies with consideration of efficacy, toxicity, and resources, with specific consideration of the conditions in low-resource settings (Anderson et al., 2003a). Recommendations must also respect the social, economic, religious, and political milieu within which they are to be applied. Involvement of social scientists, economists, religious leaders, and politicians may also be appropriate. However, the patient and delivery of evidence-based health care must remain the primary focus.

At every point of recommendation, the panel should consider not only the applicable scientific evidence, but also the implications and barriers to implementing the recommendation. It makes little sense to recommend a therapy that is available at only a few centers in the world. It is also impossible to implement even a cost-effective, simple therapy if it requires special resources that are not available.

Thus, the responsibility of the guideline panels is to develop an inclusive, objective, evidence-based guideline associated with a prioritization schema stratified by available health care resources. Further refinement of the guidelines produced will undoubtedly be necessary when actually applied to be respectful of local geographic, social, political, and religious issues, and to incorporate the actual costs in a given site.

Guideline Implementation

Developing and publishing guidelines is one step, but it does not equal implementation. The practical application of treatment guidelines in a specific site requires an honest evaluation of existing resources and expertise. This assessment must recognize which procedures are available to *all* patients, as this identifies the associated level of resources, from basic to maximal. To the extent that a sequential strategy can be followed, providing universal access to one level and then moving up, substantial inequity in the use of limited resources is prevented, and the greatest benefit can accrue to the largest number of people.

Once the level of existing resources is defined, an analysis will identify the missing elements to allow completion of that level of resource. Resources can then be allocated strategically to improve the performance of the cancer unit. This strategy can be used at the national level for allocation of resources for breast cancer. It also can help to prevent using scarce resources on the latest technologies or drugs to benefit a few at the expense of basic effective care for much larger numbers.

The checklists developed by the BHGI panels are suitable for use by health ministries or hospital administrators and provide an inventory of the minimal technical and staff requirements. The information can be used to plan the future development of a unit by prioritizing the acquisition of missing elements. The guidelines also can support a clinician's request for specific equipment and funding for breast cancer treatment. Finally, the checklists can be used as one input for accreditation of units for breast cancer diagnosis and treatment.

APPLYING THE BHGI MODEL TO OTHER CANCERS

Breast cancer was a good choice for a first effort at guideline development for low-resource areas—for whatever reasons it was actually chosen. It is among the most common cancers everywhere, a variety of effective treatments is available, and breast cancer has been the driver in patient advocacy around the world. It might have been easier to fund this effort than would have been the case for a different cancer, although funding was a challenge, particularly at the beginning (Personal communication, B. Anderson, Director, BHGI June 2006). The success of the BHGI, at least through the guideline development phase, should give potential funders confidence that tackling other cancers can also be successful.

The BHGI has built financial support from the first summit through the upcoming 3rd biennial summit, and no new such undertaking will succeed without adequate support. As a benchmark, the budget for the 2007 global summit, which will support 75 participants from around the world and 5 staff members at a 4-day meeting in Budapest, is US $400,000. An additional US $100,000 is budgeted for a journal supplement with the revised guidelines and supplementary papers, including a writer and production and printing costs. The actual guideline development work is carried out largely uncompensated, by the participants who volunteer their time. In the case of the BHGI, a full-time manager is employed, and the scientific leader has partial salary support for the project. The usual costs of operations (office, equipment, and supplies) also must be covered (Personal communication, L. Sullivan, Program Manager, BHGI, October 2, 2006). These costs will, of course, vary according to the host organizations for other initiatives.

PRIORITIZING CANCERS FOR GUIDELINE DEVELOPMENT IN LIMITED-RESOURCE COUNTRIES

Following the lead of breast cancer, the greatest benefit from additional resource-level-appropriate guidelines would be for relatively common cancers for which treatments are affordable and have proven reasonably successful in some settings. Cancers that are less common but highly curable, with treatments that can be used in a low-resource setting, could also be considered.

No purely objective, scientific method exists for prioritizing cancers for "resource-level-specific" attention. What actually happens will be a result of leaders coming forward for a specific type of cancer, and obtaining support for an international collaborative effort. It would make sense, however, not to spend a great deal of effort on cancers for which treatment is less successful, but to encourage work on those for which treatment is more successful. Cancers for which treatment is difficult and less likely to succeed would typically not warrant complex guideline development, at least initially. Guidelines for palliative care for the common cancers should be developed, and will be applicable to people dying from all types of cancer.

A major consideration in decisions about offering treatment for cancers in resource-limited settings are characteristics of the interventions themselves—the specific types of surgery or drugs, for example—needed to achieve a good outcome. Short-term toxicity and long-term sequelae are also important considerations for both medical and social reasons. The available choices of interventions, the personnel needed, and other necessary conditions are the heart of future discussions to develop resource-level-appropriate guidelines, as was done by the BHGI. For most cancers, different subtypes can be identified that are more or less amenable to treatment, and the time course and side effect profiles for the treatment choices may differ in ways that are significant medically and practically for patients. These and a host of other details will require careful consideration of every option as it applies to the types of settings that exist in LMCs.

In every case, good cancer treatment will require a multidisciplinary, coordinated team of individuals with training in the specific cancers for which treatment will be offered. One of the benefits of the BHGI-type of initiative is to make explicit the resource needs in all categories. Having this information should assist decision makers, whether at the national or facility level, to decide what can be offered, and what the next steps would be to expand treatment to patients with other types of cancers.

Table 4-10 lists the 10 cancer types responsible for the greatest numbers of deaths in developing countries in 2002. The top four—cancers of the lung, liver, stomach, and esophagus—make up nearly half of the deaths in these countries. Survival from these cancers in the United States, where most people have access to treatment, is relatively poor and has not improved a great deal since the 1970s. This is corroborated by the related (but not identical) statistic of the ratio of mortality to incidence in more developed countries, and its similarity to the same statistic in less developed countries.[1] Taking lung cancer, for example, the 5-year survival in the United States was reported as 12 percent in the 1970s. In the late 1990s, it was still only 15 percent. The mortality to incidence ratio was 86 and 88 percent in more and

[1]The ratio of mortality to incidence uses the number of deaths and the number of cases in a given year, rather than survival over time. This number is affected by short-term trends in incidence, whereas survival rates are not. For example, where lung cancer rates are increasing, the number of new cases would be greater than the number the previous year, when many of those dying would have been diagnosed. For most cancers, particularly those with poor survival, this distortion is probably not very large.

TABLE 4-10 Selected Cancers: Factors to Consider in Prioritizing Treatment in Developing Countries

	5-Year Relative Survival, U.S. 1970s (different years)	5-Year Relative Survival, U.S. 1995–2001	Deaths in Less Developed Countries, 2002 (GLOBOCAN)	Mortality/ Incidence Ratio in Less Developed Countries (%)	Mortality/ Incidence Ratio in More Developed Countries (%)
1. Lung	12	15	591,000	88	86
2. Liver	4	9	487,000	95	99
3. Stomach	15	23	486,000	78	68
4. Esophagus	5	15	320,000	83	88
5. Breast	75	88	221,000	43	30
6. Cervix uteri	70	73	234,000	57	47
7. Colon and rectum	50	64	214,000	60	47
8. Leukemia	34	48	137,000	78	68
9. Non-Hodgkin's lymphoma	47	60	97,000	66	49
10. Prostate	67	100	91,000	55	25
11. *Head and neck*			*89,000*	*61*	*42*
Oral cavity and pharynx	*54*	*59*			
Larynx	*66*	*66*			
12. *Hodgkin's lymphoma*	*71*	*85*	*15,000*	*44*	*28*
13. *Testicular*	*79*	*96*	*6,000*	*31*	*9*

SOURCES: IARC (2004); Ries et al. (2006).

less developed countries, meaning that there were nearly as many deaths as cases in 2002, regardless of resource levels.

For other cancers down the list of the 10 leading causes of cancer death, the overall survival among U.S. cancer patients is much better, and there are substantial differences between the mortality to incidence ratio between less and more developed countries, suggesting that treatment makes a significant difference in survival. This is true for the following cancers: cancers of the breast, cervix, colon and rectum, prostate, and leukemia and non-Hodgkin's lymphoma. In the case of leukemias, a substantial increase in survival occurred in the United States from the 1970s through 2000, suggesting that treatment has improved the chances of survival. One caveat in looking at changes in overall survival is that a change can be the result of improved stage distribution (i.e., more cancers detected in early stages), and therefore more amenable to long-term survival or cure.

Head and neck cancers are added to the list because they are relatively common and have a very good prognosis when treated. Hodgkin's lymphoma and testicular cancer both have very high survival rates and are among the most common cancers in young adults. Treatment of Hodgkin's lymphoma among older adults is also highly successful.

Table 4-11 looks more closely at the cancers with high survival rates in the United States and relatively large differentials in mortality to incidence ratios between less and more developed countries. It is useful to note that survival is relatively good for both localized and regionally spread cancers for all of these cancer types. This is particularly important for cancers that are more likely to be detected in early stages in more developed countries, either because of screening or because they produce symptoms early, causing people to seek medical attention.

The mortality to incidence ratio has a slightly different interpretation in the case of cervical cancer than for other cancers. This is because most of the effect of screening—which is widespread in the United States and other high-income countries—is to detect *precancerous* stages rather than early-stage cancers. This dramatically lowers the number of incident cases, so incident cervical cancers in more developed countries are only a small proportion of the cancers that *would* have occurred (and that do occur in less developed countries) in the absence of screening. The difference in the mortality to incidence ratio between less and more developed countries would be larger if these statistics were more comparable.

Cancers of Children and Young Adults

As is the case with cancers of adults, practitioners in LMCs have formally or informally prioritized cancer types of children and young adults for treatment. Several leaders in pediatric oncology in Asia, Latin America, and the Pacific contacted for this report provided insight into their schema for prioritizing childhood cancers for treatment. Leukemias and lymphomas are the most frequent childhood cancers everywhere, although the specific types and proportions vary around the world. Most also have high cure rates except in advanced stages, and require only chemotherapy. A respondent from Pakistan, in charge of pediatric oncology at a government-owned hospital, provided a table based on his experience (Table 4-12). Tradeoffs are implied in the juxtaposition of prevalence, survival, and cost. The only cancers clearly excluded from treatment are very high-cost, very poor-survival types. Other respondents gave similar priorities, except in some cases retinoblastoma was ranked higher and Wilms' tumor and neuroblastoma lower. All of these solid tumors, which are the most frequent among children in many countries (Abdullaev et al., 2000; Leal-Leal et al.,

TABLE 4-11 Stage-Specific 5-Year Survival and Main Treatment Modalities for Selected Cancers

Cancer Site	5-Year Relative Survival, U.S. 1995–2001	Main Treatment Modalities
Breast (overall)	88	***Surgery, radiotherapy, chemotherapy, hormonal therapy***
Localized	98	Surgery with or without radiotherapy
Regional	81	Surgery with or without radiotherapy and/or chemotherapy and/or hormonal therapy
Cervix uteri (overall)	73	***Radiotherapy, surgery, chemotherapy***
Localized	92	Surgery and/or radiotherapy
Regional	55	Radiotherapy or surgery
Colon and rectum (Overall)	64	***Surgery, chemotherapy, radiotherapy***
Localized	90	Surgery
Regional	68	Surgery and chemotherapy with or without radiotherapy
Non-Hodgkin's lymphoma (overall)	60	***Radiotherapy, chemotherapy***
Localized	73	Radiotherapy and/or chemotherapy
Regional	63	Radiotherapy and/or chemotherapy
Head and neck (Overall)	59–66	***Radiotherapy, surgery***
Larynx	**66**	
Localized:		Radiotherapy and/or surgery
Oral cavity and pharynx	82	
Larynx	85	
Regional:		Surgery and/or radiotherapy
Oral cavity and pharynx	51	
Larynx	50	
Testicular (overall)	96	***Surgery, chemotherapy***
Localized	100	Surgery with or without radiotherapy
Regional	71	Surgery and chemotherapy
Prostate (overall)	100	***Surgery, radiotherapy***
Local/regional	100	Surgery or radiotherapy
Hodgkin's lymphoma (overall)	85	***Chemotherapy, radiotherapy***
Local	90	Radiotherapy or chemotherapy
Regional	90	Radiotherapy and/or chemotherapy
Distant	76	Radiotherapy and chemotherapy

SOURCE: National Cancer Institute (2006).

TABLE 4-12 Priority Ranking for Treating Pediatric Cancers in a Pakistani Hospital, with U.S. Survival Rates

Disease	Percentage Distribution of Cancers (%)	Long-Term Survival (%)	Cost	5-Year Relative Survival, U.S., 1985–1994 (%)
Acute lymphoblastic leukemia	25	60	Intermediate	77
Hodgkin's lymphoma	10	90	Low	91
Non-Hodgkin's lymphoma	10	65	Intermediate	72
Germ cell tumor	3	80	Low	88
Wilms' tumor	5	80	Low	92
Retinoblastoma	6	70	Low	94
Rhabdomyosarcoma and neuroblastoma, or NBS (nonmetastatic)	5	30	High	64 (NBS)
Brain tumors: Selected nonmetastatic and low grade	3	50	Intermediate	Various
Osteosarcoma (nonmetastatic)	3	40	High	63
Would not treat:				
Acute myelogenous leukemia	*5*	*<10*	*Very high*	*41*
Stage IV neuroblastoma and sarcoma	*15*	*<10*	*Very high*	—
Relapsed disease and others	*10*	*<10*	*Very high*	—

SOURCES: Personal communication, M.S. Ashraf, Children Cancer Hospital, Karachi, Pakistan, March 2006; Ries et al. (1999).

2006) were considered worth treating. Resource-level-specific guidelines would be useful for all the prioritized tumors.

DISCUSSION AND RECOMMENDATION

The BHGI guidelines, as well as any other guidelines produced, are tools that can enable progress in cancer control, but their mere existence is unlikely to result in major changes. The BHGI is entering a new phase, assisting LMCs in putting the guidelines into practice. Feedback from this effort should be useful in moving forward with the BHGI and in new areas. The challenges include making the guidelines and supporting documentation available in languages and formats that are accessible to decision-makers.

Even acknowledging the remaining challenges in putting guidelines into practice, the value of resource-level-appropriate, evidence-based guidelines is clear. Such guidelines should be developed for other priority cancers meeting the criteria discussed in this chapter. As cancer control continues to evolve, with newer drugs, screening methods, and other cutting-edge interventions becoming available, the need will become even greater to maintain an evidence base of established, effective interventions, especially those that are less costly and less demanding of health care infrastructure than the state-of-the-art in high-income countries.

This report encourages international collaborations to address the priority cancers discussed in this chapter and international funders to support these efforts. The collaborations should be inclusive of all interested parties and should, ideally, be limited to a single collaboration per cancer type or natural grouping of cancers that represents as close to a true global consensus as possible. Each of these efforts should be viewed as a long-term commitment based on sustainable structures that can produce updated guidelines and take on the challenges of implementation.

Leadership and support will be key to the success of further initiatives to develop guidance for other priority cancers. The success of the BHGI thus far is due, in large part, to Dr. Anderson. The existing BHGI model should make it easier for parallel initiatives to get started, but the need for a dedicated leader, willing to devote substantial time to the project, is still a limiting factor. The lion's share of the technical work of the BHGI—reviewing evidence, preparing papers and guidelines—has been carried out by professionals with no extra compensation. Support is needed, however, for administrative functions (including some personnel costs), travel, and logistics, at a minimum. As is the case with the BHGI, support could come from a number of sources, including public- and private-sector organizations. Sustainability, of both personnel and funding, will be critical to the long-term success of any such initiatives.

> **RECOMMENDATION 4-1. Resource-level-appropriate guidelines should be developed for the overall management of major cancers for which treatment can make a substantial difference in a meaningful proportion of patients, and for selected pediatric cancers.** *The BHGI model could be used or others developed. The priority adult cancers for which resource-level-specific guidelines are needed are cervical cancer, colon cancer, and head and neck cancers. Pediatric priority cancers are leukemias and lymphomas. Motivated professionals from high-income countries and LMCs should work together to spearhead these efforts, with financial support from a variety of institutions.*

REFERENCES

Abdullaev FI, Rivera-Luna R, Roitenburd-Belacortu V, Espinosa-Aguirre J. 2000. Pattern of childhood cancer mortality in Mexico. *Archives of Medical Research* 31(5):526–531.

Anderson BO. 2003. Global Summit Consensus Conference on International Breast Health Care: Guidelines for countries with limited resources. *Breast Journal* 9(Suppl 2):S40–S41.

Anderson BO, Braun S, Carlson RW, Gralow JR, Lagios MD, Lehman C, Schwartsmann G, Vargas HI. 2003a. Overview of breast health care guidelines for countries with limited resources. *Breast Journal* 9(Suppl 2):S42–S50.

Anderson BO, Braun S, Lim S, Smith RA, Taplin S, Thomas DB, Global Summit Early Detection Panel. 2003b. Early detection of breast cancer in countries with limited resources. *Breast Journal* 9(Suppl 2):S51–S59.

Anderson BO, Eniu AE, Sullivan L, Carlson RW. 2005 (December). *Guidelines for Breast Cancer Detection, Diagnosis and Treatment in Limited Resource Countries as a Framework for Change: The Breast Health Global Initiative.* Unpublished.

Anderson BO, Shyyan R, Eniu A, Smith RA, Yip CH, Bese NS, Chow LW, Masood S, Ramsey SD, Carlson RW. 2006a. Breast cancer in limited-resource countries: An overview of the Breast Health Global Initiative 2005 guidelines. *Breast Journal* 12(Suppl 1):S3–S15.

Anderson BO, Yip CH, Ramsey SD, Bengoa R, Braun S, Fitch M, Groot M, Sancho-Garnier H, Tsu VD, Global Summit Health Care Systems and Public Policy Panel. 2006b. Breast cancer in limited-resource countries: Health care systems and public policy. *Breast Journal* 12(Suppl 1):S54–S69.

Carlson RW, Anderson BO, Bensinger W, Cox CE, Davidson NE, Edge SB, Farrar WB, Goldstein LJ, Gradishar WJ, Lichter AS, McCormick B, Nabell LM, Reed EC, Silver SM, Smith ML, Somlo G, Theriault R, Ward JH, Winer EP, Wolff A, National Comprehensive Cancer Network. 2000. NCCN Practice Guidelines for Breast Cancer. *Oncology (Huntington)* 14(11A):33–49.

Carlson RW, Anderson BO, Chopra R, Eniu AE, Jakesz R, Love RR, Masetti R, Schwartsmann G, Global Summit Treatment Panel. 2003. Treatment of breast cancer in countries with limited resources. *Breast Journal* 9(Suppl 2):S67–S74.

Chow LW, Ho P. 2000. Hormonal receptor determination of 1,052 Chinese breast cancers. *Journal of Surgical Oncology* 75(3):172–175.

Eniu A, Carlson RW, Aziz Z, Bines J, Hortobagyi GN, Bese NS, Love RR, Vikram B, Kurkure A, Anderson BO, Global Summit Treatment and Allocation of Resources Panel. 2006. Breast cancer in limited-resource countries: Treatment and allocation of resources. *Breast Journal* 12 (Suppl 1):S38–S53.

Gijsbers van Wijk CM, van Vliet KP, Kolk AM. 1996. Gender perspectives and quality of care: Towards appropriate and adequate health care for women. *Social Science & Medicine* 43(5):707–720.

Glassman A, Reich MR, Laserson K, Rojas F. 1999. Political analysis of health reform in the Dominican Republic. *Health Policy & Planning* 14(2):115–126.

International Agency for Research on Cancer. 2004. *GLOBOCAN 2002.* Lyon: IARC.

Leal-Leal CA, Rivera-Luna R, Flores-Rojo M, Juarez-Echenique JC, Ordaz JC, Amador-Zarco J. 2006. Survival in extra-orbital metastatic retinoblastoma:treatment results. *Clinical & Translational Oncology: Official Publication of the Federation of Spanish Oncology Societies & of the National Cancer Institute of Mexico* 8(1):39–44.

Lim GC. 2002. Overview of cancer in Malaysia. *Japanese Journal of Clinical Oncology* 32(Suppl):S37–S42.

Mathew A, Cowley S, Bliss J, Thistlewood G. 2003. The development of palliative care in national government policy in England, 1986–2000. *Palliative Medicine* 17(3):270–282.

McCabe MS, Varricchio CG, Padberg R, Simpson N. 1995. Women's health advocacy: Its growth and development in oncology. *Seminars in Oncology Nursing* 11(2):137–142.

National Cancer Institute. *Cancer Stat Fact Sheets.* [Online] Available: http://seer.cancer.gov/statfacts/ [accessed July 2, 2006].

NCCN (National Comprehensive Cancer Network). 2005. *The NCCN Breast Cancer Screening and Diagnosis Guidelines.* Jenkintown, PA: NCCN.

Pal SK, Mittal B. 2004. Fight against cancer in countries with limited resources: The post-genomic era scenario. *Asian Pacific Journal of Cancer Prevention* 5(3):328–333.

Redman BK. 1996. Ethical issues in the development and use of guidelines for clinical practice. *Journal of Clinical Ethics* 7(3):251–256.

Ries LAG, Harkins D, Krapcho M, Mariotto A, Miller BA, Feuer EJ, Clegg L, Eisner MP, Horner MJ, Howlader N, Hayat M, Hankey BF, Edwards BK (eds.). 2006. *SEER Cancer Statistics Review, 1975–2003*. Bethesda, MD: National Cancer Institute.

Ries LAG, Smith MA, Gurney JG, Linet M, Tamra T, Young JL, Bunin GR. 1999. *Cancer Incidence and Survival Among Children and Adolescents: United States SEER Program 1975–1995*. Bethesda, MD: National Cancer Institute, SEER Program.

Shyyan R, Masood S, Badwe RA, Errico KM, Liberman L, Ozmen V, Stalsberg H, Vargas H, Vass L, Global Summit Diagnosis and Pathology Panel. 2006. Breast cancer in limited-resource countries: Diagnosis and pathology. *Breast Journal* 12(Suppl 1):S27–S37.

Smith RA, Caleffi M, Albert US, Chen TH, Duffy SW, Franceschi D, Nystrom L, Global Summit Early Detection and Access to Care Panel. 2006. Breast cancer in limited-resource countries: Early detection and access to care. *Breast Journal* 12(Suppl 1):S16–S26.

Stavros AT, Thickman D, Rapp CL, Dennis MA, Parker SH, Sisney GA. 1995. Solid breast nodules: Use of sonography to distinguish between benign and malignant lesions. *Radiology* 196(1):123–134.

Vargas HI, Anderson BO, Chopra R, Lehman CD, Ibarra JA, Masood S, Vass L, Global Summit Diagnosis Panel. 2003. Diagnosis of breast cancer in countries with limited resources. *Breast Journal* 9(Suppl 2):S60–S66.

WHO (World Health Organization). 2002. *National Cancer Control Programmes: Policies and Managerial Guidelines*. 2nd ed. Geneva, Switzerland: WHO.

Winn RJ, McClure J. 2003. The NCCN Clinical Practice Guidelines in Oncology: A primer for users. *Journal of the National Comprehensive Cancer Network* 1(1):5–13.

Zotov V, Shyyan R, PATH Breast Cancer Assistance Program. 2003. Introduction of breast cancer screening in Chernihiv Oblast in the Ukraine: Report of a PATH Breast Cancer Assistance Program experience. *Breast Journal* 9(Suppl 2):S75–S80.

5

Preventing Cancers (and Other Diseases) by Reducing Tobacco Use

Cigarette smoking and other forms of tobacco use impose a large and growing global public health burden. Worldwide, tobacco use kills nearly 5 million people annually—about one third from cancer and two thirds from other diseases—accounting for 1 in every 5 male deaths, and 1 in 20 female deaths, over age 30. On current smoking patterns, annual tobacco deaths will rise to 10 million by 2030, about 3 million of which will be from cancer. If current smoking patterns persist, with about 30 percent of all young adults (50 percent of men and 10 percent of women) becoming smokers and most not giving it up, then the 21st century is likely to see 1 billion tobacco deaths, most of them in today's developing countries. In contrast, the 20th century saw 100 million deaths caused by tobacco, most of them in developed countries.

This report is about cancer control. In the case of tobacco, however, cancer is just one of the ways in which tobacco kills, and interventions to reduce tobacco use will have much broader benefits than just in terms of cancer. In this chapter the health effects of tobacco—overwhelmingly cardiovascular diseases, cancers, and respiratory diseases—and the benefits of stopping tobacco use are considered together, not separately.

Before discussing the interventions that can reduce tobacco use, the landmark Framework Convention on Tobacco Control (FCTC) is introduced. Global tobacco control efforts have been unified by the FCTC, an international treaty negotiated by the World Health Organization (WHO). The treaty calls for tobacco control measures that are firmly rooted in evidence, and creates an organization of all parties to monitor its progress and promote its implementation. This report recommends that all countries

TABLE 5-1 Estimated Smoking Prevalence (by gender) and Number of Smokers, 15 Years of Age and Over, by World Bank Region, 2000

	Smoking Prevalence (percentage)			Total Smokers	
World Bank Region	Males	Females	Overall	Millions	Percentage of All Smokers
East Asia and Pacific	63	5	34	429	38
Europe and Central Asia	56	17	35	122	11
Latin America and the Caribbean	40	24	32	98	9
Middle East and North Africa	36	5	21	37	3
South Asia	32	6	20	178	15
Sub-Saharan Africa	29	8	18	56	6
Low and middle income	49	8	29	920	82
High income	37	21	29	202	18

SOURCE: Reprinted, with permission, from Jha et al. (2006). Copyright 2006 by the World Bank.

ratify the FCTC, which requires them to implement its provisions. The evidence supporting the interventions recommended by the FCTC are reviewed later in this chapter. One caveat for this chapter is that the evidence on the effectiveness of interventions is largely from studies and programs in high-income countries. In recent years, some more research has been conducted in LMCs, but overall, the body of this evidence is relatively small. The assumption is made that behavior will be similar in LMCs and high-income countries, but clearly, direct observation and study in those countries is needed to ensure that interventions are working and, if not, new approaches are developed to respond to local conditions.

PREVALENCE AND EFFECTS OF SMOKING[1]

Smoking Prevalence

More than 1.1 billion people worldwide smoke tobacco. Smoking prevalence is highest in Europe and Central Asia (35 percent of adults), but overall, about 82 percent of smokers are in LMCs (Table 5-1) (Jha et al., 2006). Globally, male smoking far exceeds female smoking; the gender difference is smallest in high-income countries.

[1]The sections on the effects of tobacco and on interventions are based on Jha et al. (2006), the chapter on tobacco addiction from the report *Disease Control Priorities in Developing Countries*.

While overall smoking prevalence continues to increase in many LMCs, many high-income countries have witnessed decreases, most clearly in men. A study in 36 mostly western countries, from the early 1980s to the mid-1990s, suggested that the decrease in smoking prevalence among men was due both to the lower prevalence of starting smoking in younger age groups, as well as adults quitting smoking. Among women, there was little overall change in smoking prevalence because the increasing prevalence of smokers in younger age cohorts counterbalanced increasing cessation in older age groups (Molarius et al., 2001).

Health Consequences of Smoking

It is often taken for granted that the harm done by tobacco is well understood. But the magnitude of tobacco's harm is widely underestimated. More than 50 years of epidemiologic study of smoking-related diseases have led to three key messages for individual smokers and for policy makers (Doll et al., 2004; Peto et al., 2003). They are:

1. The eventual risk of death from smoking is high, with about one-half of long-term smokers eventually dying from their addiction.
2. About half of all tobacco deaths occur between ages 35 and 69—in middle age—about 20 to 25 years sooner than the deaths of nonsmokers.
3. Cessation works: Adults who quit before middle age avoid almost all the excess hazards of continued smoking.

The evidence is heavily weighted toward high-income countries, so it is not surprising that governments and individuals in LMCs have found it less relevant. However, as more studies are undertaken in those countries, a similar picture emerges, with somewhat different local details, depending on the other major risk factors and patterns of death. Studies in a wide range of countries, preferably long-term prospective studies (see Chapter 3), are needed to increase our understanding of these details and to tailor tobacco control interventions and messages.

Current Mortality from Smoking and Future Projections

An estimated 5 million deaths were caused by tobacco in 2000 (Ezzati and Lopez, 2003), about half (2.6 million) in low-income countries. Males accounted for 3.7 million deaths, three quarters of the total. About 60 percent of male and 40 percent of female tobacco deaths occurred in middle age (ages 35 to 69).

The patterns of causes of these deaths differ between high- and low-income countries. In high-income countries and former socialist economies, nearly half (450,000) of the 1 million middle-aged male tobacco deaths were from cardiovascular disease, and about half that number (210,000) from lung cancer. In contrast, in low-income countries, the leading causes of death among the 1.3 million male tobacco deaths were cardiovascular disease (400,000), chronic obstructive pulmonary disease (200,000), other respiratory disease (chiefly tuberculosis, 200,000) and lung cancer (180,000).

Future increases in tobacco deaths worldwide are expected to arise from increased smoking by men in developing countries, and by women worldwide. The increases will be a product of population growth and increased age-specific tobacco mortality rates, the latter relating to both smoking duration and the amount of tobacco smoked. Peto and others (Peto et al., 1994) have made the following calculation: If the proportion of young people taking up smoking continues to be about half of men and 10 percent of women, then there will be about 30 million new long-term smokers each year. Half of these smokers will eventually die from smoking. However, conservatively assuming that "only" about one-third of smokers die as a result of smoking, then smoking will eventually kill about 10 million people a year. Thus, for the 25-year period from 2000 to 2025, there will be about 150 million tobacco deaths or about 6 million deaths per year on average; from 2025 to 2050, there will be about 300 million tobacco deaths, or about 12 million deaths per year.

Further estimations are more uncertain, but based on current smoking trends and projected population growth, from 2050 to 2100 there will be an additional 500 million tobacco deaths. These projections for the next three to four decades are comparable to retrospective and early prospective epidemiological studies in China (Liu et al., 1998; Niu et al., 1998), which suggest that annual tobacco deaths will rise to 1 million before 2010 and 2 million by 2025, when the young adult smokers of today reach old age. Similarly, results from a large retrospective study in India suggest that 1 million annual deaths are expected from male smokers by 2025 (Gajalakshmi et al., 2003). With other populations in Asia, Eastern Europe, Latin America, the Middle East, and, less certainly, sub-Saharan Africa showing similar growth in population- and age-specific tobacco death rates, the estimate of some 450 million tobacco deaths over the next five decades appears to be plausible.

Benefits of Smoking Cessation

Smoking cessation reduces the risk of death from all tobacco-related diseases. The study of smoking habits, including cessation, with the longest follow-up is of doctors in the United Kingdom. Of those doctors who stopped smoking, the risk of lung cancer fell steeply over time (Doll et al., 2004; Peto et al., 2000) (Figure 5-1). These results are mirrored in a recent multicenter study of men in four European countries, which found that

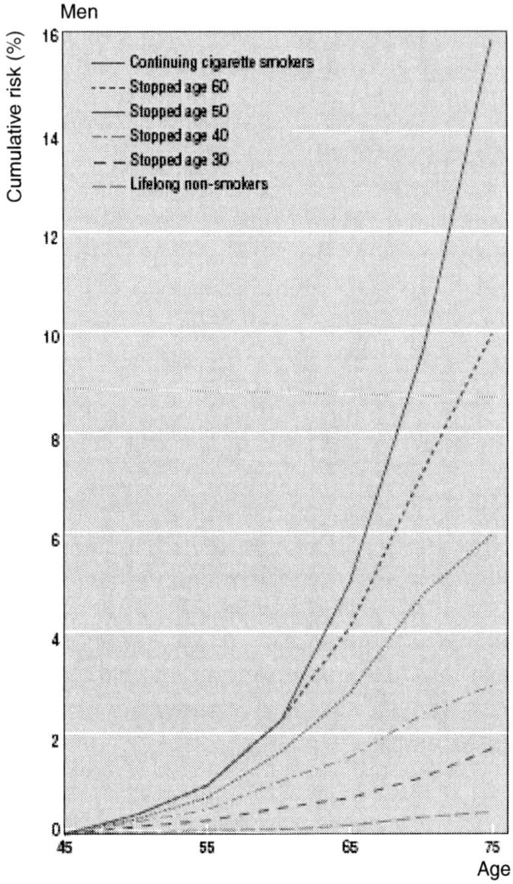

FIGURE 5-1 Stopping works: Cumulative risk of lung cancer mortality in U.K. males, 1990 rates.
SOURCE: Reprinted, with permission, from Peto et al., 2000. Copyright 2000 by the BMJ Publishing Group Ltd.

quitting smoking at age 40 avoided 80 to 85 percent of the excess risk of lung cancer (Crispo et al., 2004). Smoking cessation is uncommon in most developing countries, but there is some evidence that, among Chinese men, quitting also reduces the risks of dying from all causes together and at least from vascular disease specifically (Lam et al., 2002). Among doctors in the United Kingdom, the benefits of quitting were greatest in those who quit before middle age, but were still significant in those who quit later (Doll et al., 2004).

Current tobacco mortality statistics reflect past smoking behavior, given the long delay between the onset of smoking and the development of disease. The only way to prevent a substantial proportion of tobacco deaths before 2050 is for adult smokers to stop. For example, if the per-capita adult consumption of tobacco (mainly from people quitting entirely) could be cut in half by 2020 (akin to the declines in adult smoking in the United Kingdom), about 180 million premature tobacco deaths would be averted. Continuing to reduce the percentage of children who start to smoke will prevent many deaths, but its main effect will be on mortality rates in 2050 and beyond (Figure 5-2) (Jha and Chaloupka, 2000a; Peto and Lopez, 2002).

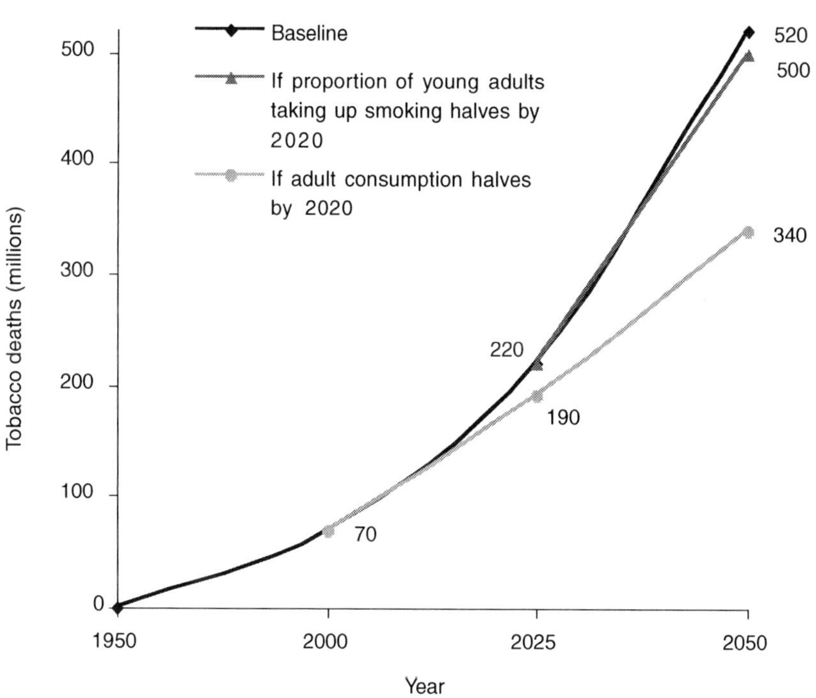

FIGURE 5-2 Tobacco deaths in the next 50 years under current smoking patterns.
SOURCE: Reprinted, with permission, from Jha and Chaloupka, 2000a. Copyright 2000 by the BMJ Publishing Group Ltd.

THE FRAMEWORK CONVENTION ON TOBACCO CONTROL

The FCTC is a pillar in tobacco control. The FCTC, adopted by the World Health Assembly (WHA), the WHO governing body, in May 2003, is the world's first global health treaty (WHO, 2003). The idea for an international instrument for tobacco control first arose at the annual WHA in 1995, in response to the globalization of tobacco and the increases in tobacco use, particularly among women and in LMCs. The following year, the WHA adopted a resolution calling for the WHO Director-General to initiate development of a Framework Convention on Tobacco Control. Work did not begin in earnest until 1999, and was adopted by the WHA and then opened for signatures in June 2003 and remained open until June 29, 2004.

The treaty came into force in February 2005, 90 days after the 40th country (Peru) had signed and ratified it. Countries that have ratified the FCTC are obligated, under international law, to enact its provisions. Countries that did not sign the treaty can still join by "accession," a one-step process equivalent to ratification. As of July 2006, 134 countries, including 108 LMCs, had become parties to it by ratification or the legal equivalent (accession, acceptance, approval, or formal confirmation). A total of 52 countries (including the United States) have signed but not ratified the FCTC (WHO, 2006).

Entering into force triggered another provision of the FCTC, which was the first meeting of the "Conference of the Parties," a formal body on which all signatories are represented, to be held within one year. The 2-week meeting took place in February 2006. The conference will meet regularly to review national reports and generally promote the FCTC, including promoting the financial aspects of treaty activities.

The FCTC includes provisions for both demand reduction and supply reduction, based on sound evidence that they are effective in reducing tobacco use. Key provisions are the following:

- **Advertising, sponsorship, and promotion**

Parties to the treaty must ban tobacco advertising, promotion, and sponsorship, as far as permitted by their constitutions. Where constitutions do not allow this, restrictions on all advertising, promotion, and sponsorship must be adopted.

- **Packaging and labeling of tobacco products**

The treaty obligates parties to adopt and implement large, clear, visible, legible, and rotating health warnings and messages on tobacco products and their outside packaging, occupying at least 30 percent of the principal display areas.

- **Protection from exposure to tobacco smoke**

Parties must adopt and implement (in areas of national jurisdiction) or promote (at other jurisdictional levels) effective measures to prevent exposure to tobacco smoke in indoor workplaces, public transport, indoor public places, and, as appropriate, other public places.

- **Illicit trade in tobacco products**

Parties must adopt and implement effective measures to eliminate illicit trade, illicit manufacturing, and counterfeiting of tobacco products.

INTERVENTIONS TO PREVENT SMOKING

Hundreds of millions of premature tobacco deaths could be avoided if effective interventions were applied widely in LMCs. The measures that have proven effective in reducing tobacco use, mainly in high-income countries thus far, are: tobacco tax increases, timely dissemination of information about health risks from smoking, restrictions on smoking in public places and workplaces, comprehensive bans on advertising and promotion, and increased access to cessation therapies. Price and nonprice interventions are, for the most part, highly cost-effective in high-income countries, with less evidence available from LMCs. The interventions discussed here are divided into those aimed at reducing the demand for tobacco and those aimed at reducing tobacco supply.

Interventions to Reduce Demand for Tobacco

The following sections review the evidence on the impact of interventions to reduce demand for tobacco, including a discussion of each intervention's effect on initiation of smoking and smoking cessation. As has been stated, much of the evidence is from high-income countries.

Tobacco Taxation

Nearly all governments tax tobacco products, but at widely varying levels. In some places, taxes are specific or per unit, and elsewhere, they are expressed as a percentage of wholesale or retail prices (*ad valorem* taxes). Taxes tend to be absolutely higher and account for a greater share of the retail price (two-thirds or more) in high-income countries (Figure 5-3). Tobacco taxes are much lower, and account for less than half of the final price of cigarettes, in most LMCs.

More than 100 studies from high-income countries clearly demonstrate that increases in taxes on cigarettes and other tobacco products lead to significant reductions in cigarette smoking and other tobacco use (Chaloupka et al., 2000). The reductions in tobacco use that result from higher taxes and prices reflect the combination of increased smoking cessation, reduced relapse, lower smoking initiation, and decreased consumption among

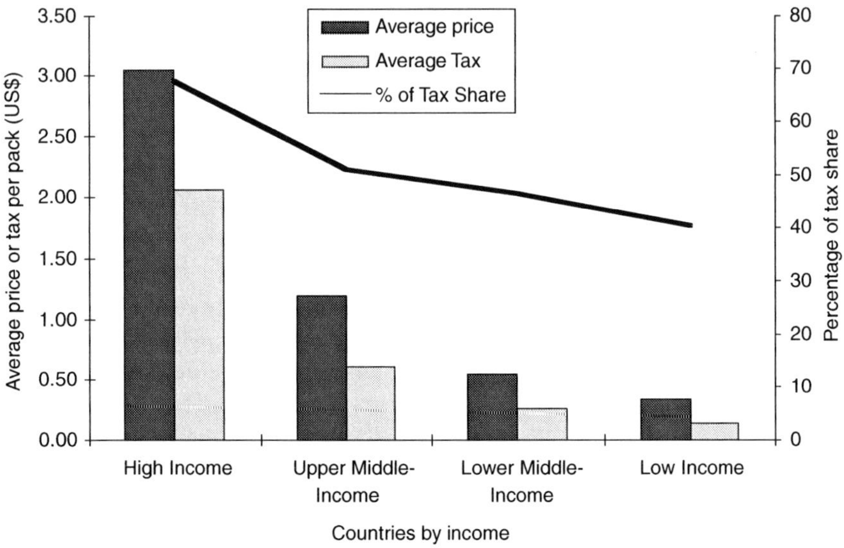

FIGURE 5-3 Average cigarette price, tax, and percentage of tax share per pack, by income group, 1996.
SOURCE: Reprinted, with permission, from Jha et al. (2006). Copyright 2006 by the World Bank.

continuing tobacco users. Studies of price elasticity of demand (i.e., how sensitive sales volume is to price) from the United States, United Kingdom, Canada, and other high-income countries have generally produced estimates that range from –0.25 up to an upper limit of –0.50, indicating that a 10 percent increase in cigarette prices could reduce overall cigarette smoking by 2.5 percent to 5 percent (Chaloupka et al., 2000; Gallus et al., 2006; U.S. DHHS, 2000).

Studies from LMCs have produced mixed results, however, some suggesting a greater price elasticity in such countries (Jha et al., 2006) while others suggest a smaller effect in some LMCs. A study in China and Russia, for example, using longitudinal data (as opposed to most studies, which have used aggregate data) found price elasticity estimates ranging from 0 to –0.15 (i.e., including a possibility of no effect) (Lance et al., 2004). Laxminarayan and Deolalikar (2004) examined the impact of tobacco prices on decisions to begin or quit smoking in Vietnam, using household survey data from the early and late 1990s. They found that decisions may be more complex than in high-income countries because a larger array of tobacco products—including nonmanufactured, local products—enlarges the choices people may make. Higher cigarette prices might divert smokers to products that are less expensive, but potentially equally detrimental to health.

Studies using survey data have concluded that half or more of the effect of price on overall cigarette demand results from reducing the number of current smokers (U.S. DHHS, 1994; Wasserman et al., 1991). Higher taxes increase both the number of attempts at quitting smoking and the success of those attempts (Tauras and Chaloupka, 2003). A study in the United States (Tauras, 1999) suggested that a 10 percent increase in price would result in an 11 to 13 percent shorter smoking duration or a 3.4 percent higher probability of cessation.

According to recent studies, there is an inverse relationship between price elasticity and age, with estimates for youth price elasticity of demand up to three times those of adults (Gruber, 2003; Ross et al., 2001). Several recent studies have begun to explore the differential impact of cigarette prices on youth smoking uptake, concluding that higher cigarette prices are particularly effective in preventing young smokers from moving beyond experimentation into regular, addicted smoking (Emery et al., 2001; Ross et al., 2001).

In the United States and the United Kingdom, increases in the price of cigarettes have had the greatest impact on smoking among the lowest income and least educated populations (Townsend et al., 1994; U.S. DHHS, 1994). Furthermore, it was estimated that smokers in U.S. households below median income level are four times more responsive to price increases than smokers in households above median income level.

Overall, the evidence strongly supports the premise that price affects behavior, in many cases very strongly. However, the evidence is still largely from high-income countries. It cannot be assumed that the impacts will be the same in LMCs, where so many aspects of life differ from those in high-income countries. As more evidence directly relevant to LMCs accumulates, patterns may emerge that reflect differences from the effects seen in high-income countries. Policy decisions should improve as more such information becomes available. The current recommendation of the FCTC, to increase tobacco taxes, is still well supported, but the magnitude of the impact and the specifics of effects appear likely to vary from place to place, possibly very considerably.

Restrictions on Smoking

Over the past three decades, as the quantity and quality of information about the health consequences of exposure to passive smoking has increased, many governments, especially in high-income countries, have restricted smoking in a variety of public places and private worksites. Increased concern about the consequences of passive smoking exposure, particularly to children, has led many workplaces to adopt voluntary restrictions on smoking. These restrictions reduce nonsmokers' exposure to passive tobacco smoke, but also reduce smokers' opportunities to smoke. Additional reductions in smoking, especially among youth, will result from the changes in social norms that are introduced by adopting these policies (U.S. DHHS, 1994).

In high-income populations, comprehensive restrictions on cigarette smoking reduced population smoking rates, possibly by as much as 5 to 15 percent (see Woolery et al. [2000] for a review of the effects of indoor smoking bans on youth smoking rates; see Levy et al. [2001]) for the results of simulation modeling of the impacts of smoking bans). As with higher taxes, both the prevalence of smoking and cigarette consumption among current smokers are reduced. According to Levy and colleagues (2001), no-smoking policies are most effective when strong social norms against smoking help to make smoking restrictions self-enforcing. The evidence is not entirely consistent with overall smoking declines as a result of smoking bans, however. A recent systematic review of workplace interventions for smoking cessation (Moher et al., 2005) included a subset of studies of indoor smoking bans that confirmed the decrease in smoking at work by smokers, and a corresponding decrease of exposure to environmental tobacco smoke. The evidence was less clear, however, about an overall decrease in smoking.

The applicability of findings related to smoking restrictions in high-income countries to conditions in LMCs is, as for other aspects, somewhat uncertain. Smoking bans are still rare in LMCs, so little to no direct evidence is yet available. To the extent that workplaces themselves differ between high-income countries and LMCs, different results might be expected. Nonetheless, the existing evidence should be sufficient to support the FCTC recommendation of smoking bans wherever feasible, with the caveat that impacts should be evaluated.

Health Information and Counteradvertising

The 1962 report by the British Royal College of Physicians and the 1964 U.S. Surgeon General's Report were landmark tobacco control events. These publications resulted in the first widespread press coverage of the scientific links between smoking and lung cancer. The reports were followed, in many high-income countries, by policies requiring health warning labels on tobacco products, which were later extended to tobacco advertising. The message did reach some LMCs as well, such as Malaysia (Box 5-1), with little delay.

Research from high-income countries indicates that these initial reports and the publicity that followed about the health consequences of smoking led to significant reductions in consumption, with initial declines of between

BOX 5-1
Tobacco Control in Malaysia

Malaysia has a long history of tobacco control campaigns, beginning in the 1970s. The Cancer and Tobacco unit in the Ministry of Health (MOH) is the government focal point for tobacco control. The vision of this unit is that by the year 2020, tobacco will no longer be a major public health concern in Malaysia, where decreasing national prevalence of tobacco use will be halved and tobacco-attributed illnesses and mortality will continuously decline. In 1972, the MOH and the Malaysian Medical Association jointly established the Action on Smoking on Health Committee (ASH).

In 1992, cigarette taxes were increased by 100 percent. Import and excise duties were doubled in 1993 to $11.44 per kg. All direct advertising of tobacco is prohibited, but brand name stretching (the use of tobacco brand names on non-tobacco merchandise or services) is still allowed, and advertising is permissible in any imported print media. Cigarette packets bear a single fixed health warning. Tobacco sales to any person under 18 years are prohibited, as are vending machines.

Smoking is banned in government offices, prisons, amusement centers, theaters, hospitals and clinics, public elevators, air-conditioned restaurants (with some exceptions), and public transportation.

Antismoking Campaigns

Since 1970, regular antismoking campaigns have been organized by schools, the Ministry of Health, and nongovernmental organizations (NGOs), such as the Malaysian Medical Association and consumer associations. Information on the dangers of smoking to pregnant women is distributed through pamphlets, posters, and health talks. Articles on smoking and health appear regularly in the media.

A national antismoking campaign—"Tak Nak Merokok" or "No to Tobacco"—was launched with fanfare by the Prime Minister in February 2004, funded by government at 20 million Malaysian Ringgits (about $5.4 million) per year for 5 years. Despite huge banners and screaming television coverage of the antismoking campaign, results have not yet been seen. While other antismoking campaigns have tried to sell the idea that smoking was unhealthy and "uncool," the "Tak Nak" campaign is about the need to look good, which is even more important to today's young people (e.g., by displaying posters of people with smoking-damaged teeth).

NGOs are also active in antismoking campaigns. In June 2004, the Malaysian Association of Youth Clubs launched the Youth Smoking Prevention Media Campaign, building on a previous government campaign. It is designed to address the misconceptions among the younger generation that smoking is hip, cool, and trendy. This campaign was sponsored by two major tobacco companies, the British-American Tobacco Company

continued

BOX 5-1 Continued

and JT International, as part of a trend in tobacco company sponsorship of antismoking campaigns.

There is no evidence that youth smoking prevention campaigns sponsored by the tobacco industry have been effective. However, the 2004 campaign was used by the tobacco companies to strengthen their waning public credibility and to influence the government.

Tobacco transnationals have been notorious for using aggressive advertising and promotional tactics not allowed at home. Malaysia, for example, has come to be known as the world capital for indirect advertising used by the transnationals. Brand-stretching activities and sponsorship of sports and entertainment events has remained legal and extremely widespread. With more aggressive control on advertising by tobacco companies, Malaysia should no longer be known for such tactics.

Smoking Prevalence

Despite antismoking activities, smoking prevalence continued to increase from 1986 through 2000, according to surveys in those years and in 1996. In 2000, just about half of all adult males smoked, as did about 5 percent of females. Peak age groups for smoking were 25–29 and 60–64. The age when their smoking began was lower among younger than older smokers, and younger among males (average age 19.5 years) than females (average age 24.7 years).

Indigenous groups (29.1 percent) and the Malays (27.9 percent) had the highest smoking prevalence, while the Indians (16.2 percent) and the Chinese

4 and 9 percent, and longer term cumulative declines of 15 to 30 percent (Kenkel and Chen, 2000; Townsend, 1993). Efforts to disseminate information about the risks of smoking and of other tobacco use in LMCs have led to similar declines in tobacco use in these countries (Kenkel and Chen, 2000). In addition, mass media antismoking campaigns, in many cases funded by earmarked tobacco taxes, have generated reductions in cigarette smoking and other tobacco usage (Kenkel and Chen, 2000; Saffer, 2000). Decreases in smoking prevalence are greatest in countries where the public is constantly and consistently reminded of the dangers of smoking by coverage of issues related to tobacco in the news media (Molarius et al., 2001).

In many LMCs, the public has not been well informed about the health risks of smoking. A national survey in China in 1996 found that 61 percent of smokers thought tobacco did them "little or no harm" (Chinese Academy of Preventive Medicine, 1997). In high-income countries, smokers are aware of the risks, but a recent review of psychological studies found that few smokers judge the size of these risks to be higher and more established

(19.2 percent) were less likely to smoke. Smoking was highest among those with only primary-level education (35.1 percent) and lowest in the highest educated group (23.1 percent). Smoking was also higher in lower income households. The professional and clerical occupational groups had the lowest rates (25.5 percent and 21 percent respectively), while the highest rates were in the agricultural occupations (56.4 percent).

Legislation

In 2005, the Cabinet approved a stand-alone Tobacco Control Act to take effect in the next 2 years. The Act will replace the Control of Tobacco Products Regulation 1993 (CTPR93) as the comprehensive tobacco control legislation in Malaysia, incorporating all relevant provisions and country obligations stated in the Framework Convention on Tobacco Control, which was signed by Malaysia in 2003. Until then, CTPR93 will remain the most important anti-smoking legislation. Among its provisions (which have been strengthened since passage) are:

- Prohibition of all advertising, promotion, and sponsorship
- Requirement of fixed health warnings on cigarette packets
- Ceiling levels of tar and nicotine
- Smoking bans in many public places
- Prohibition of tobacco sales to people under age 18, and possession of tobacco products and smoking by any person under 18

SOURCE: Hamzah (2005).

than do nonsmokers, and that smokers minimize the personal relevance of these risks (Weinstein, 1998).

Bans on Advertising and Promotion

Cigarettes are among the most heavily advertised and promoted products in the world. In 2001, cigarette companies spent $11.2 billion on advertising and promotion in the United States alone, the highest spending level reported to date (Federal Trade Commission, 2003). Tobacco advertising efforts worldwide include traditional forms of advertising through television, radio, billboards, magazines, and newspapers; favorable product placement; price-related promotions, such as coupons and multipack discounts; and sponsorship of highly visible sporting and cultural events.

The evidence is somewhat mixed about the effect of cigarette advertising and promotion on demand for cigarettes. Survey research and experiments that assess reactions to and recall of cigarette advertising find that increases in cigarette advertising and promotion directly and indirectly increase demand and smoking initiation (U.K. Department of Health, 1992; U.S. DHHS, 1994). Others have concluded that "the weight of the evidence from the academic literature suggests that advertising does not play a significant role in smoking initiation" (Taylor and Bonner, 2003). At least in part, the uncertainties arise from the difficulty of measuring the effects of advertising. One analyst points out that controlled, randomized experiments where some youth are exposed to cigarette advertising and others are not, are not possible, nor is it possible it isolate changes in advertising from other factors (e.g., societal attitudes) that are changing simultaneously (Goldberg, 2003). The types of studies that can be done, e.g., correlations between smoking behaviors and advertisement recall and awareness, are subject to different sorts of potential biases that arise from self-reported opinions and recall.

Econometric studies, mostly from the United States and the United Kingdom, have studied the effect of *marginal* changes in expenditures for advertising, concluding that at most, they have a small a small impact on demand (Chaloupka et al., 2000; Federal Trade Commission, 2003; Townsend, 1993).

Further studies of advertising and promotion bans should provide more direct evidence on the effect of these measures (Saffer, 2000). One study using data from 22 high-income countries for the period 1970 through 1992 provides some evidence that comprehensive bans on cigarette advertising and promotion led to significant reductions in cigarette smoking. The study predicted that a comprehensive set of tobacco advertising bans in high-income countries could reduce tobacco consumption by more than 6 percent, taking into account price and nonprice control interventions (Saffer and Chaloupka, 2000). The study concludes, however, that partial bans have little impact on smoking behavior, given that the tobacco industry can shift its resources from banned media to other media that are not banned.

Smoking Cessation Treatments

Near-term reductions in smoking-related mortality depend heavily on smoking cessation. There are many approaches to smoking cessation, including self-help manuals, community-based programs, and minimal or intensive clinical interventions (U.S. DHHS, 2000). In clinical settings, pharmacological treatments, including nicotine replacement therapies (NRT) and bupropion, have become much more widely available in recent years in high-income countries through deregulation of some NRTs from prescription to over-the-counter status (Curry et al., 2003; Novotny et al., 2000; U.S. DHHS, 2000). The evidence is strong and consistent that pharmacological treatments significantly improve the likelihood of quitting, with success rates two to three times better than without pharmaceutical treatments (Novotny et al., 2000; Raw et al., 1999; U.S. DHHS, 2000). The effectiveness of all commercially available NRTs seems to be largely independent of the duration of therapy, the setting in which the NRT is provided, regulatory status (over-the-counter versus prescribed), and the type of provider (Novotny et al., 2000). Over-the-counter NRTs without physician oversight have been used in many countries for a number of years with good success.

Ironically, the markets for NRT and other antismoking pharmacological therapies are more highly regulated and less affordable than are cigarettes and other forms of tobacco. Recent evidence indicates that the demand for NRT is related to economic factors, including price (Tauras and Chaloupka, 2003). A systematic review of the few studies of policies to cover (or decrease) the cost of NRT to the consumer—such as mandating private health insurance coverage of NRT, including NRT coverage in public health insurance programs, and subsidizing NRT for uninsured or underinsured individuals—does conclude that these policies increase the (self-reported) rate of quitting and sustained abstinence, but the evidence base is small (Kaper et al., 2005).

Interventions to Reduce the Supply of Tobacco

The key intervention on the supply side is the control of smuggling. Recent estimates suggest that 6 to 8 percent of cigarettes consumed globally are smuggled (Merriman et al., 2000). Of note, the tobacco industry itself has an economic incentive to smuggle, in part to increase market share and decrease tax rates (Joossens et al., 2000; Merriman et al., 2000). While differences in taxes and prices across countries create a motive for smuggling, a recent analysis comparing the degree of corruption in individual countries with price and tax levels found that corruption within countries is a stronger predictor of smuggling than is price (Merriman et al., 2000). Several governments are adopting policies aimed at controlling smuggling. In addition to harmonizing price differentials between countries, effective measures include prominent tax stamps and warning labels in local languages, better methods for tracking cigarettes through the distribution chain, aggressive enforcement of antismuggling laws, and stronger penalties for those caught violating these laws (Joossens et al., 2000). Recent analysis suggests that even in the presence of smuggling, tax increases will reduce consumption and increase revenue (Merriman et al., 2000).

The evidence that interventions aimed at reducing the supply of tobacco products are effective in reducing cigarette smoking is much weaker than it is for demand-side interventions (Jha and Chaloupka, 1999, 2000b). The U.S. experience provides mixed evidence about the effectiveness of limiting youth access to tobacco products in reducing tobacco use (U.S. DHHS, 2000; Woolery et al., 2000). In addition, the effective implementation and enforcement of these policies may require infrastructure and resources that do not exist in many LMCs. A preliminary discussion is occurring in Canada about reducing the number of retail outlets for tobacco from its current 65,000. The potential effect of such a move, and its enforcement costs, are not yet known. Crop substitution and diversification programs are often proposed as a means to reduce the supply of tobacco. However, there is little evidence that such programs would significantly reduce the supply of tobacco, given that the incentives for growing tobacco tend to attract new farmers who would replace those who abandon tobacco farming (Jacobs et al., 2000). Similarly, direct prohibition of tobacco production is not likely to be politically feasible, effective, or economically optimal. Finally, while trade liberalization has contributed to increases in tobacco use, particularly in LMCs, restrictions on trade in tobacco and tobacco products that violate international trade agreements or draw retaliatory measures (or both) may be more harmful.

Effectiveness and Cost-Effectiveness of Tobacco Control Interventions: Projections from a Model

Jha and colleagues (2006) estimated the effect that various interventions to reduce tobacco supply and demand would have on deaths due to smoking, with separate estimates for low- and for middle-income countries. The details of this model have been published previously (Ranson et al., 2002). Based on a cohort of smokers alive in 2000, they estimated the number of smoking-attributable deaths over the next few decades that could be averted by (1) price increases, (2) NRT, and (3) a package of nonprice interventions other than NRT (e.g., advertising and promotion bans, mass information, and warning labels). The data available for use in this model (and other such models) are from high-income countries. The model takes a public policy perspective in that the costs included are only those incurred by the public sector. Costs to individuals (e.g., out-of-pocket costs for such things as NRT, or the time costs of accessing interventions) are not included. The model does not take a "societal" perspective, which would include costs to all others affected. Effectiveness was estimated as years of healthy life saved, measured in disability adjusted life years (DALYs). The analysis is conservative in its assumptions about effectiveness (i.e., may underestimate effectiveness) and generous in its assumptions about the costs of tobacco control (i.e., may overestimate costs). This model is the most comprehensive of its type available, and the only one that attempts to make estimates separately for low- and middle-income countries for a range of interventions. It should be kept in mind that these are just estimates. The inputs to the model are, as stated, largely from high-income countries, where relationships may be somewhat different, so the results should be taken only as approximate indicators of what might be expected.

Potential Impact of Price Increases

The effect of increasing cigarette prices by 33 percent, 50 percent, and 70 percent were estimated. With a 33 percent increase, the model predicts that 22 million to 65 million smoking-attributable deaths would be averted worldwide, approximately 5 to 15 percent of all smoking-attributable deaths expected among those who smoke in 2000 (Table 5-2). Ninety percent of the deaths averted would be in low- and middle-income countries. Roughly 40 percent of the averted deaths would be in East Asia and the Pacific. For a 50 percent increase, worldwide smoking-attributable deaths averted range from 33 million to 92 million, and for a 70 percent price increase, 46 million to 114 million deaths (10 to 26 percent of all smoking-attributable deaths) would be averted.

Of the tobacco-related deaths that would be averted by a price increase, 80 percent would be male, reflecting the higher overall prevalence of smoking in men. The greatest relative impact of a price increase on deaths averted is among younger age cohorts. The price increases used in the model are achievable, and may even be conservative. In certain countries, such as South Africa and Poland, recent tax increases have doubled the real price of cigarettes (Guindon et al., 2002) (Box 5-2).

Potential Impact of Nicotine Replacement Therapy

The provision of NRT with an effectiveness of 1 percent is predicted to result in the avoidance of about 3.5 million smoking-attributable deaths (Table 5-3). NRT of 5 percent effectiveness will have about five times the impact. Again, LMCs would account for roughly 80 percent of the averted deaths. The relative impact of NRT (of 2.5 percent effectiveness) on deaths averted is 2 to 3 percent among individuals ages 15 to 59, and lower among those ages 60 and older (results not shown). Clearly, NRT is more expensive than interventions such as tax increases, and will not be affordable everywhere, despite being relatively cost effective.

Potential Impact of Nonprice Interventions Other Than NRT

A package of nonprice interventions other than NRT that decrease the prevalence of smoking by 2 percent is predicted to prevent about 7 million smoking-attributable deaths (more than 1.6 percent of all smoking-attributable deaths among those who smoked in 2000; see Table 5-4). A package of interventions that decreases the prevalence of smoking by 10

TABLE 5-2 Potential Impact of Price Increases of 10 Percent, 33 Percent, 50 Percent, and 70 Percent on Tobacco Mortality by World Bank Region, 2000

World Bank Region	Smoking attributable deaths in millions	Change in number of deaths in millions							
		10% price increase		33% price increase		50% price increase		70% price increase	
		Low	High	Low	High	Low	High	Low	High
East Asia and Pacific	173	–2.9	–8.7	–9.6	–27.5	–14.5	–37.5	–20.3	–46.2
(percent)		(–1.7)	(–5.0)	(–5.5)	(–15.9)	(–8.4)	(–21.7)	(–11.7)	(–26.8)
Europe and Central Asia	51	–0.9	–2.6	–2.8	–8.1	–4.3	–11.2	–6.0	–13.8
(percent)		(–1.7)	(–5.1)	(–5.6)	(–16.0)	(–8.5)	(–22.0)	(–11.8)	(–27.2)
Latin America and the Caribbean	40	–0.7	–2.1	–2.3	–6.7	–3.5	–9.5	–4.9	–11.6
(percent)		(–1.8)	(–5.3)	(–5.8)	(–16.8)	(–8.8)	(–23.7)	(–12.3)	(–29.1)
Middle East and North Africa	13	–0.2	–0.7	–0.8	–2.2	–1.2	–3.1	–1.6	–3.8
(percent)		(–1.7)	(–5.2)	(–5.8)	(–16.6)	(–8.7)	(–23.2)	(–12.2)	(–28.5)
South Asia	62	–0.9	–2.6	–2.9	–8.5	–4.4	–12.5	–6.2	–16
(percent)		(–2.4)	(–8.6)	(–9.5)	(–27.7)	(–14.3)	(–40.6)	(–20.1)	(–52)
Sub-Saharan Africa	23	–0.4	–1.1	–1.3	–3.7	–1.9	–5.5	–2.7	–6.6
(percent)		(–1.6)	(–4.9)	(–5.4)	(–15.9)	(–8.2)	(–23.6)	(–11.5)	(–28.5)
Low- and middle-income	362	–6.0	–17.9	–19.7	–56.8	–29.8	–79.2	–41.7	–98.2
(percent)		(–1.6)	(–4.9)	(–5.4)	(–15.7)	(–8.2)	(–21.9)	(–11.5)	(–27.1)
High-income	81	–0.6	–2.6	–2.1	–8.5	–3.2	–12.2	–4.5	–16.2
(percent)		(–0.8)	(–3.2)	(–2.6)	(–10.6)	(–4.0)	(–15.1)	(–5.6)	(–20.0)
World	443	–6.6	–20.5	–21.8	–65.3	–33.0	–91.5	–46.2	–114.3
(percent)		(–1.5)	(–4.6)	(–4.9)	(–14.7)	(–7.5)	(–20.7)	(–10.4)	(–25.8)

SOURCE: Reprinted, with permission, from Jha et al. (2006). Copyright 2006 by the World Bank.

BOX 5-2
Tobacco Control in Poland

Through the 1980s Poland had among the highest smoking rates in the world and higher lung cancer rates than any other country in Europe, save Hungary. Nearly three-quarters of men and 30 percent of women were regular smokers. An estimated 42 percent of cardiovascular deaths and 71 percent of deaths from respiratory diseases among middle-aged men were caused by smoking. Members of the Polish public were ill informed about the hazards of smoking, so few perceived a reason to stop.

Cigarettes in Poland were produced by a government-run enterprise and were a significant source of revenue, particularly important in lean economic times. The fall of communism in Poland led to increases in smoking, not only among adults, but among adolescents and teenagers. By the mid-1990s, the tobacco industry was almost completely in private hands, with multinational tobacco corporations playing an ever larger role. Prices were kept low as a result of agreements between the government and the tobacco companies. Cigarettes became the most heavily advertised product in the country, as companies vied for market share and a bigger smoker population, with a goal of increasing cigarette consumption by 10 percent per year. The success of these efforts was seen in increased smoking rates, particularly among adolescents and young teens (Zatonski, 1998).

The Tobacco Control Movement

Anti-tobacco forces began to organize during the 1980s as part of the first initiatives of Poland's emerging civil society. The Polish Anti-Tobacco Society and other groups formed and began to reach out domestically and internationally. The Polish mass media were increasingly active in reporting on health issues, including the dangers of tobacco. In the 1990s, when Polish society opened up, the movement took hold. A conference called "A Tobacco-Free New Europe," with health advocates from Eastern and Western Europe, was held in Kazimierz, Poland, in 1990. The policy recommendations that emerged from that meeting became the basis for legislation proposed to the Polish Senate beginning in 1991.

Several years of intense, heavily funded opposition by the tobacco industry and public debate ensued. Public opinion eventually swung toward the health advocates, and in 1995 the Senate passed—with 90 percent of the vote—the "Law for the Protection of Public Health Against the Effects of Tobacco Use." Provisions included a ban on smoking and cigarette sales in health care centers, schools, and enclosed workplaces; a ban on tobacco sales to those under 18 years; a ban on smokeless tobacco; a ban on radio and television advertising and limits on other media; large health warnings on cigarette packages; and free smoking

continued

BOX 5-2 Continued

cessation treatment. Later measures raised taxes on cigarettes by 30 percent each year in 1999 and 2000.

The Health Promotion Foundation led the legislative effort, accompanied by public education and action campaigns, including annual "smoke-outs" credited with helping 2.5 million smokers to quit over a decade.

The Results

During the 1990s, cigarette consumption fell 10 percent, smoking among adult men fell from 62 to 40 percent, and among adult women, from 30 to 20 percent. The health benefits were almost immediate: overall mortality fell by 10 percent over the same period, and about one-third of the decline is attributed to smoking reductions. Lung cancer rates also had begun to decrease, falling 30 percent in younger men (ages 20–44) and 19 percent in men ages 45–64. Positive effects on cardiovascular disease and low-birthweight babies is also attributable to the decline in smoking.

Poland and its neighbor Hungary had similar lung cancer rates in the 1980s, but Hungary did not take measures to control tobacco when Poland did. While lung cancer rates fell in Poland, they continued to rise through the 1990s in Hungary, and are now substantially higher.

SOURCE: Levine and Kinder (2004).

percent would have an impact five times greater. LMCs would account for approximately four-fifths of quitters and averted deaths. The greatest relative impact of nonprice interventions on deaths averted would be among younger age cohorts.

Figure 5-4 summarizes the potential impact of a set of independent tobacco control interventions, using 33 percent and 70 percent price increases (employing a high elasticity of –1.2 for low- and middle-income regions and –0.8 for high-income regions), a 5 percent effectiveness of NRT, and a 10 percent reduction from nonprice interventions other than NRT. In this cohort of smokers alive in 2000, approximately 443 million are expected to die in the next 50 years in the absence of interventions. A substantial fraction of these tobacco deaths are avoidable with interventions. Price increases have the greatest impact on tobacco mortality, with the most aggressive price increase of 70 percent having the potential to avert nearly one-quarter of all tobacco deaths. Even a modest price increase of 33 percent could potentially prevent 66 million tobacco deaths over the course of the next 50 years. While NRTs and other nonprice interventions are less effective than price increases, they can still avert a substantial number of tobacco deaths (18 million and 35 million deaths, respectively). The greatest impact of these

TABLE 5-3 Potential Impact of Price Increase of 33 Percent, Increased NRT Use, and a Package of Nonprice Measures, 2000

World Bank Region	Smoking attributable deaths in millions	Change in number of deaths in millions: 33% price increase, Low elasticity	33% price increase, High elasticity	NRT effectiveness 1.0%	NRT effectiveness 5.0%	Nonprice intervention effectiveness 2%	Nonprice intervention effectiveness 10%
East Asia and Pacific	173	−9.6	−27.5	−1.4	−6.9	−2.8	−13.8
(percent)		(−5.5)	(−15.9)	(−0.8)	(−4.0)	(−1.6)	(−8.0)
Europe and Central Asia	51	−2.8	−8.1	−0.4	−2.1	−0.8	−4.1
(percent)		(−5.6)	(−16.0)	(−0.8)	(−4.0)	(−1.6)	(−8.1)
Latin America and the Caribbean	40	−2.3	−6.7	−0.3	−1.7	−0.7	−3.4
(percent)		(−5.8)	(−16.8)	(−0.8)	(−4.2)	(−1.7)	(−8.5)
Middle East and North Africa	13	−0.8	−2.2	−0.11	−0.6	−0.2	−1.1
(percent)		(−5.8)	(−16.6)	(−0.8)	(−4.2)	(−1.7)	(−8.4)
South Asia	62	−2.9	−8.5	−0.4	−2.2	−0.9	−4.3
(percent)		(−9.5)	(−27.7)	(−1.4)	(−7.2)	(−2.8)	(−13.9)
Sub-Saharan Africa	23	−1.3	−3.7	−0.2	−0.9	−0.4	−1.8
(percent)		(−5.4)	(−15.9)	(−0.8)	(−4.0)	(−1.6)	(−7.9)
Low- and middle-income	362	−19.7	−56.8	−2.9	−14.3	−5.7	−28.6
(percent)		(−5.4)	(−15.7)	(−0.8)	(−4.0)	(−1.6)	(−7.9)
High-income	81	−2.1	−8.5	−0.6	−3.1	−1.2	−6.1
(percent)		(−2.6)	(−10.6)	(−0.8)	(−3.8)	(−1.5)	(−7.6)
World	*443*	*−21.8*	*−65.3*	*−3.5*	*−17.4*	*−6.9*	*−34.7*
(percent)		*(−4.9)*	*(−14.8)*	*(−0.8)*	*(−3.9)*	*(−1.6)*	*(−7.8)*

SOURCE: Reprinted, with permission, from Jha et al. (2006). Copyright 2006 by the World Bank.

tobacco control interventions would occur after 2010, but a substantial number of deaths could be avoided even before then.

No attempt has been made in this analysis to examine the impact of combining the various packages of interventions (e.g., price increases with NRT, or NRT and other nonprice interventions). A number of studies have compared the impact of price and nonprice interventions, but few empirical attempts have been made to assess how these interventions might interact. While price increases may be the most cost-effective antismoking intervention, policy makers should use all the tools at their disposal to counter smoking. Nonprice measures may be required to reach the most heavily dependent smokers, for whom medical and social support in stopping will

TABLE 5-4 Range of Cost-Effectiveness Values for Price Increase, Nicotine Replacement Therapies, and Nonprice Interventions (2002 US dollars per DALY Saved), by World Bank Region, 2000

World Bank Region	Smoking attributable deaths in millions	33% price increase		NRTs with effectiveness of 1% to 5%		Nonprice interventions with effectiveness of 2% to 10%	
		Low-end estimate	High-end estimate	Low-end estimate	High-end estimate	Low-end estimate	High-end estimate
East Asia and Pacific	173	2	30	65	864	40	498
Europe and Central Asia	51	3	42	45	633	55	685
Latin America and the Caribbean	40	6	85	53	812	109	1,361
Middle East and North Africa	13	6	89	47	750	115	1,432
South Asia	62	2	27	54	716	34	431
Sub-Saharan Africa	23	2	26	42	570	33	417
Low- and middle-income	362	3	42	55	761	54	674
High-income	81	85	1,773	175	3,781	1,166	14,572
World	443	13	195	75	1,250	233	2,916

SOURCE: Reprinted, with permission, from Jha et al. (2006). Copyright 2006 by the World Bank.

be necessary. Furthermore, these nonprice measures may be effective in increasing social acceptance and support of tobacco price increases.

Comprehensive Tobacco Control Programs

In recent years, several governments, mostly in high-income countries, have adopted comprehensive programs to reduce tobacco use, often funded by earmarked tobacco tax revenues. These programs have similar goals for reducing tobacco use, including preventing initiation among youth and young adults, promoting cessation among all smokers, reducing exposure to passive tobacco smoke, and identifying and eliminating disparities among population subgroups (U.S. DHHS, 1994). These programs have one or more of four key components: (1) community interventions engag-

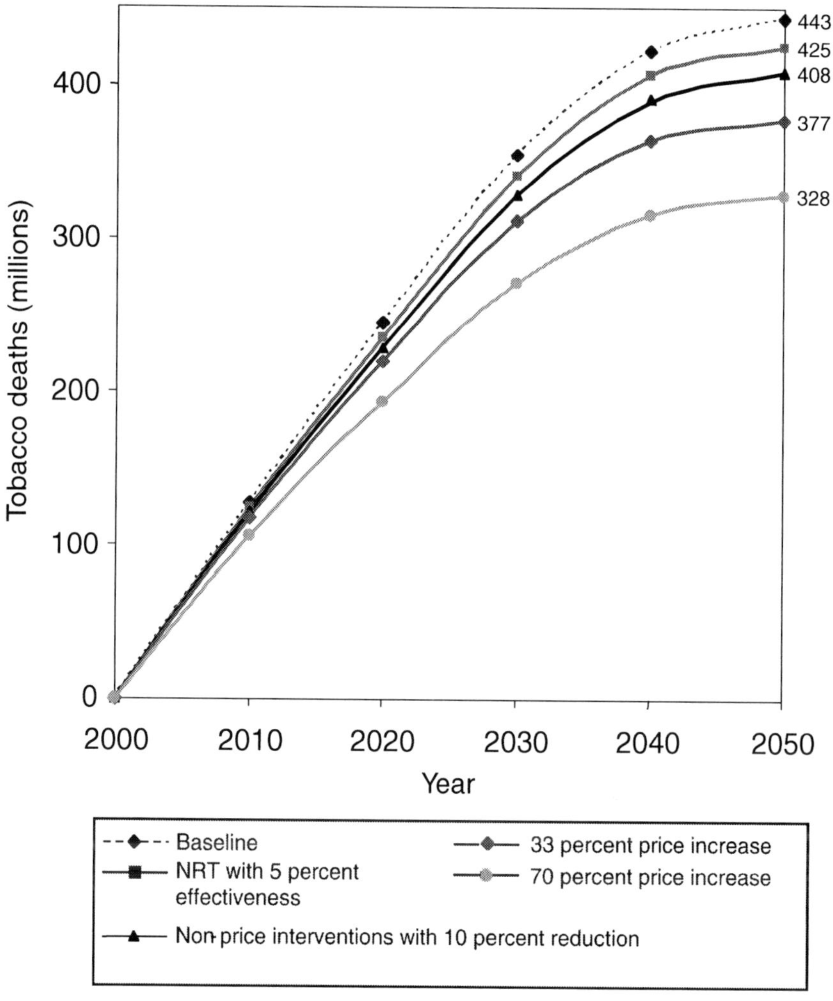

FIGURE 5-4 Potential impact of tax increases, nicotine reduction therapies, and nonprice interventions on tobacco mortality, 2000–2050, among the world's smokers in 2000.

NOTE: Price increases assume a high price elasticity (–1.2 for low- and middle-income countries and –0.8 for high-income countries).

SOURCE: Reprinted, with permission, from Jha et al. (2006). Copyright 2006 by the World Bank.

ing a diverse set of local organizations; (2) countermarketing and health information campaigns; (3) program policies and regulations (e.g., taxes, restrictions on smoking, bans on tobacco advertising, and access to better cessation treatments); and (4) surveillance and evaluation of potential issues, such as smuggling (U.S. DHHS, 1994). Programs have placed differing emphasis on these four components, with substantial diversity among the types of activities supported within each component. Recent analyses from the United States and United Kingdom clearly indicate that these comprehensive efforts have been successful in reducing tobacco use and in improving public health (Farrelly et al., 2003; Townsend et al., 1994; U.S. DHHS, 1994). In California, for example, the state's comprehensive tobacco control program has produced a rate of decline in tobacco use double that seen in the rest of the United States. As with other aspects of tobacco control, the impacts of comprehensive tobacco control may be different in LMCs than they are in high-income countries, which differ in much more than simply economic status. The following discussion is presented with the understanding that efforts to develop comprehensive tobacco control in LMCs should be accompanied by adequate monitoring and evaluation to ensure that the efforts are worthwhile.

The cost of implementing control programs is relatively low and certainly affordable for high-income countries. Table 5-5 provides the estimated total costs of implementing price and NRT interventions by World Bank region. Current estimates of the costs of implementing a comprehensive tobacco control program range from $2.50 to $10 per capita in the United States. The Centers for Disease Control and Prevention (CDC) recommends spending $6 to $16 per capita for a comprehensive tobacco control program in the United States (CDC, 1999). Canadian spending on tobacco control programs was approximately $1.65 per capita in 1996 (Pechmann et al., 1998). At the highest recommending spending level ($16 per capita) in the United States, annual funding for a comprehensive tobacco program would equal 0.9 percent of U.S. public spending, per capita, on health.

Constraints to Effective Tobacco Control Policies

Use of the effective interventions described here is uneven and limited (see a more formal analysis in Chaloupka et al., 2001). World Bank data reveal that there is ample room to increase tobacco taxes: In 1995 the average percentage of all government revenue derived from tobacco tax was 0.63. Middle-income countries averaged 0.51 percent of government revenue from tobacco taxes, while lower income countries averaged 0.42 percent. An increase in cigarette taxes of 10 percent globally would raise cigarette tax revenues by nearly 7 percent, with relatively larger increases in revenues in high-income countries, and smaller increases in revenues in LMCs (Sunley

TABLE 5-5 Estimated Cost of Price Intervention and Nicotine Replacement Therapy Programs by World Bank Region

		Cost for price increase (millions 2002 US$)		Cost of NRTs ($25 to $150) (millions 2002 US$)					
	GDP			To treat 1% of current smokers			To treat 5% of current smokers		
World Bank Region	(billions 2002 US$)	Low-end estimate	High-end estimate	$25	$50	$150	$25	$50	$150
East Asia and Pacific	1,802	360	901	1,079	2,158	6,474	5,395	10,791	32,372
Europe and Central Asia	1,136	227	568	318	635	1,906	1,588	3,176	9,529
Latin America and the Caribbean	1,673	335	836	250	500	1,500	1,250	2,500	7,499
Middle East and North Africa	694	139	347	84	169	506	422	843	2,530
South Asia	655	131	327	2,312	1,926	3,853	11,558	2,312	1,926
Sub-Saharan Africa	319	64	159	868	723	1,447	4,340	868	723
Low- and middle-income	6,256	1,251	3,128	13,565	11,305	22,609	67,827	13,565	11,305
High-income	25,992	5,198	12,996	3,034	2,529	10,114	15,172	3,034	2,529
World	32,253	6,451	16,126	16,600	13,833	32,723	82,999	16,600	13,833

GDP = Gross domestic product.

SOURCE: Reprinted, with permission, from Jha et al. (2006). Copyright 2006 by the World Bank.

et al., 2000). Despite this, price increases have been underused. Guindon and colleagues (2002) studied 80 countries and found that the real price of tobacco, adjusted for purchasing power, fell in most developing countries from 1990 to 2000.

Why is there so much variation in tobacco control policies? The political economy of tobacco control has been inadequately studied. A few plausible areas of interest are outlined here. First, the recognition of tobacco as a major health hazard appears to be the impetus for most of the tobacco control policies in many high-income countries. There is some evidence that improved national capacity and local needs assessment could increase the likelihood that tobacco control measures will be adopted. For example, econometric analyses in South Africa geared to local policy needs substantially increased the willingness of the country to implement tobacco control policies (Abedian et al., 1998). Second, tobacco control budgets are only a fraction of what is required. Funding is needed not so much to implement programs, but to counter tobacco industry tactics and to build popular support for control. Third, the most obvious constraint to tobacco control is political opposition, but this is difficult to quantify. Opposition from the tobacco industry is well organized and well funded (Pollock, 1996).

A key political tool for addressing political opposition is earmarking tobacco taxes. Earmarking has been successful in several countries, including Australia, Finland, Nepal, and Thailand. Of the 48 countries currently in the WHO European Region, 12 earmark taxes for tobacco control and other public health measures. The average level of allocation is less than 1 percent of total tax revenue (WHO, 2002). Earmarking does introduce clear restrictions and inefficiencies on public finance, and for this reason alone most macroeconomists do not favor earmarking, no matter how worthy the cause. However, earmarking tobacco taxes can be justified if governments use these funds to benefit those who pay for tobacco control policies and programs, and secure public support for new or higher tobacco taxes.

Earmarked taxes also have a political function in that they help to concentrate political winners of tobacco control, and thus influence policy. Earmarked funds that support broad health and social services (e.g., other disease programs) broaden the political and civil society support base for tobacco control. In Australia, broad political support among the Ministries of Sports and Education helped to convince the Ministry of Finance that raising tobacco taxes was possible. Indeed, once an earmarked tax was passed, the Ministry of Finance went on to raise tobacco taxes further without earmarking (Galbally, 1997). Additionally, targeting revenue from tobacco taxes to other health programs for the poorest socioeconomic groups could produce double health gains—reduced tobacco consumption combined with increased access to and use of health services. In China, a 10 percent increase in cigarette taxes would decrease consumption by 5 percent and increase government revenue by 5 percent. These increased earnings could finance a package of essential health services for one-third of China's poorest 100 million citizens in 1990 (Saxenian and McGreevey, 1996).

Monitoring the Effects of Tobacco (and Other Important Risk Factors)

Understanding trends in the use of tobacco and its consequences is important to understanding population health generally, and to determining how well interventions are working to reduce tobacco use. It is possible to do this through economical long-term studies of large samples of the population. Such prospective studies (described in Chapter 3) should be considered an integral part of cancer (and other chronic disease) control.

SUMMARY AND RECOMMENDATIONS

There is no real disagreement about the health effects of tobacco: At least half of all long-term smokers eventually die from tobacco-related disease, including, but not limited to, cancer. Also incontrovertible, but not as well appreciated, is that stopping smoking reduces the risk of tobacco-related death enormously. The question is how to get current smokers to stop (most important) and how to discourage nonsmokers (young people and adults) from taking up smoking. A relatively large body of evidence, most from high-income countries, supports both "demand-" and, to a lesser extent, "supply-" side interventions. These are the interventions that are included in the FCTC, and endorsed by this report. The most important step is ratification of the FCTC by as many countries as possible, at which time they will be obligated to adopt its provisions.

RECOMMENDATION 5-1. Every country should sign and ratify the Framework Convention on Tobacco Control and implement its provisions, most importantly:

- *Substantial increases in taxation to raise the prices of tobacco products (goal is to have taxes at 80 percent or higher of retail price)*
- *Complete advertising and promotion bans on tobacco products*
- *Mandating that public spaces be smoke free*
- *Large, explicit cigarette packet warnings in local languages (which also helps to reduce smuggling)*
- *Support of counteradvertising to publicize the health damage from tobacco and the benefits of stopping tobacco use*

REFERENCES

Abedian I, van der Merwe R, Wilkins N, Jha P. 1998. *The Economics of Tobacco Control: Towards an Optimal Policy Mix.* Cape Town, South Africa: University of Cape Town.

Centers for Disease Control and Prevention. 1999. *Best Practices for Comprehensive Tobacco Control Programs.* Atlanta: GA: Department of Health and Human Services.

Chaloupka FJ, Hu TH, Warner KE, Jacobs R, Yurekli A. 2000. The taxation of tobacco products. In: Jha P, Chaloupka F, eds. *Tobacco Control in Developing Countries.* Oxford, England: Oxford University Press. Pp. 238–272.

Chaloupka FJ, Jha P, Corrao MA, Costa e Silva V, Ross H, Czart C, Yach D. 2001. *The Evidence Base for Reducing Mortality From Smoking in Low and Middle Income Countries.* Commission on Macroeconomics and Health Working Paper Series. Geneva, Switzerland: WHO.

Chinese Academy of Preventive Medicine. 1997. *Smoking in China: 1996 National Prevalence Survey of Smoking Pattern.* Beijing, China: China Science and Technology Press.

Crispo A, Brennan P, Jockel KH, Schaffrath-Rosario A, Wichmann HE, Nyberg F, Simonato L, Merletti F, Forastiere F, Boffetta P, Darby S. 2004. The cumulative risk of lung cancer among current, ex- and never-smokers in European men. *British Journal of Cancer* 91(7):1280–1286.

Doll R, Peto R, Boreham J, Sutherland I. 2004. Mortality in relation to smoking: 50 years' observations on male British doctors. *British Medical Journal* 328(7455):1519–1528.

Emery S, White MM, Pierce JP. 2001. Does cigarette price influence adolescent experimentation? *Journal of Health Economics* 20(2):261–270.

Ezzati M, Lopez AD. 2003. Estimates of global mortality attributable to smoking in 2000. *Lancet* 362(9387):847–852.

Farrelly MC, Pechacek TF, Chaloupka FJ. 2003. The impact of tobacco control program expenditures on aggregate cigarette sales: 1981–2000. *Journal of Health Economics* 22(5):843–859.

Federal Trade Commission. 2003. *Cigarette Report for 2001.* Washington, DC: Federal Trade Commission.

Gajalakshmi CK, Jha P, Ranson K, Nguyen S. 2000. Global patterns of smoking and smoking attributable mortality. In: Jha P, Chaloupka F, eds. *Tobacco Control in Developing Countries.* Oxford, England: Oxford University Press. Pp. 11–39.

Gajalakshmi V, Peto R, Kanaka TS, Jha P. 2003. Smoking and mortality from tuberculosis and other diseases in India: Retrospective study of 43,000 adult male deaths and 35,000 controls. *Lancet* 362(9383):507–515.

Galbally RL. 1997. Health-promoting environments: Who will miss out? *Australian & New Zealand Journal of Public Health* 21(4 Spec. No.):429–430.

Gallus S, Schiaffino A, La Vecchia C, Townsend J, Fernandez E. 2006. Price and cigarette consumption in Europe. *Tobacco Control* 15(2):114–119.

Goldberg ME. 2003. Correlation, causation, and smoking initiation among youths. *Journal of Advertising Research* 43(1):431–440.

Gruber J. 2003. *Government Policy Toward Smoking: A New View From Economics.* Paper presented at the Disease Control Priorities Project Nicotine Addiction Workshop, Mumbai, India. DCPP Working Paper Series.

Guindon GE, Tobin S, Yach D. 2002. Trends and affordability of cigarette prices: Ample room for tax increases and related health gains. *Tobacco Control* 11(1):35–43.

Hamzah E. 2005. *Malaysian Case Study of Cancer Control.* Unpublished.

Hu TW, Xu X, Keeler T. 1998. Earmarked tobacco taxes: Lessons learned. In: Abedian I, van der Merwe R, Wilkins N, Jha P. *The Economics of Tobacco Control.* Cape Town, South Africa: University of Cape Town, Applied Fiscal Research Centre.

IOM (Institute of Medicine). 2003. *Fulfilling the Potential of Cancer Prevention and Early Detection.* Curry, SJ, Byers, T, Hewitt, M, eds. Washington, DC: The National Academies Press.

Jacobs R, Gale HF, Capehart TC, Zhang P, Jha P. 2000. The supply-side effects of tobacco control policies. In: Jha P, Chaloupka F, eds. *Tobacco Control in Developing Countries.* Oxford, England: Oxford University Press. Pp. 312–341.

Jha P, Chaloupka F. 2000a. *Tobacco Control in Developing Countries.* Oxford, England: Oxford University Press.

Jha P, Chaloupka FJ. 2000b. The economics of global tobacco control. *BMJ* 321(7257): 358–361.

Jha P, Chaloupka FJ. 1999. *Curbing the Epidemic: Governments and the Economics of Tobacco Control.* Washington, DC: World Bank.

Jha P, Chaloupka FJ, Moore J, Gajalakshmi V, Gupta PC, Peck R, Asma S, Zatonski W. 2006. Tobacco addiction. In: Jamison DT, Breman JG, Measham AR, Alleyne G, Claeson M, Evans DB, Jha P, Mills A, Musgrove P, eds. *Disease Control Priorities in Developing Countries.* 2nd ed. New York: Oxford University Press.

Jha P, Musgrove P, Chaloupka FJ, Yurekli A.2000. The economic rationale for intervention in the tobacco market. In: Jha P, Chaloupka F, eds. *Tobacco Control in Developing Countries.* Oxford, England: Oxford University Press. Pp. 154–174.

Joossens L, Chaloupka FJ, Merriman D, Yurekli A. 2000. Issues in the smuggling of tobacco products. In: Jha P, Chaloupka F, eds. *Tobacco Control in Developing Countries.* Oxford, England: Oxford University Press. Pp. 394–406.

Kaper J, Wagena EJ, Severens JL, Van Schayck CP. 2005. Healthcare financing systems for increasing the use of tobacco dependence treatment. *Cochrane Database of Systematic Reviews* (1):CD004305.

Kenkel D, Chen L. 2000. Consumer information and tobacco use. In: Jha P, Chaloupka F, eds. *Tobacco Control in Developing Countries.* Oxford, England: Oxford University Press. Pp. 154–174.

Lam TH, He Y, Shi QL, Huang JY, Zhang F, Wan ZH, Sun CS, Li LS. 2002. Smoking, quitting, and mortality in a Chinese cohort of retired men. *Annals of Epidemiology* 12(5):316–320.

Lance PM, Akin JS, Dow WH, Loh CP. 2004. Is cigarette smoking in poorer nations highly sensitive to price? Evidence from Russia and China. *Journal of Health Economics* 23(1):173–189.

Levine R, Kinder M. 2004. *Millions Saved: Proven Successes in Global Health.* Washington, DC: Center for Global Development.

Levy DT, Friend K, Polishchuk E. 2001. Effect of clean indoor air laws on smokers: The clean air module of the SimSmoke computer simulation model. *Tobacco Control* 10(4):345–351.

Lightwood J, Collins D, Lapsley H, Novotny TE. 2000. Estimating the costs of tobacco use. In: Jha P, Chaloupka F, eds. *Tobacco Control in Developing Countries.* Oxford, England: Oxford University Press. Pp. 63–103.

Liu BQ, Peto R, Chen ZM, Boreham J, Wu YP, Li JY, Campbell TC, Chen JS. 1998. Emerging tobacco hazards in China: Retrospective proportional mortality study of one million deaths. *BMJ* 317(7170):1411–1422.

Merriman D, Yurekli A, Chaloupka FJ. 2000. How big is the worldwide cigarette smuggling problem? In: Jha P, Chaloupka F, eds. *Tobacco Control in Developing Countries.* Oxford, England: Oxford University Press.

Molarius A, Parsons RW, Dobson AJ, Evans A, Fortmann SP, Jamrozik K, Kuulasmaa K, Moltchanov V, Sans S, Tuomilehto J, Puska P, WHO MONICA Project. 2001. Trends in cigarette smoking in 36 populations from the early 1980s to the mid-1990s: Findings from the WHO MONICA Project. *American Journal of Public Health* 91(2):206–212.

Niu SR, Yang GH, Chen ZM, Wang JL, Wang GH, He XZ, Schoepff H, Boreham J, Pan HC, Peto R. 1998. Emerging tobacco hazards in China: Early mortality results from a prospective study. *BMJ* 317(7170):1423–1424.

Novotny TE, Cohen JC, Yurekli A, Sweaner D, de Beyer J. 2000. Smoking cessation and nicotine-replacement therapies. In: Jha P, Chaloupka F, eds. *Tobacco Control in Developing Countries.* Oxford, England: Oxford University Press.

Pechmann C, Dixon P, Layne N. 1998. An assessment of U.S. and Canadian smoking reduction objectives for the year 2000. *American Journal of Public Health* 88(9):1362–1367.

Peto R, Darby S, Deo H, Silcocks P, Whitley E, Doll R. 2000. Smoking, smoking cessation, and lung cancer in the UK since 1950: Combination of national statistics with two case-control studies. *BMJ* 321(7257):323–329.

Peto R, Lopez A, Boreham J, Thun M. 1994. *Mortality from Smoking in Developed Countries, 1950–2000.* Oxford, England: Oxford University Press.

Peto R, Lopez A, Boreham J, Thun M. 2003. *Mortality from Smoking in Developed Countries.* 2nd ed. Oxford, England: Oxford University Press.

Peto R, Lopez AD. 2002. Future worldwide health effects of current smoking patterns. In: Koop EC, Pearson CE, Schwarz MR, eds. *Critical Issues in Global Health.* New York: Jossey-Bass.

Pollock D. 1996. Forty years on: A war to recognise and win. How the tobacco industry has survived the revelations on smoking and health. *British Medical Bulletin* 52(1):174–182.

Ranson MK, Jha P, Chaloupka FJ, Nguyen SN. 2002. Global and regional estimates of the effectiveness and cost-effectiveness of price increases and other tobacco control policies. *Nicotine & Tobacco Research* 4(3):311–319.

Raw M, McNeill A, West R. 1999. Smoking cessation: Evidence based recommendations for the healthcare system. *BMJ* 318(7177):182–185.

Ross H, Chaloupka FJ, Wakefield M. 2001. *Youth Smoking Uptake Progress: Price and Public Policy Effects.* Research Paper No. 11. Chicago, IL: University of Illinois at Chicago, Health Research and Policy Centers, ImpacTeen.

Saffer H. 2000. Tobacco advertising and promotion. In: Jha P, Chaloupka F, eds. *Tobacco Control in Developing Countries.* Oxford, England: Oxford University Press.

Saffer H, Chaloupka F. 2000. The effect of tobacco advertising bans on tobacco consumption. *Journal of Health Economics* 19(6):1117–1137.

Saxenian H, McGreevey B. 1996. *China: Issues and Options in Health Financing.* World Bank Report No. 15278-CHA. Washington, DC: World Bank.

Sloan FA, Ostermann J, Conover C, Taylor DH Jr., Picone G. 2004. *The Price of Smoking.* Cambridge, MA: MIT Press.

Sunley EM, Yurekli A, Chaloupka FJ. 2000. The design, administration, and potential revenue of tobacco excises. In: Jha P, Chaloupka F, eds. *Tobacco Control in Developing Countries.* Oxford, England: Oxford University Press. Pp. 410–426.

Tauras JA. 1999. *The Transition to Smoking Cessation: Evidence From Multiple Failure Duration Analysis.* NBER Working Paper No. 7412. Cambridge, MA: National Bureau of Economic Research.

Tauras JA, Chaloupka FJ. 2003. The demand for nicotine replacement therapies. *Nicotine & Tobacco Research* 5(2):237–243.

Tauras JA, Chaloupka FJ, Farrelly MC, Giovino GA, Wakefield M, Johnston LD, O'Malley PM, Kloska DD, Pechacek TF. 2005. State tobacco control spending and youth smoking. *American Journal of Public Health* 95(2):338–344.

Taylor CR, and Bonner PG. 2003. Comment on "American media and the smoking-related behavior of Asian adolescents." *Journal of Advertising Research* 43:419–430.

Taylor A, Chaloupka FJ, Guindon E, Corbett M. 2000. The impact of trade liberalization on tobacco consumption. In: Jha P, Chaloupka F, eds. *Tobacco Control in Developing Countries.* Oxford, England: Oxford University Press. Pp. 344–364.

Townsend J. 1993. Policies to halve smoking deaths. *Addiction* 88(1):37–46.

Townsend J, Roderick P, Cooper J. 1994. Cigarette smoking by socioeconomic group, sex, and age: Effects of price, income, and health publicity. *BMJ* 309(6959):923–927.

UK Department of Health. 1992. *Effect of Tobacco Advertising on Tobacco Consumption: A Discussion Document Reviewing the Evidence.* London, England: UK Department of Health, Economics and Operational Research Division.

U.S. DHHS (U.S. Department of Health and Human Services). 1994. *Preventing Tobacco Use Amongst Young People.* A Report of the Surgeon General. Atlanta, GA: U.S. Department of Health and Human Services, Public Health Service, Centers for Disease Control and Prevention, Center for Chronic Disease Prevention and Health Promotion, Office on Smoking and Health.

U.S. DHHS. 2000. *Reducing Tobacco Use.* A Report of the Surgeon General. Atlanta, GA: U.S. Department of Health and Human Services, Public Health Service, Centers for Disease Control and Prevention, Center for Chronic Disease Prevention and Health Promotion, Office on Smoking and Health.

Wasserman J, Manning WG, Newhouse JP, Winkler JD. 1991. The effects of excise taxes and regulations on cigarette smoking. *Journal of Health Economics* 10(1):43–64.

Weinstein ND. 1998. Accuracy of smokers' risk perceptions. *Annals of Behavioral Medicine* 20(2):135–140.

WHO (World Health Organization). 2002. *The European Report on Tobacco Control Policy.* WHO European Ministerial Conference for a Tobacco-Free Europe. Warsaw, Poland. Document EUR/01/5020906/8. Copenhagen, Denmark: WHO Regional Office for Europe.

WHO. 2003. *Framework Convention on Tobacco Control.* [Online] Available: http://www.who.int/tobacco/framework/WHO_FCTC_english.pdf [accessed 1/2/06].

WHO. 2006. *Updated Status of the WHO Framework Convention on Tobacco Control.* [Online]. Available: http://www.who.int/tobacco/framework/countrylist/en/index.html [accessed July 19, 2006].

Woolery T, Asma S, Sharp D. 2000. Clean indoor-air laws and youth access. In: Jha P, Chaloupka F, eds. *Tobacco Control in Developing Countries.* Oxford, England: Oxford University Press.

Zatonski W. 1998. *Evolution of Health in Poland Since 1988.* Warsaw, Poland: Marie Sklodowska-Curie Memorial Cancer Center and Institute of Oncology.

6

Compelling Opportunities in Global Cancer Control

Where cancer control is currently limited and resources are scarce for all health and social expenditures, decisions about expanding services has to be pragmatic and focus on interventions that are guaranteed to provide substantial benefit. Priority setting among the sectors, within the health sector, and within cancer, all require consideration of economic, political, and ethical perspectives, as well as the qualities of equity and fairness. Different countries with similar circumstances may make very different decisions. This stream of priority setting is not a focus of this report, although the report does attempt, through presentation of evidence, to make a strong case for considering the expansion of cancer control in every country. This chapter discusses interventions that would provide such benefit in most, if not all, countries.

In this report, we have seconded the already-strong efforts in tobacco control, for all the reasons discussed in Chapter 5. Palliative care, the subject of Chapter 7, represents a set of services that will benefit large numbers of people at reasonable cost, and will never become obsolete. In this chapter we identify three additional areas of opportunity with the potential to save lives now and in the future and to build capacity in cancer control where it is currently limited. They are:

- Increased coverage with hepatitis B virus (HBV) vaccine to prevent most liver cancer globally
- Cervical cancer prevention through cost-effective screening and treatment, and planning for the expeditious adoption of human papillomavirus

(HPV) vaccine to prevent infection with the viral agents that cause cervical cancer

• Expansion of global capacity to treat the highly curable cancers of children and young adults

HBV vaccines have been available for 20 years and are now inexpensive, but still not being used in areas with some of the highest liver cancer rates. The reasons are detailed in the first section of this chapter. This is the most straightforward and obvious cancer control intervention that requires added support from the global community. One vaccine for HPV just entered the market in 2006 and another is soon to follow. A global consortium has given this intervention high visibility, and it, too, deserves continued support toward implementation. In the meantime, advances in understanding the natural history of cervical cancer have led to approaches to screen for and treat precancerous changes in adult women who will not benefit from vaccines. These approaches have proven feasible in some low- and middle-income countries (LMCs), and should be expanded. The final opportunity is to expand the availability of treatment for highly curable cancers of children and young adults. The number of children with cancer is small, but the lives saved can be long and productive. Of all the interventions described, treating children with cancer will give immediate positive results, demonstrating the curability of cancer.

REDOUBLED EFFORTS TO INCREASE THE UPTAKE OF HEPATITIS B VACCINATION

Liver cancer—hepatocellular carcinoma (HCC)—is the cause of more than 500,000 deaths each year worldwide, making it the third most frequent cause of cancer deaths in LMCs. It is currently the most preventable cancer caused by an infectious agent, chronic infection with HBV. Chronic HBV also causes significant numbers of deaths from liver cirrhosis and liver failure (Lavanchy, 2004), and an estimated 40,000 worldwide die from acute hepatitis infection (Goldstein et al., 2005). The prevalence of HBV varies widely among regions. About 45 percent of the world's population lives where HBV prevalence is high, with the highest endemicity being in Asia, sub-Saharan Africa, and the Pacific. Other areas where infection rates are high include the southern parts of Eastern and Central Europe, the Amazon basin, the Middle East, and the Indian subcontinent. About 350 million chronic carriers are alive today, of whom 15 to 40 percent will die as a result of HBV, many in middle age. HBV is the 10th leading cause of death worldwide, and HCC is the 5th leading cause of cancer deaths, of which about 80 percent occur in developing countries (Lavanchy, 2004).

Infection with HBV and Other Hepatitis Viruses

Viral hepatitis—an inflammation of the liver—can be caused by at least six mostly unrelated viruses in humans. Some cause only acute disease (e.g., hepatitis A) and others, like HBV, can cause acute and chronic disease (although an acute phase is not a prerequisite for chronic infection). HBV is the predominant cause of chronic infection and chronic liver disease in the world, but the hepatitis C virus (HCV) is also responsible for one-quarter or more cases. HBV, because of its importance and the existence of an effective vaccine, is the focus of the remainder of this section. HCV vaccine development is ongoing and, if successful, would provide a way to prevent another part of the liver cancer burden.

Where HBV is widespread, babies may be infected perinatally by their mothers in the period shortly before and after birth, or during early childhood from contact with other children. Where HBV is less prevalent, more new infections occur among adults, from needle sharing among infected individuals, unprotected sexual contact with an infected person, and blood transfusions of infected blood. HBV is highly infectious and robust, and can survive outside the body.

Acute clinical hepatitis may or may not develop at the time of HBV infection. Few babies (about 1 percent of those infected perinatally) develop acute disease, but it becomes more common at older ages (about 30 percent of new infections). Regardless of the development of clinically apparent disease, people who clear their infections become immune for life. However, the earlier the infection occurs, the more likely it is to become chronic. As many as 90 percent of babies infected perinatally, and 30 percent of children infected before age 5, become chronically infected carriers, while the same is true of only about 6 percent of those infected as adults.

The Role of Co-Carcinogens in the Development of HCC

People with chronic HBV infection are at much higher risk of HCC when they are also exposed to a co-carcinogen that is synergistic with the virus. The most widespread known co-carcinogens are "aflatoxins," which are chemicals produced by a genus of fungus (*Aspergillus*) that grows on many types of stored grains and other foods. Groundnuts (peanuts) and corn, dietary staples for millions of people, are particularly susceptible. People with exposures to both HBV and certain common aflatoxins have about a 60-fold increased risk of HCC compared with exposure to neither (Kensler et al., 2003). Other mycotoxins (products of other fungi) contaminate stored foods, mainly in developing countries with hot, humid climates. Up to one-quarter of the world's food supply may be contaminated with mycotoxins (Turner et al., 2002). Aflatoxin contamination can be reduced by low technology techniques such as drying crops in the sun, discarding moldy kernels before storing, and storing in natural fiber sacks on wooden pallets. Such efforts may be worthwhile, although they are more complex and difficult to achieve than vaccination (Hall and Wild, 2003).

The relationship of HBV, aflatoxins, and HCC is probably the best studied example of a virus–chemical interaction acting synergistically to vastly increase the risk of a cancer. The relationships have been established definitively in epidemiologic studies and in animal models. Both HBV and exposure to aflatoxin (through ingesting contaminated food) are detectable in blood samples, a factor that has added to the ability to study their relationship to HCC and other liver diseases (Turner et al., 2002).

Preventing Deaths from Hepatocellular Carcinoma (and Other HBV-Related Liver Diseases)

If new HBV infections could be prevented, most deaths from HCC and other HBV-related liver diseases would be avoided. Of the 350 million living HBV carriers, some proportion of deaths could also be avoided by modifying exposure to co-carcinogens. There are also treatments for chronic HBV, but they are expensive, toxic, and only partially effective. The intervention with the greatest potential for controlling HBV-related cancer and other deaths is HBV vaccination. For people already infected, reducing exposure to aflatoxin or modifying its effect through diet and reducing excessive alcohol consumption can help.

HBV Vaccination

An HBV vaccine suitable for widespread public use has been available for more than 20 years. Currently, both a plasma-derived and a recombinant DNA vaccine are available for \$0.25–.50 per dose (\$0.75–1.50 for the series). The three-dose series of HBV vaccine is 90 to 95 percent efficacious in preventing infection (Centers for Disease Control and Prevention, 2003). The first nationwide vaccination program began in Taiwan in 1984. It was a phased program that first vaccinated babies of carrier mothers, then all newborns, then unvaccinated preschool and elementary children. Since 1991, catch-up vaccinations have been given to unvaccinated children in first grade. Overall HBV prevalence (as measured by hepatitis B surface antigen, or HBsAg, in blood) declined from about 10 percent in 1984 to less than 1 percent in 1999 (Lavanchy, 2004). Similar declines where chronic infection rates were historically high have been documented in the Gambia, China, Indonesia, Senegal, Thailand, and among Alaska natives.

Strategies for vaccine use and vaccination schedules may vary by HBV endemicity levels (Table 6-1). The higher the prevalence, the higher the perinatal transmission; this means that giving a first dose within 24 hours

TABLE 6-1 Preferred Strategies Based on Economic Evaluation, According to the Level of Chronic Hepatitis B Endemicity

Level of Endemicity	Preferred Strategy Based on Recent Economic Evaluations[a]	Cost Saving to the Health Care Sector[a]	Cost Saving to Society[a]
High	Universal neonatal vaccination	ND[b]	Yes
Intermediate	Universal neonatal, infant, or adolescent vaccination[c]	No	Yes
Low	Universal adolescent or infant vaccination[c]	No	Yes
Very low	Selective risk group[d]	No	ND

ND = not determined.

[a]Generalizations, based on baseline calculations of recent evaluations.
[b]Dependent on the level of available treatment.
[c]Dependent on local economic and epidemiologic situation and efficiency of vaccine delivery system.
[d]Most likely more cost-effective than universal vaccination, provided coverage in risk groups is sufficiently high.

SOURCE: Reprinted, with permission, from Beutels (2001). Copyright 2001 by John Wiley & Sons Limited.

of birth is most important in high-prevalence areas. Other doses can coincide with regular childhood vaccine schedules. Where transmission is less intense, all three doses can be given along with the other routine childhood vaccines. The United States, a low-endemicity country, adopted universal infant vaccination in 1991, supplemented with targeted vaccinations for older children and adults at highest risk of infection. The recommendations have been revised over time toward ever greater coverage, with the aim of eliminating HBV transmission entirely.

Cost-Effectiveness of Hepatitis B Immunization

Hepatitis B immunization has been the subject of many economic evaluations, nearly all in industrialized countries. These countries also tend to have relatively low prevalence of HBV, with relatively little perinatal or early childhood transmission, but the availability of hepatitis B vaccines has meant that policy makers have had to make active decisions about what should be recommended. A comprehensive review of studies published worldwide between 1994 and 2000 identified 16 cost-effectiveness analyses, 4 cost-benefit analyses, and 3 combined cost-effectiveness and cost-benefit analyses. Among these were only one study in a middle-income country,

Romania, and one in a low-income country, China. Romania is categorized as "intermediate endemicity" and China, "high endemicity."

The Romanian analysis was carried out from two perspectives: the health care payer only, and society as a whole. The main analysis used a relatively high discount rate, 7 percent. In a country like Romania—similar to other middle-income countries and certainly all low-income countries—there is little potential to "save" health care costs because virtually no treatment is offered for either the acute or chronic effects of hepatitis B. Not surprisingly, the Romanian analysis found that the vaccination program was not cost saving to the health care system. It was very sensitive to the discount rate, however. At discount rates lower than 4 percent, universal infant immunization would be cost saving for the health care system, and at rates lower than 6.3 percent, it would be cost saving to society.

How Many Deaths Could Be Prevented with HBV Vaccination?

Using information on infection rates by age, Goldstein and colleagues (Goldstein et al., 2005) developed a relatively simple model to estimate HBV infection rates and mortality from both acute and chronic disease, and the effect that HBV vaccination would have on these outcomes. The model is electronically accessible and is set up to produce estimates for individual countries (Centers for Disease Control and Prevention, 2003).

The model In the model, infection was assumed to occur in one of three age periods: perinatal (at birth); early childhood (after birth through 5 years); and late (>5 years). Deaths from cirrhosis and HCC deaths among chronic HBV carriers were presumed to be HBV related, and were estimated from age-specific, HBV-related cirrhosis and HCC mortality curves, adjusted for background mortality.

A complete HBV vaccination series (≥3 doses of hepatitis B vaccine, including the first dose within 24 hours of birth) was estimated to be 95 percent effective in preventing perinatal HBV infection (postexposure immunization) and early childhood and late infection (preexposure immunization), and was assumed to provide lifelong protection. Where the first dose was given more than 24 hours after birth, infants were considered susceptible to perinatal infection, but protected from early childhood and late infection. Values were varied in several sensitivity analyses. The central estimates are discussed here.

Calculations using the model Results based on the 2000 birth cohort were calculated. With complete global immunization, including a birth dose, it should be possible to prevent 95 percent of all HBV-related deaths. Without a birth dose, the estimate is 75 percent of HBV-related deaths prevented.

With coverage increasing from 50 to 80 to 90 percent, the proportion of deaths prevented increased from 38 to 60 to 68 percent. With 90 percent complete vaccine series coverage, administration of a birth dose to 50 percent and 90 percent of the vaccinated birth cohort increased the proportion of deaths prevented to 77 percent and 84 percent, respectively.

This is basically a static model looking at a single birth cohort. As immunization rates rise and prevalence falls, the effect of vaccination will be greater in later cohorts.

Results by World Health Organization (WHO) region (Table 6-2) show the greatest potential gains in the Western Pacific, Southeast Asia, and Africa. At the highest coverage, including a birth dose, more than 1 million premature deaths of the 2000 birth cohort could be prevented. Most of these would be deaths from HCC.

Global Vaccine Coverage

As the price of HBV vaccine declined, universal vaccination became a realistic goal. In 1992, WHO recommended that all countries with a high hepatitis B disease burden introduce HBV vaccine into their routine immunization programs by 1995, and that all countries do so by 1997. These targets were not met, however. The greatest shortfalls were in the poorest countries, most of which have high HBV burdens. Before 2000, only seven

TABLE 6-2 Reduction in Future Hepatitis B-Related Deaths: Hepatitis B Disease Burden Model

WHO Region	Number of Deaths in 2000 Birth Cohort without Vaccination	Proportional Reduction in Deaths with Three Doses of Hepatitis B Vaccine: No Birth Dose	50% Birth Dose[a]	90% Birth Dose[a]
Africa	276,000	70%	78%	84%
Americas	28,000	66%	76%	84%
Eastern Mediterranean	96,000	74%	80%	84%
Europe	56,000	72%	79%	84%
Southeast Asia	368,000	71%	78%	84%
Western Pacific	581,000	63%	74%	83%
Global	*1,405,000*	*68%*	*77%*	*84%*

[a]Proportion of the vaccinated cohort receiving the first dose of vaccine within 24 hours of birth.

SOURCE: Reprinted, with permission, from Goldstein et al. (2005). Copyright 2005 by the International Epidemiological Association.

BOX 6-1
The Global Alliance for Vaccines and Immunization and the Vaccine Fund

The Global Alliance for Vaccines and Immunization (GAVI) was established in 2000 with the goal of increasing immunization rates in the poorest countries and reversing widening global disparities in access to vaccines. Countries with gross national income (GNI) levels below $1,000 are eligible for assistance from GAVI through the associated Vaccine Fund. GAVI partners include governments in industrialized and developing countries, UNICEF, the World Health Organization, the World Bank, nongovernmental organizations, foundations, vaccine manufacturers, and public health and research institutions. The Vaccine Fund has been financed by the Bill & Melinda Gates Foundation and by 10 governments to date—Canada, Denmark, France, Ireland, Luxembourg, the Netherlands, Norway, Sweden, the United Kingdom, and the United States—as well as the European Union and private contributors.

Countries eligible on the basis of GNI must submit proposals to GAVI for Vaccine Fund support. Proposals are reviewed by a panel of experts from around the world. Currently, The Vaccine Fund offers the following support to qualifying governments:

- New and underused vaccines, currently hepatitis B virus (HBV), Hib, and yellow fever;
- Funding to help governments strengthen their basic immunization services; and
- Safe injection equipment in the form of auto-disable syringes and safe disposal boxes.

As of December 2003, more than 42 million children had been vaccinated with GAVI-supported HBV vaccine.

(less than 10%) of the poorest countries were using HBV vaccine in their routine immunization programs. When the Global Alliance for Vaccines and Immunization (GAVI) (Box 6-1) was established in 2000, HBV vaccine was one of the underused vaccines in its portfolio. The GAVI partners set a new milestone, which is for HBV vaccine to be introduced in all countries with adequate delivery systems by 2007.

Childhood HBV vaccination has now been adopted by many countries, but there is still a wide gap between rich and poor countries. In 2001, 137 of 191 WHO Member States had universal infant or childhood HBV vaccination programs. An estimated 32 percent of infants were fully vaccinated, with a range of 65 percent in the Western Pacific, to 58 percent in the Americas, to less than 10 percent in Southeast Asia and Africa. By May 2003, the number of countries with a universal childhood HBV vaccination policy had risen to 151, but that included only about half (24 out of 46) of the African countries (Centers for Disease Control and Prevention, 2003). Eighty-nine WHO Member States have historically high HBV prevalence (HBsAg $\geq$ 8%), where infant vaccination is of particular importance. Of these, 64 have adopted universal infant vaccination, and of these, 34 have a policy to administer the first dose at birth, which is the best way to prevent perinatal transmission.

Fifty of the more than 70 countries eligible for support from the Vaccine Fund, the financing arm of GAVI, had approval for HBV vaccine funding as of December 2004 (although implementation varies). Coverage of at least 50 percent for the basic infant vaccines (three doses of DTP: diphtheria, tetanus, polio) is required before a country can request support for HBV vaccine. For countries with less than 50 percent DTP3 coverage, GAVI offers assistance to improve the immunization infrastructure and boost basic coverage.

The Vaccine Fund will cover the purchase of hepatitis B vaccine and safe injection equipment for 5 years, together with a single payment of $100,000 to facilitate the introduction of the new vaccine. GAVI will then work with countries to develop a financial sustainability plan to ensure continued financing for hepatitis B vaccine once Vaccine Fund support ends.

Can More Be Done to Increase HBV Vaccine Coverage?

The global community can continue to encourage countries to include HBV vaccination with their childhood immunization programs, and particularly in high-prevalence countries, to start with a birth dose. Both a financing mechanism (at least in the short term) and technical assistance are on offer from GAVI and the Vaccine Fund. If some countries have been reluctant to request funds to begin because of the longer term cost, GAVI could extend financing for a longer period (as they are doing with the Hib vaccine in some places). Overall, further gains will depend on improving the vaccination infrastructure and implementation, both of which are likely to be slow processes in the countries that are already lagging. With poor coverage of even the standard childhood vaccines, HBV will not be the main driver for improvement.

REDUCING THE TOLL OF CERVICAL CANCER IN LMCS

Nearly half a million women around the world develop cervical cancer each year and 270,000 die from it. More than 80 percent of the cases and

TABLE 6-3 Incidence and Mortality from Cervical Cancer by Income Group of Countries

Country Income Group	Cases Per Year	Deaths Per Year
High income	54,000	22,000
Upper middle income	37,000	17,000
Lower middle income	161,000	87,000
Low income	238,000	147,000
World	***490,000***	***273,000***

SOURCE: Barton et al. (2005).

a slightly higher percentage of the deaths are women in LMCs (Table 6-3) (IARC, 2004). The burden of disease is highest in Africa, Latin America, and South and Southeast Asia.

Virtually all cases of cervical cancer are caused by persistent infection with certain oncogenic strains of HPV, a very common sexually transmitted virus. For most women initially infected with HPV, the infection clears with no intervention; these women are no longer at risk for cervical cancer. For those who remain infected, cervical cancer can develop through a long—usually decades-long—process of cellular change. Even before the details of this progression were understood completely, most cervical cancer in high-income countries was being prevented by frequent screening for abnormal (but not yet cancerous) cells on the surface of the cervix, which can be removed using relatively simple, minimally invasive procedures.

The more detailed understanding of how cervical cancer develops, and the role of HPV, has led to new screening and treatment approaches, as well as the development of vaccines to protect against HPV infection, one of which just entered the market in 2006. These new approaches, still relatively early in development, are discussed later in this section.

Cervical Cancer and HPV

The epidemiologic study of cervical cancer dates to the 18th century and Bernardino Ramazzini's observation that "cancer of the womb" was uncommon among Catholic nuns, but common among married women (American Cancer Society, 2005). A link with sexual activity was long suspected, eventually leading to the discovery that cervical cancer is caused by a sexually transmitted infection.

It is now understood that 90 percent of women infected with HPV will clear their infections within a few years. HPV infection will persist in the remaining 10 percent, who make up the population at risk of cervical

TABLE 6-4 Distribution of HPV Types in Invasive Cervical Cancer in All Studies

HPV Type	Estimated Number of Cases Observed	Percentage of All Cases Observed	Percentage of Cases (cumulative)
16	251,200	53.5	53.5
18	80,900	17.2	70.7
45	31,600	6.7	77.4
31	13,700	2.9	80.3
33	12,100	2.6	82.9
52	11,000	2.3	85.2
58	10,000	2.2	87.4
35	6,600	1.4	88.8
59	6,100	1.3	90.1
56	5,800	1.2	91.3
51	4,600	1.0	92.3
39	3,200	0.7	93.0
68	2,700	0.6	93.6

SOURCE: Adapted from Munoz et al. (2004).

cancer (Bosch and Muñoz, 2002). A vast body of evidence supports this understanding and is now fully accepted.

To summarize, studies worldwide have consistently found HPV in 95 to 100 percent of cervical cancer cells, and in virtually all cases of cervical intraepithelial neoplasia (CIN) (Bosch et al., 2002). More than 90 percent of cervical cancers have the same 10 to 15 types of HPV (Table 6-4) (Bosch et al., 1995), and metastases contain the same types as in primary sites (Lancaster et al., 1986). Morphological changes in oncogenic HPV studied in cells in the laboratory (in vitro) closely resemble the changes seen during the progression from normal to cancerous tissue in women (Meyers and Laimins, 1994; Steenbergen et al., 1996). In cervical lesions, the HPV viral genome is always active, increasing in viral numbers as the lesion increases in severity (Stoler et al., 1992). In 1995, the International Agency for Research on Cancer (IARC) categorized HPV (types 16 and 18; see below) as "carcinogenic to humans" ("Group 1"), which denotes IARC's highest level of evidence for a causal association (IARC, 1995).

Transmission of HPV

HPV is transmitted almost entirely through sexual intercourse. The risk of acquiring HPV increases with the number of sexual partners and with early age at first sexual activity (IARC Working Group, 2005). A history of sexually transmitted infections (STIs) of women and their partners, male circumcision, and the presence of penile HPV have also been shown to be significant risk factors in acquiring HPV (Bosch et al., 1994; Juarez-Figueroa et al., 2001; Kjaer et al., 1991; Palacio et al., 1993; Thomas et al., 2001b, cited by IARC Working Group, 2005). The natural history and persistence of HPV in men has not been well documented; however, a 4-year National Institutes of Health-funded study with that goal is under way, with results expected in 2008.

HPV Types and Their Association with Cervical Cancer

Only a handful of the 100 known types of human papillomaviruses are associated with a high risk of cervical cancer (IARC Working Group, 2005). Types 16 and 18 have accounted for 70 percent of cervical cancer cases in studies around the world (Table 6-4). Thirteen high-risk carcinogenic HPV types account for almost 95 percent of all cases studied (Muñoz et al., 2004, cited by IARC Working Group, 2005).

Once a firm causal link was drawn between HPV and cervical cancer, it became clear that many of the risk factors observed for cervical cancer—such as the number of sexual partners and age at first intercourse—were actually the risk factors for acquiring HPV. It was also recognized that certain factors might, in the presence of HPV infection, increase the chances of cancer developing, and this has been borne out by studies of infection and these risk factors. Cigarette smoking raises the risk of cervical cancer two- to three-fold among HPV-positive women (IARC Working Group, 2005; Plummer et al., 2003; Szarewski and Cuzick, 1998). HPV infections are maintained significantly longer and are less likely to clear in smokers compared to nonsmokers (Giuliano et al., 2002, cited by IARC Working Group, 2005).

Both *Herpes simplex* virus type 2 (HSV2) and the bacterium *Chlamydia trachomatis*, two common STIs, both may enhance the oncogenic potential of HPV (IARC Working Group, 2005). HIV infection appears to potentiate the risk of cervical cancer among HPV-positive women, and invasive cervical cancer is an AIDS-defining illness. Women infected with HIV are more likely to be infected with oncogenic types of HPV and have higher rates of progression to cervical dysplasia than those without HIV (IARC Working Group, 2005; Massad et al., 1999; Thomas et al., 2001b).

The number of pregnancies a woman has had may also increase the risk of cervical cancer. The risk among HPV-positive women rises with the number of full term pregnancies, reportedly as much as four times higher with seven or more full-term pregnancies, compared with no children (IARC Working Group, 2005).

The evidence linking oral contraceptives (OCs) to cervical cancer in HPV-positive women is inconclusive. Several studies have found weak to no associations (Kruger-Kjaer et al., 1998; Lacey et al., 1999; Thomas et al.,

2001a), and others have found strong associations with long-term OC use (Bosch et al., 2002; Castellsague and Munoz, 2003; Moreno et al., 2002; Smith et al., 2003). Studies of this topic continue (Bosch et al., 2002; IARC Working Group, 2005; Smith et al., 2003).

Natural History of HPV and Cervical Cancer

In 1908, Schanenstein proposed the idea that invasive cervical cancer develops only after progressing through preinvasive lesions (Chirenje, 2004). Two decades later, Papanicolaou and Babes introduced a method to examine cells from the surface of the cervix (the Papanicolaou, or "Pap," smear) to identify women with early-stage invasive cancer, with the aim of providing curative treatment. They recognized the long period during which preinvasive lesions could exist, and that they regressed in many women. This meant that women could be treated while the condition was still in a preinvasive lesion stage, preventing the development of cervical cancer.

As now understand, the progression toward cervical cancer begins with prolonged HPV infection, i.e., an HPV infection that is not eliminated by an immune response. After HPV clearance, infections have rarely been detected during the follow-up period in cohort studies, suggesting that immunity is acquired against reinfection with the same HPV type (Shah et al., 1997, cited by IARC Working Group, 2005). However, this evidence is incomplete and the question continues to be studied (IARC Working Group, 2005).

HPV Transience

Average levels of HPV prevalence vary and several distinct patterns of age-specific prevalence have been found in different areas of the world. In many areas, including most high-income countries (but also including some LMCs), HPV prevalence declines sharply after 30 years of age (Molano et al., 2002; Pham et al., 2003; Ronco et al., 2005). In other areas, prevalence is more constant across age groups (Shin et al., 2003; Thomas et al., 2004; Pham et al., 2003). In at least one place (Shania Province, China), prevalence was low in young women and rose with age (Dai et al., 2006). Repeated sampling of younger women in follow-up studies where prevalence declines with age has shown a median duration of transient HPV infection of 8 months for high-risk types, and 4.8 months for low-risk types. Approximately 90 percent of infections are eliminated within about 2 years (IARC Working Group, 2005). Of the remaining 10 percent of women with persistent infection with a high-risk type of HPV, some will develop abnormal cervical cells, most of which will revert to normal. A small percentage will progress to advanced-stage cervical neoplasia and cancer (Bosch et al., 2002; IARC Working Group, 2005).

TABLE 6-5 International Federation of Gynecology and Obstetrics Staging for Cervical Cancers

Stage	Description
Stage 0	Carcinoma in situ, preinvasive carcinoma (advanced CIN 3)
Stage I	Invasive carcinoma strictly confined to cervix
Stage II	Carcinoma extending beyond cervix but not to pelvic sidewall; carcinoma involves vagina, but not lower third
Stage III	Carcinoma extending onto pelvic wall; tumor involves lower third of vagina
Stage IV	Carcinoma extends beyond true pelvis or clinically involves mucosa of bladder or rectum

SOURCE: IARC Working Group on the Evaluation of Cancer Preventive Strategies (2005).

Stages of Cervical Dysplasia and Cancer

Several classification systems are used to describe the stages of cervical changes leading to cervical cancer. *Cervical intraepithelial neoplasia 1 (CIN 1)*, also known as low-grade squamous intraepithelial lesion (LSIL) and mild dysplasia, tends to be benign and transient, and detected as borderline or mild cytological abnormalities (IARC Working Group, 2005). *CIN 2*, known also as high-grade squamous intraepithelial lesion (HSIL) and moderate dysplasia, represents a true premalignant lesion (Schiffman and Brinton, 1995), usually associated with high-risk HPV types. *CIN 3* is also known as severe dysplasia, carcinoma in situ, and HSIL. CIN 3 lesions are virtually always associated with high-risk HPV types. CIN 3 is considered Stage 0 in the commonly accepted cervical cancer staging system (Table 6-5) and lasts an average of 5 to 11 years (IARC Working Group, 2005). About half of women with CIN 3 lesions will progress to invasive cervical cancer if not treated (<1 percent of all original HPV infections) (IARC Working Group, 2005).

Stage I invasive cervical cancer has several phases, depending on the rate of growth of the lesion(s), but are small (less than 5 mm) with minimal invasion. Cervical cancer at this stage is highly curable. Stage II is considered advanced cervical cancer, with extension of the carcinoma beyond the cervix to the pelvic wall but not beyond. Stage III carcinoma extends into the lower vagina. Stage IV carcinoma involves the spread of cancer to adjacent organs, including the bladder and rectum.

Intervening to Prevent Cervical Cancer

The important message from the current understanding of the natural history of cervical cancer is this: Cervical cancer is the end stage of a series of cellular changes that occur over a period of decades (usually), in the presence of specific strains of HPV. Eliminating the HPV and the altered cells when they are still precancerous through one of a few relatively simple procedures stops the progression to cancer. At every stage, however, only a portion of women testing positive (i.e., with cellular changes or HPV present) would eventually develop cervical cancer. This means that the earlier in the course of progression treatment is given, the greater the number of women treated who would never have developed cancer, but also the simpler the treatment and the higher the success rate.

The challenges in designing prevention programs are in selecting the most appropriate detection and treatment methods and defining the target population in terms of age at screening, as well as screening intervals. The opportunities for doing this today are unprecedented because of the more complete scientific knowledge about the development of cervical cancer and because the newer methods have been studied systematically, alongside the older ones. Data are still emerging from a variety of studies, which means that not all questions can be answered immediately, but substantial information is available already.

Methods for Detecting Cervical Precancer and Cancer and Providing Treatment

Three basic methods are used to detect precancerous (or cancerous) cellular changes. The Pap smear and related laboratory examination of cells (cytology) is the oldest and the current standard in high-income countries. The second approach is some form of direct visualization, in which the examiner looks directly at the cervix with the naked eye (or with magnification) to search for patches of abnormal cells, which have been made evident by the use of a chemical, either dilute acetic acid or iodine. The third approach is to test for the presence of HPV through DNA testing.

Treatment of all precancerous stages of cervical cancer involves either excision (cutting out) or ablation (destruction in place) of suspect lesions. The most frequent excision technique is loop electrosurgical excision procedure (LEEP), which uses an electrified wire to excise the abnormal area. A skilled provider is needed, as is a reliable electrical supply. The excised tissue can be evaluated for a specific diagnosis, where laboratory services are available. The most commonly used ablative procedure is cryotherapy, which involves freezing the areas that appear abnormal using compressed carbon dioxide or nitrous oxide as the refrigerant. A wide range of health workers can be trained in cryotherapy. Because the tissue is destroyed, it cannot be further analyzed.

The detection test that is used dictates certain aspects of follow-up and treatment, including the number of visits needed and the technologies used. A Pap smear traditionally requires a minimum of three visits for a positive test. The first is for the sample to be taken during a pelvic examination. If the

Pap smear is read in the laboratory as positive, colposcopy will be carried out during a second visit. This involves a direct examination at the cervix with magnification, with and without acetic acid, during which biopsies are taken of abnormal areas. If the biopsied material is positive, treatment to eliminate the abnormality is provided at a third visit.

With direct visualization, detection and treatment can be carried out in a single visit, or in two visits. In the single-visit approach, if the examiner finds a lesion, it can be treated immediately with cryotherapy, or that can be carried out at a second visit (possibly at a different site). HPV testing requires two visits because samples must be processed in specialized laboratories. Women with positive tests are called back and a direct visualization procedure of some sort is used to localize the lesion, which is then treated.

These variations—the numbers of visits, the types of procedures, and infrastructure and personnel needs—take on greater significance in resource-poor settings. Each major screening approach is described briefly in the next sections.

Pap Smear and Cervical Cytology

"Conventional cervical cytology"[1] is the process of collecting cell specimens from two areas of the cervix: the transformation zone, using a specially shaped wooden or plastic spatula; and the endocervix (endocervical canal), using a conical cervical brush. The cells are then spread onto a glass slide and stained for examination under the microscope.

Liquid-based cytology (LBC), a more expensive process, was introduced in the 1990s to improve test performance. Following conventional cytology methods to the point of cell transfer, LBC allows the cells to be transferred to a liquid preservative for transport to the laboratory, where a slide is then prepared for microscopic reading. Both of these methods are largely automated. Results are classified according to one of several systems to distinguish the different stages of dysplasia and cancer, described above. A laboratory is required for cytology, including internal and external quality controls, for processing slides and microscopy. These systems include continuous monitoring of recordkeeping, review of abnormal cases by a cytopathologist, and review of negative cases by rapid rescreening of all cases or a percentage of randomly chosen samples, with correlation of cytological and histological results when possible, as well as proficiency programs (IARC Working Group, 2005).

---

[1]Conventional cytology is the most widely used cervical cytological method. For purposes of clarity in this report, whenever Pap smear or cytology is used, it is referring to conventional cytology. Liquid-based cytology, including ThinPrep and other brands, will be referred to specifically by name.

Visual Inspection with Acetic Acid or Lugol's Iodine

Before the advent of the Pap smear and routine cytology-based screening in the 1950s, direct visualization of the cervix with the naked eye and no enhancement was used to detect precancerous lesions (Ferreccio and Gage, 2003). When it became clear that the Pap smear and cytology was better for this purpose, direct visualization was largely abandoned (Sehgal et al., 1991). The application of an agent—acetic acid or iodine—to the cervix, however, greatly improves detection with direct visual inspection (DVI), also known as cervicoscopy, and aided visual inspection (WHO, 2002). The immediate excision of areas of abnormal cells, using cryotherapy or LEEP, allows screening and treatment in a single visit.

With visual inspection of any kind, results are interpreted solely by the screener based on what is seen during the examination; no permanent record exists to verify or review interpretations (except in study situations, where photographs may be taken). Accurate interpretation with either technique requires training and experience.

Visual inspection with acetic acid (VIA) In VIA dilute acetic acid (vinegar) is applied to the cervix. The acetic acid causes areas of CIN to glow white temporarily, an effect called acetowhitening (Ferreccio and Gage, 2003). No laboratory processing is required and results are immediate (ACCP, 2004). VIA has been used as both a triage method for colposcopy and as a primary screening method (IARC Working Group, 2005).

A study published in 1982 laid the groundwork for further development of VIA. In the study, 2,400 women were examined both with colposcopy and VIA. Using colposcopy as the gold standard, VIA had a high sensitivity and specificity (i.e., it correctly categorized most women either positively or negatively). With colposcopy, 312 patients were identified as having abnormalities; 98 percent were identified similarly with VIA. Of the 1,584 women diagnosed as normal by colposcopy, 99 percent were also normal by VIA (Ottaviano and La Torre, 1982, cited by Ferreccio and Gage, 2003).

In most studies of VIA, nurses or nurse-midwives have conducted the screening, although in one study (Sankaranarayanan et al., 1998), assessments were made by cytotechnicians, and in two studies (Ottaviano and La Torre, 1982; Slawson et al., 1992), the screeners were physicians. Paramedical workers, such as traditional birth attendants and community health workers, also can be trained in VIA techniques (Ferreccio and Gage, 2003).

Visual inspection with Lugol's iodine (VILI) Application of iodine solution to the normal cervix results in dark staining of mature squamous epithelium, which has a high glycogen content. Areas of neoplasia contain very little glycogen and do not stain, instead taking on a bright mustard or saffron yellow color. Although described as early as 1933 by Schiller ("Schiller's iodine test"), VILI fell into disuse as the Pap smear and cytology became standard (IARC Working Group, 2005). Interest has recently been renewed, although it has not yet been studied as extensively as has VIA.

Screening for HPV

Research on HPV DNA assays as a cervical cancer screening tool began in the late 1980s (IARC Working Group, 2005). "Hybrid Capture" nucleic acid hybridization (HC) and polymerase chain reaction (PCR) methods have been used to detect HPV DNA in screening studies over the past decade. Currently, the most commonly used commercial test includes 13 high-risk HPV types and is approved by the U.S. Food and Drug Administration (FDA) (Sankaranarayanan et al., 2005). The assay indicates that an included type is present, but does not identify the specific type. The sample to be tested is collected in much the same way as a liquid-based Pap smear sample, with cells stored in specimen transport medium (STM). Specimens in STM can be stored at room temperature for up to 2 weeks, for an additional week at 4°C, and up to 3 months at –20°C (IARC Working Group, 2005).

Accuracy and Reliability of the Screening Methods

How well do these methods work as primary screening tests? The question is more complex than simply asking whether a particular lesion is detected by a single test. It involves the natural history of the disease, including how strongly the endpoint being measured predicts eventual cancer without intervention, and the likelihood that cancer will occur in the absence of the endpoint the test is designed to detect. These, in turn, are influenced by the age of the person being screened and other individual factors. The outcome also depends on the quality of the service, and the competence of the practitioners involved.

Pap Smears and Cytology

The accuracy of Pap smears and cytology based on recent work was reviewed in 2005 (IARC Working Group, 2005) and is summarized in Table 6-6. The studies varied in design, particularly the proportion of negative tests that were verified, ranging from verification of all negative tests to verification of a sample of variable size. For a screening method that is used so widely, little evaluative information is available. This can be explained by the fact that the tests evolved and came into use before the type of evaluation

TABLE 6-6 Performance of Cervical Cytology in Various Large Research Studies

Year	Country	Age Range	Study Size	Sensitivity[a] (percentage)	Specificity[b] (percentage)	Histological Cut-off
1999	United Kingdom	34+	2,988	86	98	CIN 2+
1999	Costa Rica	18+	8,636	55	98	CIN 2+
2000	Canada	18–69	2,098	56	62	CIN 2+
2000*	South Africa	35–65	2,944	70	85	CIN 2+
2002*	South Africa	35–65	2,754	40	96	CIN 1+
2003	United Kingdom	30–60	11,085	77	96	CIN 1+
2003	Germany	30+	8,466	44	98	CIN 2+
2003	Mexico	15–85	7,868	59	98	CIN 1+
2004	India	25–65	10,591	65	92	CIN 2+

NOTE: Threshold for referral was ASCUS cytology except the South Africa studies (*), where it was LSIL.

[a]Sensitivity is defined as the proportion of truly diseased persons, as measured by the gold standard, who are identified as diseased by the test under study. It is calculated by this formula: True Positives/(True Positives + False Negatives).

[b]Specificity is the proportion of truly nondiseased persons, as measured by the gold standard, who are so identified by the diagnostic test under study. It is calculated by this formula: True Negatives/(False Positives + True Negatives).

SOURCE: Adapted from IARC Working Group on the Evaluation of Cancer Preventive Strategies (2005).

expected today was routine, and at a much earlier stage in the understanding of cervical cancer.

Results vary from a sensitivity of 40 percent to 86 percent. Several large meta-analyses have indicated that cytology sensitivity and specificity are lower than previously thought (Fahey et al., 1995; McCrory et al., 1999; Nanda et al., 2000, cited by IARC Working Group, 2005). However, a reevaluation of these meta-analyses concluded that sensitivities as low as 60–70 percent were unlikely in a modern cytological screening practice (IARC Working Group, 2005).

A critical factor for the lack of success or suboptimal performance of cytology-based screening in less developed countries is poor quality of testing. Test performance of cytology in routine conditions in many laboratories is likely to be inferior to that observed under study conditions.

Visual Inspection (VIA and VILI)

Visual inspection methods have had similar or better sensitivity than cytology for detecting CIN 2 or 3 or invasive cancer in most studies, but specificity in most studies is lower than cytology (Table 6-7) (Ferreccio and Gage, 2003; IARC Working Group, 2005). This means that a greater proportion of abnormalities are detected correctly, but that many women without abnormalities are identified as having them.

The sensitivity of VIA to detect high-grade precancerous lesions and invasive cervical cancer varied widely, from 29 to 95 percent, and specificity varied from 68 to 98 percent (IARC Working Group, 2005).

VILI has been tested in fewer studies than VIA, but they suggest a possibly improved sensitivity over VIA. In a review of cross-sectional studies involving 49,080 women aged 25–65 years in several African nations and India (Sankaranarayanan et al., 2004b), the sensitivity of VILI was 92 percent and of VIA, 77 percent for CIN 2 or 3 lesions. Specificity was about 85 percent for both techniques.

TABLE 6-7 A Comparison of VIA and Cytology Accuracy in Published Studies

		Positivity Rate (percentage)[a]		Sensitivity (percentage)		Specificity (percentage)	
Location, Year	Sample Size	VIA	Cytology	VIA	Cytology	VIA	Cytology
United States, 1992	2,690	3	6	29	87	97	95
Italy, 1993	2,036	25	4	88	63	75	96
South Africa, 1996	2,426	3	13	65	100	98	88
India, 1997	372	53	6	78	22	49	95
India, 1998	2,935	10	10	87	86	91	91
Zimbabwe, 1999	2,148	40	13	77	44	64	91
India, 1999	1,268	36	16	95	62	68	87
South Africa, 2000	2,944	18	15	67	80	83	87
South Africa, 2001	6,298	18	2	50	19	84	99
India, 2001	402	42	42	87	81	82	79
South Africa, 2002	2,754	25	70	57	79	96	n/a
Philippines, 2003	3,316 (VIA) 3,195 (Pap)	10	2	37	14	91	98
Pakistan, 2003	501	31	16	94	47	78	89
South Africa, 2003	1,093	53	9	79	53	49	95
India, 2004	22,663	17	9	72	65	84	92

NOTES: Cytology threshold: ASCUS+. Outcome threshold: CIN 2–3.

[a]Positivity rate is defined by IARC as the proportion of diagnoses of cancer in all positive results of the screening test: A process measure.

SOURCE: Reprinted, with permission, from IARC Working Group on the Evaluation of Cancer Preventive Strategies (2005). Copyright 2005 by the International Agency for Research on Cancer.

Wide variability in test performance characteristics for visual inspection methods and the lack of universally accepted definitions of VIA or VILI test results have made their evaluation difficult. Standardization of test result definitions would increase the ability to interpret results, and would likely increase reproducibility, a problem that has also hampered the use of cytology in comparison studies (IARC Working Group, 2005).

HPV DNA Testing

As a primary screening method in women older than 30 years of age, HPV testing has a sensitivity of about 95 percent for detecting CIN 2 or more severe lesions compared with 75 percent for cytology at the ASCUS cut-off level, and 70 percent for cytology at the LSIL cut-off level (IARC Working Group, 2005). HPV testing specificity is about 94 percent for women over 30 years of age, compared with 95 percent for cytology at the ASCUS level, and 98 percent at the LSIL level. The specificity of HPV testing in younger women, not surprisingly, is lower. No studies have yet prospectively investigated the impact of HPV DNA testing on subsequent cancer rates (IARC Working Group, 2005).

Comparing Testing Methods

Accuracy

HPV testing and the visual inspection methods are more sensitive than Pap smears and cytology at a single screening, at least under study conditions. However, both also have a lower specificity. In a single screening, more of the women actually at risk will be picked up, at a cost of identifying as positive more women who would not develop cancer. Where screening is readily available and carried out regularly, as in most wealthy countries, low sensitivity may not have major health consequences Lesions develop very slowly and can be detected in any of several years, still at a preclinical, curable stage. Overtreatment because of low specificity is most worrisome when the treatment carries significant risk. With cryotherapy, short-term complications are minimal, but less is known about possible long-term sequelae. No red flags have yet appeared but the issue will require continued monitoring.

Conditions of Use

Pap smear, HPV testing, and DVI each require basic essential facilities and supplies to examine women in a private space and collect samples safely and correctly. The equipment needs for DVI are simpler and less expensive than for the other methods. For VILI, Lugol's iodine may not be easily found in most developing countries, but acetic acid for VIA is available everywhere (ACCP, 2004). The conditions under which DVI can be performed are variable, and need not be in a clinic setting. HPV testing and Pap smear require laboratory facilities or transport systems to take samples to a laboratory, and a stable supply of electricity, while visual inspection techniques do not. In addition to these requirements is the need to make arrangements for treating conditions detected, from precancerous conditions to invasive cancer. For DVI, treatment of early lesions must be at or very close to the site of screening if treatment is to be provided at the same visit. For the other methods, treatment must be accessible to all women screened, which could involve referral and transport to another area.

Some problems of access could be alleviated with the use of mobile clinics, as has been tried in Thailand, for example (Swaddiwudhipong et al., 1995). A 6-year study in 54 Thai villages was successful in raising the proportion of women who had ever had a Pap smear from 20 percent in 1991, to 58 percent in 1994, to 70 percent in 1997 (Swaddiwudhipong et al., 1999). Women were invited to be screened and village health communicators provided information about screening and cervical cancer before the study started (Swaddiwudhipong et al., 1999). Mobile services are an option for all screening methods.

Acceptability of Methods

Key factors in patient acceptability of any screening program include distance to travel, number of visits, and cost. Other important factors include a good patient–physician relationship, a female screening provider, and a screening setting that assures patient privacy (IARC Working Group, 2005).

Cytology and HPV testing require facilities and personnel that make implementation difficult in most LMCs, except in some urban areas. Women in rural areas may be compelled to travel long distances, at personal expense, to be screened, and may have to return for test results and treatment. These factors are cited as contributors to a failure to decrease cervical cancer incidence and mortality (Lazcano-Ponce et al., 1999).

HPV testing presents a unique acceptability issue, distinct from the other screening methods, because it involves testing for a sexually transmitted infection. STIs can be stigmatizing in any country, developed or developing. Several studies have found significant patient dropout after initial testing; when contacted, patients indicated fear of finding out that they had contracted an STI (IARC Working Group, 2005). This points to a need for health professionals to be trained in HPV counseling of test-positive patients and their sexual partners to ensure treatment and follow-up (IARC Working Group, 2005).

Cervical Cancer Prevention Implementation

Experience with Pap Smear and Cytology Programs

By the 1960s, Pap smears were available in many developed countries from physicians on a case-by-case basis. Later, screening programs were organized, notifying women at 1- to 5-year intervals. An exception is the United States, where Pap smear services are widely available, but notification is not mandatory. Cervical cancer incidence has been reduced by as much as 80 percent in developed countries through these programs (IARC Working Group, 2005). Attempts to establish Pap smear and cytology programs have not been successful in LMCs, with a few exceptions, mainly in urban areas with appropriate hospitals and laboratory facilities.

Mexico's national screening program, for example, initiated in 1974, offers annual cytology smears to women 25 to 65 years of age (Sankaranarayanan et al., 2001). In some Mexican states, fewer than 30 percent of women have ever been screened, and no systematic organization exists for call, recall, and follow-up of screened women. Evaluations of cytology test results within Mexico's program found wide variations in test performance across screening facilities, and a random sample review indicated 64 percent of the smears were of poor quality (Lazcano-Ponce et al., 1997). Cervical cancer mortality has not declined in Mexico as a result of the program (Lazcano-Ponce et al., 1996, cited by Sankaranarayanan et al., 2001 and Arillo-Santillan et al., 2001).

Other countries have been somewhat more successful. The Colombian National League Against Cancer, a component of the public health system, has offered cytology screening alongside private organizations in several regions since the 1970s (Sankaranarayanan et al., 2001). Costa Rica has provided nationwide cytology services to women older than 15 years since 1970, with 85 percent of eligible women having been screened at least once. In Cuba, where a biennial cytology screening program was implemented as part of primary health care services in 1968, more than 80 percent of women aged 20–60 years have been screened at least once (Garrote et al., 1996).

Experience with Visual Inspection Techniques

No national or large-scale programs using visual inspection techniques have yet been established. It is unlikely that the (mainly) wealthy countries that already have functioning Pap smear and cytology programs will revamp the systems responsible for what might be the most successful cancer prevention efforts in history. However, in LMCs where the primary health care infrastructure is weak or fragile (including limited laboratory capacity) and basic health care needs are not being met, visual inspection programs may be more feasible than Pap smear-based programs. This reality is the driver behind efforts to determine the value and feasibility of alternative screening methods.

A recent multicountry study was organized by the Alliance for Cervical Cancer Prevention (ACCP), a consortium supported by the Bill & Melinda Gates Foundation to assess the feasibility and acceptability of introducing a VIA screen-and-treat (with cryotherapy) program into reproductive health services in India, Kenya, Peru, South Africa, and Thailand (ACCP, 2003; 2004). The visual inspections were performed by qualified nurses. Women who came to district hospital and local health centers for other reasons were invited to participate, and others were recruited through local publicity. The services were offered successfully everywhere, and women were generally pleased with them. The study did not compare visual inspection with other types of screening programs, so it is not a source of information on the accuracy of the method. (However, see the next section for a model that uses the data from the study.)

Work is continuing by ACCP partners to complete research and demonstration projects in Ghana, India, Peru, South Africa, and Thailand, and to summarize all ACCP findings when country projects are complete, expected in 2007 (ACCP, 2006).

Cost-Effectiveness of Different Screening Strategies

Goldie and colleagues (Goldie et al., 2005) used the results of the ACCP multicountry screen-and-treat study in India, Kenya, Peru, South Africa, and Thailand, supplemented with data from the literature, to model the cost-effectiveness of several cervical cancer screening and treatment strategies. The analysis was improved over earlier modeling studies by including more actual costs (e.g., laboratory equipment and supplies, transportation of specimens, training, administration, and others measured directly) and allowing direct comparisons among countries at different economic levels of development.

The computer-based model simulates the natural history of HPV infection through the development of cervical cancer, and superimposes on it various screening strategies. The costs (in year 2000 international dollars) and the gains in life expectancy generated by the model were used to calculate cost-effectiveness ratios. Costs and benefits were discounted by 3 percent.

The screening tests included in the model were:

- Visual inspection of the cervix with acetic acid
- Pap smear and cytologic examination of cervical cells
- HPV testing with hybrid-capture method
- HPV testing followed by visual inspection for positive tests

Each test was modeled according to a minimum and a higher number of visits, from one to three visits, varying according to test characteristics. Age at screening and number of lifetime screenings (at 5-year intervals) were also investigated. The base case was a single, lifetime screening at age 35. Key variables used in the model are in Table 6-8.

In the model, screening and most treatment took place at a primary care-level facility. More extensive cytologic abnormalities, cancers, or women with anatomic abnormalities of the cervix were referred to secondary-level facilities for further diagnosis and treatment. Cryosurgery was used to treat women with abnormal findings at the primary facilities.

Costs included in the analysis are:

- Direct medical costs (e.g., staff, disposable supplies, equipment, specimen transport)
- Women's time (time traveling and waiting for and receiving care)
- Direct transportation costs
- Program-related costs

Costs of false-positive results and the costs incurred by women in the model who were referred to higher level facilities were also included.

Results

Effectiveness All strategies reduced the lifetime risk of invasive cervical cancer. The effect of a single screening, at age 35, was greatest with HPV one- and two-visit screening (30 to 36 percent reduction in lifetime cervical cancer risk), followed by one- and two-visit visual inspection (25 to 31 percent reduction), and finally two- and three-visit Pap smear and cytology (18 to 22 percent reduction). Two screenings, at ages 35 and 40, brought all strategies up to about 40 percent reduction in lifetime cervical cancer risk, and an additional screening at age 45 reduced the risk a further 15 percent.

The number of visits was a critical factor: the more visits needed, the poorer the follow-through with all strategies. Single-visit HPV (followed closely by visual inspection) was most effective. The least effective strate-

TABLE 6-8 Selected Variables of the Models Used in the Comparative Analysis for the Five Countries

Variable[a]	Base Case (%)	Range (%)
Characteristics of Screening Tests		
VIA		
Sensitivity[b]	76	60–90
Specificity	81	66–96
HPV DNA		
Sensitivity[b]	88	65–95
Specificity	93	70–96
Cytology (Pap smear)		
Sensitivity[b]	63	45–85
Specificity	94	80–98
Characteristics of Screening Program		
Participation[c]	100	25–100
Loss to follow-up (per visit)[d]	15	0–50
Criterion for Ineligibility for Cryosurgery According to Disease Status[e]		
DNA is normal or positive for HPV, without CIN	5	0–50
CIN, grade 1	15	0–50
CIN, grade 2 or 3	25	0–50
Cryosurgery[f]		
Effectiveness in women with CIN, grade 1	85	50–90
Effectiveness in women with CIN, grade 2 or 3	75	50–90
Major complications	1	0–3
Minor complications	5	0–15

[a]The variables shown represent only those values used in the comparative analysis for all five countries; see original paper, for additional variables. Each variable used in the base case analysis was varied over the range of values shown for the sensitivity analysis.

[b]Sensitivity is defined as the probability of a positive test given the presence of CIN 2 or higher.

[c]In order to compare results with those of other published analyses, the authors assumed that screening participation was 100 percent in the base case. Sensitivity analyses varied coverage according to the assumption that the population has either a homogeneous or a heterogeneous risk of cervical cancer (i.e., women who are not screened are at higher risk than women who receive screening).

[d]The authors assumed that loss to follow-up occurred for each clinical contact. For example, for a three-visit strategy, there would be an overall loss to follow-up of approximately 45 percent.

[e]The values are the proportions of women in each underlying disease category who would be ineligible for cryosurgery on the basis of visual inspection of the cervix and would be referred to a district or tertiary clinical care site for appropriate evaluation. Among those with grade CIN 1, one-third would undergo a loop electrosurgical excision procedure, one-third a cold-knife conization, and one-third a simple hysterectomy; among those with CIN 2 or 3, half would undergo cold-knife conization and half a simple hysterectomy.

[f]Treatment for CIN 2 or 3 with cryosurgery resulted in a rate of immediate failure of 10 percent; a 10 percent recurrence of CIN after 6 months; and a 5 percent recurrence after 1 year.

SOURCE: Reprinted, with permission, from Goldie et al. (2005).

gies were two- and three-visit Pap smear cytologic examinations, and the two-visit HPV testing and visual inspection sequence.

Costs The total costs (discounted) for a single lifetime screening varied by country. India had the lowest costs and South Africa, the highest. Among the strategies, single-visit visual inspection was the least expensive and three-visit Pap smear cytology the most expensive. For every strategy, most of the cost was attributable to cancer treatment, so additional screenings tended to raise costs only minimally.

Cost-effectiveness Single lifetime screening with either visual inspection or HPV testing was most cost-effective, depending on the country. One-visit visual inspection at age 35 cost $10 per year of life saved in India and $134 in Kenya. In South Africa, single-visit HPV testing with same-day treatment was most cost-effective, at $467 per year of life saved. In Peru and Thailand, one-visit visual inspection ($124 and $109 per year of life saved, respectively) and one-visit HPV testing ($152 and $170 per year of life saved, respectively) were most cost-effective. The least attractive strategies were three-visit Pap smear cytology or HPV testing, which cost more and gave poorer results than strategies that involved fewer visits.

Sensitivity analysis The model was tested for sensitivity to values for a number of variables. All strategies were sensitive to the costs of treating invasive cancers and to the age at screening. Screening women in their mid-30s was always optimal. When choosing among screening strategies, the results were most sensitive to the costs and characteristics (sensitivity, specificity, predictive value) of the tests. This is particularly relevant to HPV testing because the test materials and laboratory facilities constitute a larger proportion of the total costs than for visual inspection or Pap smear with cytology. If the price of HPV testing—the approach with the best performance—comes down, it would become an even more attractive option.

Conclusions from the Modeling

According to this model, a single lifetime screening of women in their mid-30s with either visual inspection or HPV testing in one or two visits should reduce the lifetime risk of developing cervical cancer by 25 to 36 percent. A second screen after 5 years would increase the benefit to about a 40 percent reduction in lifetime cervical cancer risk.

Both costs and cost-effectiveness vary several-fold across the five countries, but in all cases, the best strategies (including screening two or three times in a lifetime, depending on country) had cost-effectiveness ratios in a range generally accepted as "very cost-effective" (WHO, 2001) in the context of per-capita gross domestic product. These approaches also compare favorably, in terms of cost-effectiveness, with widely adopted interventions, including hepatitis B vaccination in India, second-line treatment for chronic tuberculosis in Peru, and the use of insecticide-treated bed netting to prevent malaria in Kenya.

HPV VACCINES

GlaxoSmithKline (GSK) and Merck & Co., Inc. have each developed vaccines to prevent infection with the most prevalent types of HPV associated with cervical cancer—types 16 and 18 (associated with 70 percent of cervical cancers). The Merck vaccine is also designed to protect against types 6 and 11, the most common agents of genital warts (responsible for 90 percent of genital warts). Merck's vaccine, GARDASIL®, was approved by the FDA in June 2006, based on clinical trials that included about 21,000 women and 4,000 men around the world. GSK, whose vaccine has been tested in 30,000 women in Phase III trials, is seeking approval first by the European Union, also anticipated before the end of 2006.

Both the Merck and GSK vaccines have shown complete efficacy in preventing persistent infection by HPV types 16 and 18 (Harper et al., 2004; Koutsky et al., 2002; Villa et al., 2005). Currently, there are no predictions regarding prevention of cancer among women who have already experienced an infection to determine whether the vaccines might have some effectiveness (WHO, 2005).

Vaccine Targeting and Scheduling

Young women aged 15–25 have been the target audience of most vaccine studies, though immunogenicity and safety studies are also being conducted in groups down to 9 years of age to demonstrate tolerability in younger girls and boys (WHO, 2005). Large trials are also planned by both Merck and GSK to determine efficacy against CIN in women aged 24 to 45 years.

Merck has also begun trials among HIV-infected people in the United States, as well as in young men aged 16 to 23 years to evaluate immunogenicity and efficacy against genital warts, HPV infection, and anal precancer (WHO, 2005). Vaccinating males, who would benefit from the protection against genital warts, would also protect women from transmission of the cervical cancer-causing types of HPV.

HPV vaccination is likely to be most effective if given prior to the onset of sexual activity, before possible exposure to HPV. Delivery of the vaccine would be simplest if it could be given in conjunction with other childhood vaccines. Determining the potential to integrate HPV vaccine into routine infant or childhood immunization schedules is a long-term objective stated by WHO. However, safety data supporting integration will take many years to generate (WHO, 2005). There are theoretical reasons to expect that the response to vaccination would be better in infants than in adults, though response data for adults cannot be extrapolated to infants. Inclusion of one or two doses of HPV vaccine in infant immunization schedules might mean that only one dose (rather than three anticipated) is needed in the preteen or early teen years, which would be simpler to deliver programmatically (WHO, 2005).

Information about immunization schedules is still forthcoming. The companies have not made known their intentions regarding spacing of doses and the need for booster doses. Safety and immunogenicity in pregnant women also has not been established (WHO, 2005). Some of this information will emerge over time.

Vaccine Financing and Delivery

No reliable estimates of cost of HPV immunization have been made public yet. Both Merck and GSK have confirmed that they will offer tiered pricing, with lower prices for developing countries. A $12.9 million grant from the Bill and Melinda Gates Foundation was recently awarded to WHO, IARC, the Program on Appropriate Technology for Health (PATH), and Harvard University toward a collaborative effort to bring HPV vaccines to developing countries. WHO's Initiative for Vaccine Research is investigating the potential of HPV vaccine delivery to girls under the age of 10, and conducting demonstration projects in low- and middle-income countries on the feasibility of vaccinating adolescent girls. PATH will likely oversee the demonstration projects and secure funding, currently planned for four LMCs. PATH has also begun early planning to enter into vaccine price negotiations with Merck and GlaxoSmithKline on behalf of the world's poorest countries.

Most LMCs are likely to need external financial support to purchase the vaccine and possibly to develop delivery programs (particularly if the vaccine cannot be incorporated into the existing infant and childhood schedules). Mechanisms that could be used for this purpose exist, such as the Global Alliance for Vaccines and Immunization, the new International Finance Facility for Immunization (launched in 2005 and supported by the United Kingdom, France, and Sweden), or the Vaccines for the New Millennium Act of 2005, launched by the U.S. Congress. These or other avenues should be found to help LMCs to implement HPV vaccination where cervical cancer is of major concern.

SAVING CHILDREN WITH CANCER

The ability to cure most children with cancer stands as a great medical achievement of the last half of the 20th century. Within oncology, it is even more remarkable, given the far smaller gains against most cancers of adults. Another contrast with cancers in adults is that the gains are almost exclusively attributable to treatment alone, because no strategies for preventing childhood cancers have yet been identified (with the exception of rare childhood cancers of the liver, prevented by hepatitis B vaccination). For some relatively common cancers of childhood (e.g., certain brain tumors), treatment results remain poor, and for others, adverse effects occurring decades after treatment prod the research enterprise to find treatments that cure but do less harm (Hewitt et al., 2003). Nonetheless, in the United States and other resource-rich countries, 75–80 percent of children with cancer survive for 5 years and most live out full lifetimes. But nearly 80 percent of the world's children who develop cancer are in resource-poor countries. Those without access to treatment, which is most in poor countries, do not survive.

In high-income countries, cancer is the leading cause of disease-related death (i.e., excluding accidents) in children, even given the high cure rates. In low-resource countries, the rank order varies, with cancer becoming more important as the level of economic development rises. In some middle-income countries, cancer is the leading cause of death from disease among children and young adults (e.g., in Mexico, where cancer is second to accidents as a cause of death among young people age 5–14), although in others, infectious diseases may still predominate (Figure 6-1).

Why Should Pediatric Cancer Be Given Priority in LMCs?

The numbers of childhood cancers and deaths (below age 15) are modest in the poorest countries, and low compared with the corresponding figures for cancer in adults. In 2002, 160,000 children worldwide developed cancer, 134,000 of them in less developed countries (IARC, 2004). Including 15- to 19-year-olds increases the numbers by 25–33 percent, and adding the 20- to 24-year age group adds a similar percentage. The proportion of children with cancer who die is much higher in less developed countries (Figure 6-2), but still amounts to fewer than 100,000 per year.

Nonetheless, the number of childhood cancers, and in particular, the proportion of childhood deaths due to cancer, is rising in low-income countries as the number of children increases and other causes of childhood death diminish. Data from China illustrate this point: Between 1960 and 2002, the death rate among children under 5 from all causes had fallen from 225 to 39 per 1,000 live births, with cancer assuming greater importance as deaths from infectious diseases declined. With more than 300 million children un-

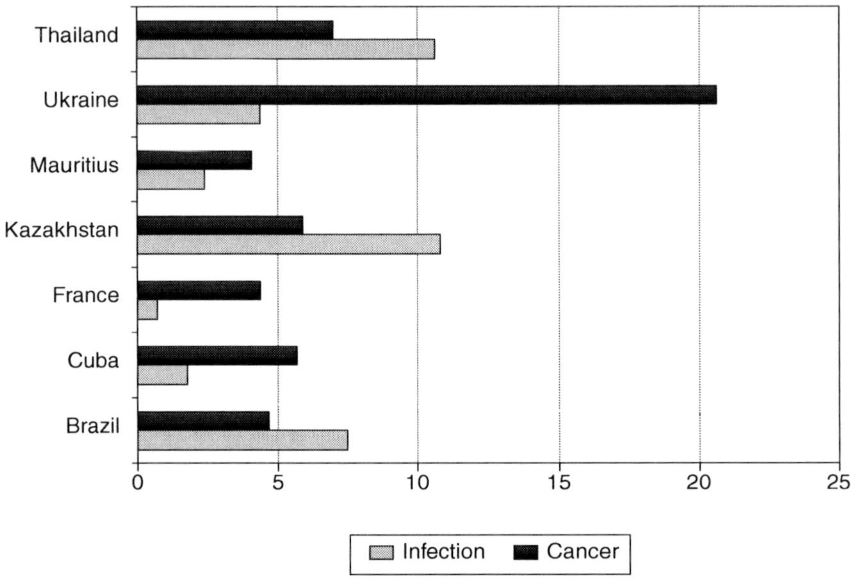

FIGURE 6-1 Number of registered deaths per 100,000 among ages 1–24 years, selected countries, in 2000.
SOURCE: Personal communication, I. Magrath, INCTR, May 2006.
Data available at http://www3.who.int/whosis/mort/table1.

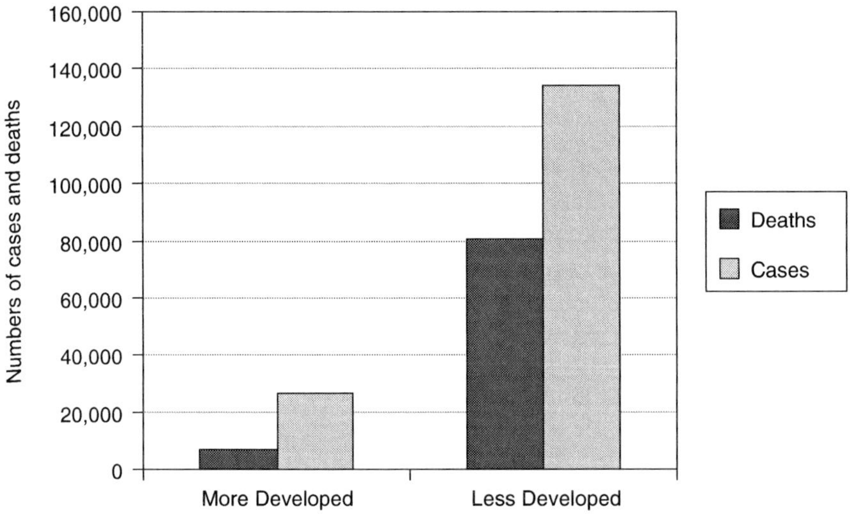

FIGURE 6-2 Annual numbers of cases and deaths from cancer, ages 0–14.
SOURCE: IARC (2004).

der 15 now in China, on the order of 45,000 new cases of childhood cancer can be expected annually (Ribeiro and Pui, 2005).

The relatively small numbers of childhood cancers in low-income countries could argue against giving them priority, or alternatively, the argument can be made that for a relatively modest investment, most of these children could be saved. There are additional benefits of a successful, visible cancer treatment program for children above and beyond curing individual children. In countries where cancer is often seen as a death sentence—because most adults and children do, in fact, die of their cancers, even if they eventually seek treatment at an advanced stage—demonstrating to the public and to health professionals that healthy survival is possible would boost the chances of adopting further achievable cancer treatment goals.

Children have long been the focus of global health efforts, but the major international organizations dealing with child health—mainly WHO and UNICEF—have not yet focused on cancer. Other parts of this report argue for effective interventions to save middle-aged and older people, and to provide comfort through palliative care for everyone, children included. But children are also a compelling focus for the reasons given: assured success for a large number if given appropriate treatment, which can be relatively uncomplicated and relatively inexpensive; living cancer survivors; and some development of cancer treatment infrastructure that forms a core for expanded services.

Differences Between Childhood and Adult Cancers

The cancers that arise in children are, by and large, different from cancers of adults, everywhere in the world. In general, they are different entities clinically and biologically, and each has its own age-specific pattern of incidence. Tumors of infants are extremely rare in adults, particularly above the age of 30 years, and vice versa, but in adolescents and young adults, there is a more mixed picture.

About 90 percent of adult cancers are carcinomas that arise from epithelial tissue. These include the familiar cancers of the prostate, breast, lung, colon and rectum, uterus, and ovary. In children, leukemias and lymphomas alone comprise some 40–50 percent of cancers. The rest are mainly cancers arising in the central nervous system; embryonal cells of the eye, kidney, and adrenal glands; and sarcomas of bone and soft tissues. These differences in tissue origin affect cancer development and the response to treatment.

Even cancers with the same name in children and adults can be significantly different in their biology and in the response to treatment. The 5-year survival rate for children with acute lymphoblastic leukemia (ALL), the most common childhood malignancy in much of the world, is about 80 percent. Among adults under age 65 with the same diagnosis, only 20 to 30 percent survive for 5 years (Ries et al., 2002). Better outcomes in children are likely due to differences in the underlying molecular abnormalities responsible for the cancer's biological characteristics, and possibly in the physiology and immune system of the patient. For example, a factor associated with poor prognosis is the "Philadelphia chromosome," a cytogenetic defect found in 30 to 40 percent of adults with ALL but less than 5 percent of children with that diagnosis (Look and Kirsch, 2002).

Patterns of Childhood Cancer in Less and More Developed Countries

While leukemias and lymphomas comprise about 40–50 percent of all new cases of cancer in children worldwide, the frequencies of other cancers—and of the specific types of leukemias and lymphomas—have distinct geographic distributions. The pattern is particularly distinct in sub-Saharan Africa, where the incidence of Burkitt's lymphoma and Kaposi's sarcoma (the latter related to HIV infection) are much higher than anywhere else in the world (Parkin et al., 2003). Retinoblastoma is also much more common in developing countries generally, and brain tumors less common than in high-income countries. The incidence of leukemias in sub-Saharan Africa is also remarkably low, in the few places in which it can be accurately measured, and the pattern of immunological subtypes differs from that observed in countries of higher socioeconomic status. The differences in the patterns of cancer are almost certainly due to environmental and lifestyle differences associated with lower socioeconomic status. Infectious causes that are more common in low-income countries (e.g., Epstein-Barr virus and malaria in Burkitt's lymphoma; HIV in Kaposi's sarcoma) may be of particular importance. These descriptions of the broad patterns of cancer in children throughout the world are relatively clear despite scanty data (Parkin et al., 2003).

Children with cancer in developing countries are much more likely than their counterparts in the United States and other wealthy countries to have late-stage cancer when diagnosed and to have additional health problems. A report from the Shaukat Khanum Memorial Cancer Hospital in Pakistan illustrates this. Of the children in the mid-1990s with ALL, 71 percent met the WHO criteria for malnutrition. One-quarter were positive for hepatitis B surface antigen or hepatitis C, and 40 percent presented with high-risk ALL (hyperleukocytosis and massive hepato-splenomegaly). Even with treatment, 40 percent of the children did not survive 5 years, most because of infection, hepatitis, and intracranial hemorrhage, a pattern similar to that reported from a number of developing countries (Usmani, 2001).

Barriers to Childhood Cancer Treatment in Low-Income Countries

Many of the factors that limit children's access to cancer care are similar to those in adults, but some are unique to children, or even to specific cancers. The major factors are discussed below.

Socioeconomic Factors

Socioeconomic factors often override all others. Particularly in rural areas, children and their parents must travel long distances to reach a facility able to treat childhood cancers, which are fewer even than those where an adult might receive treatment. Even proximity to a center, located mainly in urban areas, does not equal access. The expense of what would be considered a very modestly priced cancer treatment in a high-resource setting is out of reach for poor families, where health insurance is nonexistent and traditional treatment is less expensive and more available. As is true for adult cancers, no traditional treatments are known to be effective against childhood cancers. In addition to the purely economic and practical constraints, social and psychological support for children and families going through the arduous and prolonged process of cancer treatment is limited. Illiteracy and a general lack of understanding of the complex process further alienate people from seeking treatment in the first place, and from completing treatment and follow-up. A finding from studying retinoblastoma may be generalizable: the less educated the father, the more likely the child is to have advanced disease and delay in diagnosis (International Network for Cancer Treatment and Research, 2004).

Social and Cultural Factors

Other social and cultural factors may weigh against a child receiving treatment for a curable cancer. Cancer is stigmatized in many cultures, and patients may be rejected, even after cure. Where cure alters the body in visible ways—such as loss of an eye to retinoblastoma—children may pay an even higher price. A girl who has lost an eye may not be marriageable. Culture may also dictate consulting a traditional healer, delaying formal medical care until a cancer is far advanced. The family may be dissuaded from seeking treatment at all by some healers.

To put this in human terms, a mother may have to choose between staying with her child with cancer in a distant hospital or being with her family who may, without her, have very limited ability to fend for themselves. She may choose to provide food for her healthy children, or the family choice may be stark—money for anticancer treatment, or food and schooling for the other children.

Lack of Cancer Treatment Infrastructure

The lack of infrastructure for cancer management is pervasive in LMCs. Many children probably die from cancer without it ever being recognized and without receiving even palliative care. This is especially likely for leukemias, the early symptoms of which are fever, swollen lymph glands, and anemia, which may easily be mistaken for infectious conditions. Indeed, children in early stages of leukemia are particularly susceptible to infections that lead to death without the underlying leukemia being recognized (Usmani, 2001). Both leukemias and lymphomas in young children can progress rapidly to death in the absence of appropriate medical attention (Parkin et al., 2003).

Lack of Medical Professionals with Pediatric Cancer Training

The differences between childhood cancers and adult cancers mean that treating them appropriately requires specialized knowledge as well as drugs and other supplies and equipment. There are few trained pediatric oncologists in low-income countries, and that situation is not likely to improve significantly given the numbers of children affected and the reality of medical care in poor economies. Compounding the problem is a lack of knowledge about the signs and symptoms of childhood cancer among nonspecialists, including pediatricians, family practitioners, and others on the medical front lines. Even once in the system, other skills may be lacking. Pathologists often have not had the training needed for pediatric cancers; there may be no pediatric or specialist surgeons experienced in the diagnosis or treatment of eye and bone cancers, or even specialized pediatric surgeons, or radiotherapists with pediatric cancer training or facilities suitable for the treatment of children.

Importance of Locally Relevant Research

Treatments for childhood cancers have been optimized for the patients and infrastructure of high-income countries. The basics—key drugs and procedures—should be applicable in most settings, but the details, if treatment is to be optimized to the setting, are almost sure to differ. One feature of childhood cancer treatment in the United States and other high-income countries is worth emulating: the highly collaborative and cooperative character of the pediatric oncology community. Since the 1960s, when treatments began to make a real difference in the survival of children with cancer, the majority of pediatric oncologists and their patients have participated in clinical trials, and patients have benefited. The Children's Oncology Group (organized through the U.S. National Cancer Institute) is, in this sense, the envy of those who conduct adult cancer clinical trials (Adamson et al., 2005).

Clinical trials are needed in LMCs not only to adapt the treatments developed in high-income countries, but also to address clinical questions of local relevance. Children in high-income countries rarely present with advanced retinoblastoma or Kaposi's sarcoma, yet these are common in sub-Saharan Africa, in particular. Adapting treatment is also important. Treatment protocols from high-income countries are designed for an advanced infrastructure that does not exist in resource-poor countries. Finally, patients in LMCs may differ: in disease biology, in the way drugs are metabolized (e.g., because of nutritional differences), and because of different co-morbidities. Through clinical trials in a variety of low-resource settings, it can be determined which of the differences are important clinically, and how treatment can be modified accordingly (Personal communication, I. Magrath, International Network for Cancer Treatment and Research, November 2005).

The benefits of locally relevant clinical trials go beyond an answer to a research question. Children treated in clinical trials are likely to get treatment more in line with some current recommendations, and staff receive training and education through participation in clinical trials. Pragmatically, limited resources may be more accessible as funds are more likely to be made available for research than for routine treatment.

Programs and Alliances for Childhood Cancers Relevant to LMCs

Two global initiatives for childhood cancer (described below) have recently begun. In addition, the International Network for Cancer Treatment and Research (INCTR) has established networks of various types around several childhood cancers: acute lymphocytic leukemia, retinoblastoma (Box 6-2), and Burkitt's lymphoma. INCTR also has helped to establish "cooperative groups" that have agreed to work together toward specific goals. These include the Leukemia Study Group of India, the Middle East Children's Cancer Group, and the Retinoblastoma Group of Mexico.

Global Alliance for the Cure of Children with Cancer

A "Global Alliance for the Cure of Children with Cancer" was formed in 2001 at a meeting organized by INCTR. The meeting included the European Organization for Research and Treatment of Cancer, the International Agency for Research on Cancer, the International Society of Pediatric Oncology (SIOP), the National Cancer Institute, the Monza International School of Pediatric Oncology (MISPHO), the International Consortium for the Cure of Childhood Cancer in China, and the Oncology Center,

BOX 6-2
International Network for Cancer Treatment and Research: Public and Professional Awareness Programs for Retinoblastoma: Recent Examples

As part of a retinoblastoma awareness campaign in Brazil, a public service announcement was broadcast on television throughout the country and has been made available in multiple languages. The public responded with telephone calls, letters, and photographs of children, asking for guidance. In addition to the television campaign, 1 million telephone cards with information about retinoblastoma—including pictures—were distributed in Brazil, where such cards are used by a high fraction of the population. The results of the two campaigns are under evaluation.

The Mexican Retinoblastoma Group has formed, with ophthalmologists and pediatric oncologists working together to study individual cases, better understand the pattern of the disease in Mexico, develop uniform treatment approaches, and develop and standardize methods for better early detection of retinoblastoma. To increase public awareness, a poster about retinoblastoma has been distributed widely and a public service announcement has aired on a popular TV channel.

SOURCE: International Network for Cancer Treatment and Research (2004).

Antwerp, with other organizations expressing interest in joining. A project on Burkitt's lymphoma in Africa was the first undertaking, but the alliance otherwise has not been activated. As of late 2006, plans to revitalize the effort are under way.

"My Child Matters"

"My Child Matters" was launched in 2005 by the International Union Against Cancer (known as the UICC), in collaboration with drug manufacturer Sanofi-Aventis, as part of UICC's World Cancer Campaign to improve the treatment of children with cancer in resource-poor countries. The three major activities of the campaign are: (1) funding projects in 10 countries in the first year, based on competitively selected proposals; (2) a worldwide mobilization and awareness campaign to highlight the effects of childhood cancers; and (3) a comprehensive report on childhood cancers, which was released on World Cancer Day, February 4, 2006 (International Union Against Cancer, 2006).

Proposals for the first projects were solicited from Bangladesh, Egypt, Honduras, Morocco, the Philippines, Senegal, Tanzania, Ukraine, Venezuela, and Vietnam, as pilot countries. The list for the second year will be expanded. Project goals were:

- Raising awareness and disseminating timely information about childhood cancers to health professionals, parents, children's organizations, and the general public;
- Improving early diagnosis and access to care and treatment for children living with cancer; and
- Strengthening the social welfare aspects of caring and support for children living with cancer and their families.

Fourteen projects, which began in early 2006, were selected from more than 80 applications, funded at a total of $700,000 (with additional support from the U.S. National Cancer Institute).

Improving Childhood Cancer Treatment in LMCs

Children with cancer in LMCs can be treated and cured—and appropriate psychosocial and family support provided—under conditions that are feasible even in resource-poor settings. The pediatric cancer unit (PCU) model that has worked well in high-income countries is also considered the best approach in LMCs (see Box 6-3, which lists SIOP recommendations for the organization of a PCU). An example is the success of dedicated PCU within a pediatric hospital established in Recife, Brazil beginning in the mid-1990s. The 5-year event-free survival rate for children with ALL rose from 32 percent before the PCU to 63 percent in the most recent period (Howard et al., 2004).

The initial challenges in improving pediatric cancer care are gaining public recognition of childhood cancer as an important and addressable health problem, and sustainable funding to support treatment. The "twinning" approach, which has been successful in a number of LMCs both in establishing good treatment and financing mechanisms, is described in the next part of this chapter.

"Twinning": An Approach to Developing PCUs in Resource-Poor Settings

The "twinning" approach—partnerships between institutions in high-resource and low-resource settings—has been particularly effective in pediatric cancer treatment. Twinning programs usually involve the development or upgrading of dedicated units within cancer centers, pediatric hospitals, or other major health care institutions for the purpose of expanding access

BOX 6-3
International Society for Pediatric Oncology (SIOP)

Working Committees on Standards of Care and Training, and Psychosocial Issues in Pediatric Oncology
Recommendations for the Organization of a Pediatric Cancer Unit (PCU)

1. All children with cancer should be offered child-oriented diagnoses, treatment, after-care, and follow-up. Special attention is also required for adolescents and young adults to the age of 20.
2. A PCU functions on a multidisciplinary teamwork principle. It can be a special unit integrated in a pediatric department or be located in a large general oncology centre. In the latter case there should be close links with pediatric services and separate facilities for hospitalized children including psychosocial, social, and educational services.
3. A PCU is part of, or linked to, a national and/or international multidisciplinary organization for pediatric oncology, in order to facilitate communication and coordination of new treatment methods and research. Sufficient data management staff and equipment should be available to participate in clinical trials and to supply data to cancer registries.
4. A PCU provides centralized primary treatment to enough patients (50 or more new patients/year) to warrant specific structures for pediatric oncology in surgery, radio-oncology, pathology, intensive care, supportive care, and rehabilitation. All of these facilities should be onsite or close-by. It may be necessary to centralize further the primary treatment of brain tumors or other malignancies requiring highly specialized treatment.

to care for children with cancer and improving cure rates. A long-term commitment of both partners is essential and must include all aspects of a successful program: trained personnel; basic drugs, equipment, and supplies; and relationships with parents' groups, the extended medical community, and the community at large.

Twinning programs have been in place around the world, a few for as long as 10 or 15 years. Their success is measured in the number of children treated, the proportion who complete treatment—abandonment of treatment is a problem in most low-income countries, where families cannot afford the medical and nonmedical costs of having a child in treatment—and finally, the number successfully treated and going on to live full lives. All these factors have been demonstrated in successful programs (Ribeiro and Pui, 2005). Two major twinning programs are described below.

5. A PCU is operated by appropriately trained specialists, including pediatric oncologist/hematologists, pediatric surgeons with a special interest in oncology, pediatric oncology nurses, pediatric psychologists, social workers, teachers, and others. These specialists ensure a round-the-clock service, recruit new PCU personnel, and provide adequate training in pediatric oncology.

A PCU comprises the following facilities:

A ward for in-patients sufficiently staffed and equipped (including proper isolation facilities) to:

- Execute complex medical orders;
- Establish central lines;
- Monitor long-term infusions;
- Care and support critically ill, myelo-/immunosuppressed, or dying children and their parents;
- Handle and prepare the administration of cytostatic drugs;
- Keep adequate records;
- Provide accommodation on the ward or close by for parents; and
- Provide religious/ministerial support.

A day-clinic for short-term investigations, short-term infusions, or short-term surveillance of patients;

An outpatient clinic closely linked to imaging and laboratory facilities, providing rapid service for ambulatory treatment and control; and

An administration for organizing and coordinating the long-term follow-up and evaluation of former cancer patients.

La Mascota Hospital (Managua, Nicaragua) and Monza PCU (Milan, Italy)

In the mid-1980s, most children with cancer in Nicaragua died from lack of appropriate treatment, even in the country's one pediatric hospital, Hospital Infantil Manuel de Jesus Rivera "La Mascota." At that time, La Mascota was, in the words of a new director, "inundated beyond capacity with health issues at the primary and secondary levels." Children with cancer were largely abandoned. The Director resolved to establish a PCU and sought technical assistance to do so (Masera et al., 2004).

A physician at the Mario Negri cancer research organization in Milan responded, and eventually brought The Hemato-Oncology Center of Milan-Bicocca University at Saint Gerardo Hospital, Monza, Italy (Monza

PCU) into a collaboration with La Mascota. The stated objective from the beginning was to begin “a comprehensive, long term program to establish a national PCU capable of offering a reasonable possibility of cure to Nicaraguan children with cancer.”

Staff development La Mascota initially had no staff with training in pediatric oncology. From the beginning, pediatricians, and later nurses and other specialists (urologists, nephrologists, pulmonologists, surgeons, laboratory scientists), were sent to Monza and other Italian centers for training. The relationships have been maintained by support to attend international meetings and periodic short training stints in Italy. The reality of low health care salaries led to physicians’ (and later nurses’) salaries being supplemented to reduce the need for them to practice outside the hospital.

Sources of funding La Mascota now has some support from the Nicaraguan government and other governments (Italy, Japan, Luxembourg), but the program was begun without such support. The initial budget came from two small philanthropic groups in Monza. A “National League Against Leukemia and Cancer in Children” was established jointly by the Directors of the Managua and Monza centers, and the Oncology Department at S. Giovanni Hospital in Bellinzona, Switzerland, which has also played a continuing role in the twinning program. Most of the financing comes from private institutions and private citizens. Between 1986 and 2001, the annual investment from the Italian and Swiss partners totaled $150,000–200,000. The share of local funding in Nicaragua has grown over the years.

Results The number of children treated annually at La Mascota has increased from about 50 in 1990 to more than 150 in 2001, estimated at 50 to 60 percent of all children with cancer in Nicaragua. Many more of them are completing treatment than previously. Early on, 30 to 40 percent of children who were diagnosed with cancer at the center either were not treated or abandoned treatment before it was completed, largely because the family could not bear the economic hardship of the nonmedical costs involved. A program begun in 1995 paired newly diagnosed children and their families with a family in Italy or Switzerland, which provides financial support for these nonmedical costs, including travel and other expenses. More than 750 children and their families have been part of this program, which has brought down the rate of treatment refusal or abandonment to less than 10 percent. The parents’ associations of the institutions have played an indispensable role in this and other aspects of the program.

Long-term survival for acute lymphocytic leukemia patients (the most frequent diagnosis) rose from 20 percent before the program to 40 to 50 percent in the late 1990s. Overall, the 3-year survival rate was 56 percent for children treated at La Mascota through the late 1990s, which compares favorably with countries in the region at higher economic levels, and is better than in similarly resourced countries.

Results for Wilms' tumor and Hodgkin's disease are more impressive, and represent treatment advances developed in clinical trials at La Mascota, demonstrating excellent results without radiotherapy.

Key elements for success The La Mascota–Monza twinning program has succeeded for a number of reasons, beginning with the long-term commitment of cooperation on both sides, based on mutual respect of "autonomy, culture, and local traditions" and "assuring an active but noninvasive role of supervision and scientific advice" from the high-income institution (Masera et al., 2004).

The collaboration involves all aspects of treatment, as described. A therapeutic alliance has developed among the physicians, nurses, psychosocial workers, and parents' associations. Successful continued financing has been possible because of the diversity of organizations and individuals providing support, without total reliance on a single entity.

Outgrowths of La Mascota The success of La Mascota encouraged Monza to create a structured program to foster additional twinning relationships between Latin American countries and other centers in Italy. At least four other collaborations were spawned in the first few years of effort, involving Bolivia, Cuba, Paraguay, and the Dominican Republic in Latin America, and Bergamo, Parma, Padova, Modena, and Bologna, in addition to Monza, in Italy. Health professionals from these as well as a number of other countries have been trained at Monza.

St. Jude Children's Research Hospital International Outreach Program

St. Jude Children's Research Hospital ("St. Jude"), opened in 1962, is well known in the United States as the leading institution in advancing the treatment of children with cancer and other catastrophic diseases. It serves mainly children from the United States, but children from all over the world are admitted, regardless of ability to pay (St. Jude Children's Research Hospital, 2006). St. Jude's research and treatment are supported by the third largest health care charity in the United States. The International Outreach Program (IOP) was formally established in 1991 after years of growing interest in children from poor countries (St. Jude Children's Research Hospital, 2003).

The IOP develops twinning partnerships with (mainly) public hospitals in middle-income countries and with other local agencies and organizations. The purpose of the partnerships is to build regional capacity in diagnosis and treatment of pediatric cancer. The aim is to create a critical mass of professionals who can support existing and developing programs. At the same time, relationships are developed with local fundraising organizations to support the programs. Current program and fundraising affiliates, predominantly in Latin America, are listed in Table 6-9 (St. Jude Children's Re-

TABLE 6-9 St. Jude International Outreach Program Partners

Country and City	Institutions	Fundraising Foundation
Brazil: Recife	Centro de Hematologia e Oncologia Pedatrica, Instituto Materno Infantil de Pernambuco	Nucleo de Apoio as Crianças com Cancer
Chile: Santiago	Hospital Luis Calvo Mackenna, Universidad de Chile	
China: Shanghai	Shanghai Children's Medical Center, Shanghai 2nd Medical University	Partner in HOPE Foundation, Limited, Hong Kong, China
China: Beijing	Beijing Children's Hospital	
Costa Rica: San Jose	Hospital Nacional de Niños, Centro De Ciencias Médicas de la C.C.S.S.	Asociación Lucha Contra el Cáncer Infantil
Ecuador: Quito	Centro Médico Meditropoli	Foundation SOLCA: La Sociedad de Lucha Control el Cancer
El Salvador: San Salvador	Hospital de Niños Benjamín Bloom	Fundacion Ayudame a Vivir
Guatemala: Guatemala City	Unidad Nacional de Oncologia Pediatrica, Hospital Roosevelt	Fundacion Ayudame a Vivir
Honduras: Tegucigalpa	Hospital Escuela Bloque Materno Infantil, Hospital Viera	Fundacion Hondureña Para El Niño con Cancer
Jordan: Amman	King Hussein Cancer Centre	King Hussein Cancer Foundation
Lebanon: Beirut	The Children's Cancer Center of Lebanon, Faculty of Medicine and Medical Center, American University of Beirut	The Children's Cancer Center of Lebanon
Mexico: Sinaloa	Hospital Pediatrico de Sinaloa, Culiacan	Amigos de Niños Afectados de Cancer A.C.
Mexico: Guadalajara	Hospital Civil de Guadalajara	
Morocco: Rabat	Hospital d'Enfants Rabat-Maroc	de L'Avenir, Association des Parents et Amis de Enfants
Morocco: Casablanca	Hospital 20 Aout 1953	Agir, Association Marocaine de Soutien
Russia: Moscow	Research Institute of Pediatric Hematology	
Venezuela: Caracas	Hospital de Ninos J.M. de Los Rios	Asociacion Venezolana de Padres de Niños con Cancer
Venezuela: Maracaibo	Hospital de Especialidades Pediatricas	Fundacion Amigos del Niño con Cáncer

SOURCE: St. Jude Children's Research Hospital (2006).

search Hospital, 2003). IOP partners are treating about 3,200 new patients per year (with about 10,000 under treatment) (St. Jude Children's Research Hospital, 2005), with good results. In El Salvador, the 5-year survival for ALL rose from 10 percent to 65 percent between 1993 and 2001, and in Brazil, from 29 percent to 60 percent between 1997 and 2001.

Two new IOP initiatives, relying on advanced telecommunications technologies, were begun in 1999: Cure4Kids and the International Training Center for Hematology-Oncology Nurses in Central America, in collaboration with the professional nursing society in El Salvador, to train nurses in the pediatric subspecialty of hematology/oncology.

Cure4Kids

Cure4Kids is an Internet-based distance-learning program provided free to physicians, nurses, scientists, and health care workers who treat children with catastrophic illnesses. The Internet tools include:

- Online education about catastrophic childhood illnesses
- Collaborative work spaces for document sharing and online meetings
- Access to consultation and mentoring by St. Jude faculty
- Technology and training for better management of patient information

The education component includes a digital library of reference material (full-text access to medical journals and papers), a discussion area for physician exchange of advice and information, and access to online seminars and lectures. The technology is also being used for live meetings and lectures through the Internet. Discussion of research protocols and specific cases being treated also take place. Partners from Brazil, Lebanon, Morocco, Guatemala, El Salvador, Honduras, and Mexico regularly participate in these virtual meetings.

More than 8,400 professionals in 155 countries (as of November 2006) are currently registered Cure4Kids users (St. Jude Children's Research Hospital, 2006). Its 200 online seminars about catastrophic childhood illnesses are available in seven languages.

Regional Initiatives in Latin America

With the network of partners having grown in a number of countries, the IOP has developed more regional programs, including workshops for medical professionals and fundraisers. A Central American Pediatric Oncology Infrastructure Program has also been proposed through the Association of Central American Pediatric Hematologists-Oncologists. The program would involve collaboration with other international partners already working in the region, including MISPHO and others.

The Role of Local Foundations

Local nonprofit foundations play two vital roles for IOP partners: they raise funds to support the work of the partners and they run public awareness campaigns about childhood cancers. Governments do not typically provide the resources needed for childhood cancer care, so funds must be supplemented. The IOP, in collaboration with the fundraising arm of St. Jude, sponsors training for members of the local foundations to help ensure their success. The foundations typically develop and support:

- Care, treatment, and psychosocial support of patients
- Salaries and training for key personnel
- Construction and renovation of facilities
- Efforts to increase government support for childhood cancer treatment
- Activities to raise public awareness that childhood cancers are curable at early stages

The 19 foundations affiliated with IOP partners have raised a total of $12.5 million over the past several years through donations and by soliciting funds from grant-making organizations. These funds have been used to provide housing for patients and families at or near the hospitals, to support salaries of key personnel, and to pay for medications. Paying for medications has proven to be a continuing challenge in most centers. Six foundations reported that some children went without some scheduled treatment because of a lack of funding for medications.

Recent Progress

St. Jude compiles reports from each IOP partner every year to assess progress. The 2005 report shows progress in a number of major areas for which goals had been set, including the following:

- Nurse training had been provided to all partner clinical programs over the previous 3 years
- 18 of 19 programs report a functioning infection control program
- All partners have immunophenotyping tests (tests that help determine the origin of leukemic cells) routinely available, partially paid for by St. Jude IOP

- All programs report treatment teams that include four or more subspecialties (pediatric oncologists, oncology nurses, social workers, psychologists, surgeons, dietitians or nutritionists, pharmacists, intensivists)
- Nearly all report that the hospital has an ethics committee or review board
- 79 percent of the programs instituted measures to reduce abandonment of treatment (guest houses, food supplements, subsidized transportation, parent support groups, satellite clinics, home visits by social workers)
- Most sites report active ALL protocols and more than half also have active protocols for a number of other cancers
- 1,543 patients were treated on protocols from May 2004 to May 2005
- Solid tumor diagnosis has been improved in most programs through tumor boards or other special programs

The IOP has also encouraged other institutions around the world to collaborate with the IOP-associated programs.

New Initiatives

Major new initiatives of the IOP include the Central American Retinoblastoma Program to improve survival rates, the Joint ALL Protocol for Beijing and Shanghai, and the Pediatric Oncology Networked Database (POND, a shared electronic database for programs in 10 countries).

Improving the Quality of Pediatric Cancer Treatment Through Clinical Trials and Centers of Excellence

By the early 1980s, major advances had already raised long-term survival from ALL in the United States and Europe to 70 percent. In LMCs, this was not the case. By way of example, at the Cancer Institute, Madras (now Chennai), India, fewer than 20 percent of the children and adolescents with ALL achieved long-term survival. As a means to improve this situation, a collaboration was established between WIA and the U.S. NCI, and later the NCI-funded INCTR (Shanta, 2000).

In the case of the NCI–India collaboration, a more intensive treatment protocol than what had been in use at the time was designed. Although this carried a risk of increased toxicity, in view of the poor results and the extensive disease in most patients, the added risks appeared worth taking. In addition, treatment elements believed to be difficult to administer or particularly costly in India (e.g., high-dose methotrexate) were avoided. An initial trial confirmed that the regimen was feasible and likely to result in much better long-term survival, with high but manageable toxicity. The protocol was taken to two additional major hospitals in India in 1986 and 1992.

The process has worked with the use of a locally affordable protocol that has manageable toxicity. During the 1990s, 60 percent of children with ALL treated at the Tata Memorial Hospital (in Mumbai, formerly Bombay) and 41–43 percent of those treated at the All India Institute of Medical Sciences (New Delhi) and the Cancer Institute of Chennai were cured. In addition, deaths from drug toxicity have gradually been reduced as the medical staffs have learned to better manage toxicities. The treatments used do not include unavailable or expensive technologies and could be replicated throughout the country. Results from the three centers differ, and those differences are the basis of further study. The work suggests that not only are there significant differences between Indian populations and patients in the United States and Europe, but among centers in India as well.

The India ALL experience demonstrates that although the general principles learned from clinical research in developed countries provide a foundation for treatment strategies, the differences in the populations treated, both genetic and environmental, differences in leukemia cell biology, and differences in the quality of care received can be expected to bring about differences in results when using a standard regimen. It is clear that therapies developed through clinical trials in the relevant populations are essential to quality care.

Clinical trials in these settings result in immediate patient benefits. They also contribute to basic scientific knowledge, including gene expression profiling of leukemic cells from patients in these settings, which lead to a better understanding of the genetic and environmental factors relevant both to the pathogenesis of ALL and to the identification of prognostic factors. In the process, three centers of excellence for pediatric cancer have been developed in India that form a strong nucleus for expanding treatment to other centers.

Examples of centers of excellence improving the success of pediatric cancer treatment can be found elsewhere. In centers of excellence in Brazil, the 5-year survival rate for childhood ALL is higher than 60 percent, but much lower outside these centers. Another successful model is the national pediatric oncology program in Chile. The Chilean government requires that patients receive their diagnosis and initial treatment in a certified pediatric cancer unit, with follow-up care from more numerous satellite clinics.

SUMMARY AND RECOMMENDATIONS

Three compelling opportunities to reduce the cancer burden in LMCs have been presented. The first two opportunities, vaccination against HBV to prevent liver cancer and cervical cancer prevention by screening adult women and vaccinating young girls, address two of the three major infection-related cancers. The first, which takes place through existing childhood vaccination programs, is the simplest to implement and is already in place in many countries. The focus there is on many of the poorest countries, where coverage is still poor and liver cancer burdens are high. Cervical cancer prevention, in contrast, is not widely practiced in LMCs. Screening does require a significant infrastructure, not only for the screening itself, but to provide treatment for women who are found with advanced cancers. In some countries, however, the availability of single-visit or two-visit screening (either visual inspection or HPV) may make the opportunity more attractive than it had been.

The third opportunity is to establish or improve treatment for the curable cancers of children and young adults. Doing so will build cancer management capacity more generally, and if done properly, will result in a rare class in many LMCs—cancer survivors, whose survival belies an all-too-common belief that cancer is inevitably fatal. Experience has shown that childhood cancer treatment can be financed through a combination of local and foreign sources in countries where it has been seriously attempted. As treatment for children with cancer becomes available, outreach to the public and the medical community can be promoted to develop awareness of childhood cancer and the positive outlook with treatment.

RECOMMENDATION 6-1. GAVI and other international partners should continue to assist countries to incorporate HBV vaccination into their childhood immunization programs as quickly as possible, with support from the global cancer community.

RECOMMENDATION 6-2. Countries with a high liver cancer burden and significant aflatoxin contamination of foodstuffs should examine the options for aflatoxin exposure reduction. *Development partners should help to implement those measures that are feasible and cost-effective.*

RECOMMENDATION 6-3. Countries should actively plan for the introduction of HPV vaccination as more information becomes available about the vaccines and as they become affordable. The international community should support a global dialogue on HPV vaccine policy and pricing.

RECOMMENDATION 6-4. Countries and global partners should follow the evolving information on newer screening approaches and determine the feasibility of adoption, given local resources and infrastructure.

RECOMMENDATION 6-5. Countries should aim to provide access to treatment and psychosocial services for children and young adults with highly curable cancers in pediatric cancer units in cancer centers or children's hospitals.

REFERENCES

ACCP (Alliance for Cervical Cancer Prevention). 2003. Effectiveness, safety, and acceptability of cryotherapy: A systematic literature review. *Cervical Cancer Prevention Issues in Depth*. Volume 1. [Online]. Available: http://www.path.org/files/RH_cryo_white_paper.pdf [accessed 11/12/05].

ACCP. 2004. *Planning and Implementing Cervical Cancer Prevention and Control Programs.* Seattle, WA: ACCP.

ACCP. 2006. *Home Page.* [Online]. Available: http://www.alliance-cxca.org/ [accessed June 13, 2006].

Adamson PC, Weiner SL, Simone JV, Gelband H. 2005. *Making Better Drugs for Children With Cancer.* Washington, DC: The National Academies Press.

American Cancer Society. 2005. *The History of Cancer.* [Online]. Available: http://www.cancer.org/docroot/cri/content/cri_2_6x_the_history_of_cancer_72.asp?sitearea=cri [accessed June 5, 2005].

Arillo-Santillan E, Nigenda G, Sanchez-Prado VM, Alonso De Ruiz P, Najera-Aguilar P, Lazcano-Ponce EC. 2001. Mexico City physicians' awareness about cervical cancer prevention: Implications for cancer screening. *Journal of Cancer Education* 16(2):75–79.

Association of Reproductive Health Professionals. *HIV Infection and Cervical Intraepithelial Neoplasia.* [Online]. Available: http://www.arhp.org/healthcareproviders/cme/onlinecme/hpvcp/infection.cfm [accessed March 15, 2005].

Barton M, Frommer M, Shafiq J. 2005. *The Role of Radiotherapy in Cancer Control in Low- and Middle-Income Countries.* Background paper commissioned by the Institute of Medicine.

Beutels P. 2001. Economic evaluations of hepatitis B immunization: A global review of recent studies (1994–2000). *Health Economics* 10(8):751–774.

Bosch FX, Lorincz A, Muñoz N, Meijer CJLM, Shah KV. 2002. The causal relation between human papillomavirus and cervical cancer. *Journal of Clinical Pathology* 55(4):244–265.

Bosch FX, Manos MM, Muñoz N, Sherman M, Jansen AM, Peto J, Schiffman MH, Moreno V, Kurman R, Shah KV, Alihonou E, Bayo S, Mokhtar HC, Chichareon S, Daudt A, De los Rios E, Ghadirian P, Kitinya JN, Koulibaly M. 1995. Prevalence of human papillomavirus in cervical cancer: A worldwide perspective. *Journal of the National Cancer Institute* 87(11):796–802.

Bosch FX, Muñoz N. 2002. The viral etiology of cervical cancer. *Virus Research* 89(2): 183–190.

Bosch FX, Muñoz N, De Sanjose S, Guerrerro E, Chaffari AM, Kaldor J, Castellsague X, Shah KV. 1994. Importance of human papillomavirus endemicity in the incidence of cervical cancer: An extension of the hypothesis on sexual behavior. *Cancer Epidemiology, Biomarkers & Prevention* 3(5):375–379.

Burd EM. 2003. Human papillomavirus and cervical cancer. *Clinical Microbiology Reviews* 16(1):1–17.

Castellsague X, Muñoz N. 2003. Cofactors in human papillomavirus carcinogenesis—role of parity, oral contraceptives, and tobacco smoking. *Journal of National Cancer Institute Monographs* (31):20–28.

Centers for Disease Control and Prevention. 2003. Global progress toward universal childhood hepatitis B vaccination, 2003. *Morbidity & Mortality Weekly Report* 52(36):868–870.

Chi DS, Perez CA, Lanciano RM, Kavanagh J. 2005. Cervical Cancer. In: Pazdur R, Coia LR, Hoskins WJ, Wagman LD, Editors. *Cancer Management: A Multidisciplinary Approach.* 9th ed. New York: CMP Healthcare Media. Pp. 445–476.

Chirenje ZM. 2004. *Cervical Cancer Screening and Treatment Strategies.* [Online]. Available: http://64.233.179.104/search?q=cache:qQQKmb6dqzsJ:www.hptn.org/research_studies/HPTN035MeetingsAndTrainings.htm+%22cervical+cancer+screening+and+treatment+strategies%22&hl=en&start=2. [accessed March 15. 2005].

Dai M, Bao YP, Clifford GM, Vaccarella S, Snijders PJF, Huang RD, Sun LX, Meijer CJLM, Qiao YL, Franceschi S. 2006. Human papillomavirus infection in Shanxi Province, People's Republic of China: A population-based study. *British Journal of Cancer* 95:96–101.

DeVita VT Jr., Hellman S, Rosenberg SA. 2001. *Cancer: Principles and Practice of Oncology.* 6th ed. Philadelphia, PA: Lippincott, Williams & Wilkins.

Durst M, Gissmann L, Ikenberg H, Zur Hausen H. 1983. A papillomavirus DNA from a cervical carcinoma and its prevalence in cancer biopsy samples from different geographic regions. *Proceedings of the National Academy of Sciences of the United States of America* 80(12 I):3812–3815.

Fahey MT, Irwig L, Macaskill P. 1995. Meta-analysis of Pap test accuracy. *American Journal of Epidemiology* (141):680–689.

Ferreccio C, Gage J. 2003. *Visual Inspection of the Uterine Cervix with Acetic Acid (VIA): A Critical Review and Selected Articles.* Washington, DC: Pan American Health Organization.

Ferreccio C, Prado RB, Luzoro AV, Ampuero SL, Snijders PJ, Meijer CJ, Vaccarella SV, Jara AT, Puschel KI, Robles SC, Herrero R, Franceschi SF, Ojeda JM. 2004. Population-based prevalence and age distribution of human papillomavirus among women in Santiago, Chile. *Cancer Epidemiology, Biomarkers & Prevention* 13(12):2271–2276.

Franceschi S, Dal Maso L, Arniani S, Crosignani P, Vercelli M, Simonato L, Falcini F, Zanetti R, Barchielli A, Serraino D, Rezza G. 1998. Risk of cancer other than Kaposi's sarcoma and non-Hodgkin's lymphoma in persons with AIDS in Italy. *British Journal of Cancer* 78(7):966–970.

Garrote LF, Anta JJL, Cruz EC, Romero T, Camacho R. 1996. Evaluation of the cervical cancer control program in Cuba. *Bulletin of the Pan American Health Organization* 30(4):387–391.

Giuliano AR, Sedjo RL, Roe DJ, Harris R, Baldwin S, Papenfuss MR, Abrahamsen M, Inserra P. 2002. Clearance of oncogenic human papillomavirus (HPV) infection: Effect of smoking (United States). *Cancer Causes & Control* 13(9):839–846.

Goldie SJ, Gaffikin L, Goldhaber-Fiebert JD, Gordillo-Tobar A, Levin C, Mahe C, Wright TC, Alliance for Cervical Cancer Prevention Cost Working Group. 2005. Cost-effectiveness of cervical-cancer screening in five developing countries. *New England Journal of Medicine* 353(20):2158–2168.

Goldstein ST, Zhou F, Hadler SC, Bell BP, Mast EE, Margolis HS. 2005. A mathematical model to estimate global hepatitis B disease burden and vaccination impact. *International Journal of Epidemiology* 34(6):1329.

Hall AJ, Wild CP. 2003. Liver cancer in low and middle income countries. *BMJ* 326(7397):994–995.

Harper DM, Franco EL, Wheeler C, Ferris DG, Jenkins D, Schuind A. 2004. Efficacy of a bivalent L1 virus-like particle vaccine in prevention of infection with human papillomavirus types 16 and 18 in young women: A randomised controlled trial. *Lancet* 364(9447):1757–1765.

Hewitt M, Weiner SL, Simone JV. 2003. *Child Cancer Survivorship: Improving Care and Quality of Life.* Washington, DC: The National Academies Press.

Hildesheim A, Schiffman MH, Gravitt PE. 1994. Persistence of type-specific human papillomavirus infection among cytologically normal women. *Journal of Infectious Diseases* 169:235–240.

Howard SC, Pedrosa M, Lins M, Pedrosa A, Pui CH, Ribeiro RC, Pedrosa F. 2004. Establishment of a pediatric oncology program and outcomes of childhood acute lymphoblastic leukemia in a resource-poor area. *JAMA* 291(20):2471–2475.

IARC (International Agency for Research on Cancer). 1995 (updated in 1997). *Human Papillomaviruses/IARC Monographs on the Evaluation of Carcinogenic Risks to Humans.* Lyon, France: IARC.

IARC. 2004. *GLOBOCAN 2002.* Lyon, France: IARC

IARC Working Group on the Evaluation of Cancer Preventive Strategies. 2005. *Cervix Cancer Screening.* IARC Handbooks of Cancer Prevention. Oxford, England: Oxford University Press.

International Network for Cancer Treatment and Research. 2004. Meeting of The Retinoblastoma Strategy Group, INCTR, Brussels, Belgium, April 29–30. *NETWORK* 4(4).

International Union Against Cancer. 2006. *Making a World of Difference.* [Online]. Available: http://uicc.org/index.php?id=516 [accessed 7/03/06].

Juarez-Figueroa LA, Wheeler CM, Uribe-Salas FJ, Conde-Glez CJ, Zamilpa-Mejia LG, Garcia-Cisneros S, Hernandez-Avila M. 2001. Human papillomavirus: A highly prevalent sexually transmitted disease agent among female sex workers from Mexico City. *Sexually Transmitted Diseases* 28(3):125–130.

Kensler TW, Qian GS, Chen JG, Groopman JD. 2003. Translational strategies for cancer prevention in liver. *Nature Reviews. Cancer* 3(5):321–329.

Kjaer SK, De Villiers EM, Dahl C, Engholm G, Bock JE, Vestergaard BF, Lynge E, Jensen OM. 1991. Case-control study of risk factors for cervical neoplasia in Denmark. Role of the "male factor" in women with one lifetime sexual partner. *International Journal of Cancer* 48(1):39–44.

Koutsky LA, Ault KA, Wheeler CM, Brown DR, Barr E, Alvarez FB. 2002. A controlled trial of a human papillomavirus type 16 vaccine. *New England Journal of Medicine* 347(21):1645–1651.

Kruger-Kjaer S, Van Den Brule AJC, Svare EI, Engholm G, Sherman ME, Poll PA, Walboomers JMM, Bock JE, Meijer CJLM. 1998. Different risk factor patterns for high-grade and low-grade intraepithelial lesions on the cervix among HPV-positive and HPV-negative young women. *International Journal of Cancer* 76(5):613–619.

Lacey JV Jr, Brinton LA, Abbas FM, Barnes WA, Gravitt PE, Greenberg MD, Greene SM, Hadjimichael OC, McGowan L, Mortel R, Schwartz PE, Silverberg SG, Hildesheim A. 1999. Oral contraceptives as risk factors for cervical adenocarcinomas and squamous cell carcinomas. *Cancer Epidemiology, Biomarkers & Prevention* 8(12):1079–1085.

Lancaster WD, Castellano C, Santos C. 1986. Human papillomavirus deoxyribonucleic acid in cervical carcinoma from primary and metastatic sites. *American Journal of Obstetrics & Gynecology* 154(1):115–119.

Lavanchy D. 2004. Hepatitis B virus epidemiology, disease burden, treatment, and current and emerging prevention and control measures. *Journal of Viral Hepatitis* 11(2):97–107.

Lazcano-Ponce EC, De Ruiz PA, Lopez-Carrillo L, Najera-Aguilar P, Avila-Ceniceros R, Escandon-Romero C, Cisneros MT, Hernandez-Avila M. 1997. Validity and reproducibility of cytologic diagnosis in a sample of cervical cancer screening centers in Mexico. *Acta Cytologica* 41(2):277–284.

Lazcano-Ponce EC, Moss S, Alonso de Ruiz P, Salmeron Castro J, Hernandez Avila M. 1999. Cervical cancer screening in developing countries: Why is it ineffective? The case of Mexico. *Archives of Medical Research* 30(3):240–250.

Lazcano-Ponce EC, Rascon-Pacheco RA, Lozano-Ascencio R, Velasco-Mondragon HE. 1996. Mortality from cervical carcinoma in Mexico: Impact of screening, 1980–1990. *Acta Cytologica* 40(3):506–512.

Look AT, Kirsch IR. 2002. Molecular basis of childhood cancer. In: Pizzo PA, Poplack DG, eds. *Principles and Practice of Pediatric Oncology.* 4th ed. Philadelphia, PA: Lippincott, Williams & Wilkins. Pp. 45–88.

Manos MM, Kinney WK, Hurley LB, Sherman ME, Shieh-Ngai J, Kurman RJ, Ransley JE, Fetterman BJ, Hartinger JS, McIntosh KM, Pawlick GF, Hiatt RA. 1999. Identifying women with cervical neoplasia: Using human papillomavirus DNA testing for equivocal Papanicolaou results. *Journal of the American Medical Association* 281(17):1605–1610.

Masera G, Baez F, Biondi A, Cavalli F, Chiesa R, Conter V, Fossati-Bellani F, Marinoni M, Sala A, Valsecchi MG, Tognini G. 2004. Bridging the childhood cancer mortality gap between economically developed and low-income countries: Lessons from the MISPHO experience. In: Tannenberger S, Cavalli F, Pannuti F, Editors. *Cancer in Developing Countries: The Great Challenge for Oncology in the 21st Century.* Munich, Germany: W. Zuckschwerdt Verlag GmbH. Pp. 42–60.

Massad LS, Riester KA, Anastos KM, Fruchter RG, Palefsky JM, Burk RD, Burns D, Greenblatt RM, Muderspach LI, Miotti P. 1999. Prevalence and predictors of squamous cell abnormalities in Papanicolaou smears from women infected with HIV-1. *Journal of Acquired Immune Deficiency Syndromes & Human Retrovirology* 21(1):33–41.

McCrory DC, Matchar DB, Bastian L, Datta S, Hasselblad V, Hickey J, Meyers E, Nanda K. 1999. *Evaluation of Cervical Cytology—Evidence Report/Technology Assessment Number 5.* AHCPR Publication No. 99-E010. Durham, NC: Agency for Healthcare Research and Policy.

Meyers C, Laimins LA. 1994. In vitro systems for the study and propagation of human papillomaviruses. *Current Topics in Microbiology & Immunology* 186:199–215.

Molano M, Posso H, Weiderpass E, van den Brule AJ, Ronderos M, Franceschi S, Meijer CJ, Arslan A, Munoz N, HPV Study Group. 2002. Prevalence and determinants of HPV infection among Colombian women with normal cytology. *British Journal of Cancer* 87(3):324–333.

Moreno V, Bosch FX, Muñoz N, Meijer CJLM, Shah KV, Walboomers JMM, Herrero R, Franceschi S. 2002. Effect of oral contraceptives on risk of cervical cancer in women with human papillomavirus infection: The IARC multicentric case-control study. *Lancet* 359(9312):1085–1092.

Moscicki AB, Shiboski S, Broering J. 1998. The natural history of human papillomavirus infection as measured by repeated DNA testing in adolescent and young women. *Journal of Pediatrics* 132:277–284.

Muñoz N, Xavier Bosch F, Castellsague X, Diaz M, De Sanjose S, Hammouda D, Shah KV, Meijer CJLM. 2004. Against which human papillomavirus types shall we vaccinate and screen? The international perspective. *International Journal of Cancer* 111(2):278–285.

Nanda K, McCrory DC, Myers ER, Bastian LA, Hasselblad V, Hickey JD, Matchar DB. 2000. Accuracy of the Papanicolaou test in screening for and follow-up of cervical cytologic abnormalities: A systematic review. *Annals of Internal Medicine* 132(10):810–819.

Oguchi M, Komura J, Tagami H. 1981. Ultrastructural studies of spontaneously regressing plane warts: Macrophages attack verruca-epidermal cells. *Archives of Dermatological Research* 270:403–411.

Ottaviano M, La Torre P. 1982. Examination of the cervix with the naked eye using acetic acid test. *American Journal of Obstetrics & Gynecology* 143(2):139–142.

Palacio V, De Sanjose S, Vazquez S, Puente M, Vazquez F, Bosch FX. 1993. Cervical neoplasia and sexually transmitted diseases among prostitutes in Oviedo, Spain. *International Journal of STD & AIDS* 4(2):121–122.

Parkin DM, Ferlay J, Hamdi-Cherif M, Sitas F, Thomas JO, Wabinga H, Whelan SL. 2003. *Cancer in Africa: Epidemiology and Prevention.* Lyon, France: IARC Press.

Pham TH, Nguyen TH, Herrero R, Vaccarella S, Smith JS, Nguyen Thuy TT, Nguyen HN, Nguyen BD, Ashley R, Snijders PJ, Meijer CJ, Munoz N, Parkin DM, Franceschi S. 2003. Human papillomavirus infection among women in South and North Vietnam. *International Journal of Cancer* 104(2):213–220.

Plummer M, Herrero R, Franceschi S, Meijer CJLM, Snijders P, Bosch FX, De Sanjose S, Muñoz N. 2003. Smoking and cervical cancer: Pooled analysis of the IARC multi-centric case-control study. *Cancer Causes & Control* 14(9):805–814.

Ribeiro RC, Pui CH. 2005. Saving the children—improving childhood cancer treatment in developing countries. *New England Journal of Medicine* 352(21):2158–2160.

Ries LAG, Eisner MP, Kosary KL, Hankey BF, Miller BA, Clegg L, Edwards BK, eds. 2002. *SEER Cancer Statistics Review, 1973–1999.* Bethesda, MD: National Cancer Institute, SEER Program.

Ronco G, Ghisetti V, Segnan N, Snijders PJ, Gillio-Tos A, Meijer CJ, Merletti F, Franceschi S. 2005. Prevalence of human papillomavirus infection in women in Turin, Italy. *European Journal of Cancer* 41(2):297–305.

Sankaranarayanan R, Basu P, Wesley RS, Mahe C, Keita N, Mbalawa CCG, Sharma R, Dolo A, Shastri SS, Nacoulma M, Nayama M, Somanathan T, Lucas E, Muwonge R, Frappart L, Parkin DM. 2004a. Accuracy of visual screening for cervical neoplasia: Results from an IARC multicentre study in India and Africa. *International Journal of Cancer* 110(6):907–913.

Sankaranarayanan R, Budukh AM, Rajkumar R. 2001. Effective screening programmes for cervical cancer in low- and middle-income developing countries. *Bulletin of the World Health Organization* 79(10):954–962.

Sankaranarayanan R, Gaffikin L, Jacob M, Sellors J, Robles S. 2005. A critical assessment of screening methods for cervical neoplasia. *International Journal of Gynecology & Obstetrics* 89(Suppl 2):S4–S12.

Sankaranarayanan R, Thara S, Sharma A, Roy C, Shastri S, Mahe C, Muwonge R, Fontaniere B. 2004b. Accuracy of conventional cytology: Results from a multicentre screening study in India. *Journal of Medical Screening* 11(2):77–84.

Sankaranarayanan R, Wesley R, Somanathan T, Dhakad N, Shyamalakumary B, Amma NS, Parkin DM, Nair MK. 1998. Visual inspection of the uterine cervix after the application of acetic acid in the detection of cervical carcinoma and its precursors. *Cancer* 83(10):2150–2156.

Sankaranarayanan R, Wesley R, Thara S, Dhakad N, Chandralekha B, Sebastian P, Chithrathara K, Parkin DM, Nair MK. 2003. Test characteristics of visual inspection with 4% acetic acid (VIA) and Lugol's iodine (VILI) in cervical cancer screening in Kerala, India. *International Journal of Cancer* 106(3):404–408.

Schiffman MH, Brinton LA. 1995. The epidemiology of cervical carcinogenesis. *Cancer* 76(10 Suppl):1888–1901.

Sehgal A, Singh V, Bhambhani S, Luthra UK. 1991. Screening for cervical cancer by direct inspection. *Lancet* 338(8762):282.

Serraino D, Carrieri P, Pradier C, Bidoli E, Dorrucci M, Ghetti E, Schiesari A, Zucconi R, Pezzotti P, Dellamonica P, Franceschi S, Rezza G. 1999. Risk of invasive cervical cancer among women with, or at risk for, HIV infection. *International Journal of Cancer* 82(3):334–337.

Shah KV, Viscidi RP, Alberg AJ, Helzlsouer KJ, Comstock GW. 1997. Antibodies to human papillomavirus 16 and subsequent in situ or invasive cancer of the cervix. *Cancer Epidemiology Biomarkers and Prevention* 6(4):233–237.

Shanta V. 2000. *Partner Profile: Cancer Institute (WIA), Chennai, India.* [Online]. Available: http://www.inctr.org/publications/2000_v01_n01_a07.shtml [accessed January 25, 2006].

Shin HR, Lee DH, Herrero R, Smith JS, Vaccarella S, Hong SH, Jung KY, Kim HH, Park UD, Cha HS, Park S, Touze A, Munoz N, Snijders PJ, Meijer CJ, Coursaget P, Franceschi S. 2003. Prevalence of human papillomavirus infection in women in Busan, South Korea. *International Journal of Cancer* 103(3):413–421.

Slawson DC, Bennett JH, Herman JM. 1992. Are Papanicolaou smears enough? Acetic acid washes of the cervix as adjunctive therapy: A HARNET study. *Journal of Family Practice* 35(3):271–277.

Smith JS, Green J, Berrington De Gonzalez A, Appleby P, Peto J, Plummer M, Franceschi S, Beral V. 2003. Cervical cancer and use of hormonal contraceptives: A systematic review. *Lancet* 361(9364):1159–1167.

Sodhani P, Gupta S, Singh V, Sehgal A, Mitra AB. 2004. Eliminating the diagnosis atypical squamous cells of undetermined significance: Impact on the accuracy of the Papanicolaou test. *Acta Cytologica* 48(6):783–787.

St. Jude Children's Research Hospital. 2003. *About International Outreach.* [Online]. Available: http://www.stjude.org/international-outreach/0,2564,455_3206_5160,00.html [accessed February 8, 2006].

St. Jude Children's Research Hospital. 2005. *International Outreach Program—I.O.P. Annual Report 2005.* Memphis, TN: St. Jude Children's Research Hospital.

St. Jude Children's Research Hospital. 2006. *About St. Jude.* [Online]. Available: http://www.stjude.org/aboutus [accessed February 8, 2006].

Steenbergen RDM, Walboomers JMM, Meijer CJLM, Van der Raaij-Helmer EMH, Parker JN, Chow LT, Broker TR, Snijders PJF. 1996. Transition of human papillomavirus type 16 and 18 transfected human foreskin keratinocytes towards immortality: Activation of telomerase and allele losses at 3p, 10p, 11q and/or 18q. *Oncogene* 13(6):1249–1257.

Stoler MH, Rhodes CR, Whitbeck A, Wolinsky SM, Chow LT, Broker TR. 1992. Human papillomavirus type 16 and 18 gene expression in cervical neoplasias. *Human Pathology* 23(2):117–128.

Sun XW, Kuhn L, Ellerbrock TV, Chiasson MA, Bush TJ, Wright TC Jr. 1997. Human papillomavirus infection in women infected with the human immunodeficiency virus. *New England Journal of Medicine* 337(19):1343–1349.

Swaddiwudhipong W, Chaovakiratipong C, Nguntra P, Mahasakpan P, Lerdlukanavonge P, Koonchote S. 1995. Effect of a mobile unit on changes in knowledge and use of cervical cancer screening among rural Thai women. *International Journal of Epidemiology* 24(3):493–498.

Swaddiwudhipong W, Chaovakiratipong C, Nguntra P, Mahasakpan P, Tatip Y, Boonmak C. 1999. A mobile unit: An effective service for cervical cancer screening among rural Thai women. *International Journal of Epidemiology* 28(1):35–39.

Szarewski A, Cuzick J. 1998. Smoking and cervical neoplasia: A review of the evidence. *Journal of Epidemiology and Biostatistics* 3:229–256.

Thomas DB, Ray RM, Koetsawang A, Kiviat N, Kuypers J, Qin Q, Ashley RL, Koetsawang S. 2001a. Human papillomaviruses and cervical cancer in Bangkok. Risk factors for invasive cervical carcinomas with human papillomavirus types 16 and 18 DNA. *American Journal of Epidemiology* 153(8):723–731.

Thomas DB, Ray RM, Kuypers J, Kiviat N, Koetsawang A, Ashley RL, Qin Q, Koetsawang S. 2001b. Human papillomaviruses and cervical cancer in Bangkok. The role of husbands and commercial sex workers. *American Journal of Epidemiology* 153(8):740–748.

Thomas JO, Herrero R, Omigbodun AA, Ojemakinde K, Ajayi IO, Fawole A, Oladepo O, Smith JS, Arslan A, Munoz N, Snijders PJ, Meijer CJ, Franceschi S. 2004. Prevalence of papillomavirus infection in women in Ibadan, Nigeria: a population-based study. *British Journal of Cancer* 90(3):638–645.

Turner PC, Sylla A, Diallo MS, Castegnaro JJ, Hall AJ, Wild CP. 2002. The role of aflatoxins and hepatitis viruses in the etiopathogenesis of hepatocellular carcinoma: A basis for primary prevention in Guinea-Conakry, West Africa. *Journal of Gastroenterology & Hepatology* 17(Suppl):S441–S448.

Usmani GN. 2001. Pediatric oncology in the third world. *Current Opinion in Pediatrics* 13(1):1–9.

Villa LL, Costa RL, Petta CA, Andrade RP, Ault KA, Giuliano AR, Wheeler CM, Koutsky LA, Malm C, Lehtinen M, Skjeldestad FE, Olsson SE, Steinwall, Brown DR, Kurman RJ, Ronnett BM, Stoler MH, Ferenczy A, Harper DM, Tamms GM, Yu J, Lupinacci L, Railkar R, Taddeo FJ, Jansen KU, Esser MT, Sings HL, Saah AJ, Barr E. 2005. Prophylactic quadrivalent human papillomavirus (types 6, 11, 16, and 18) L1 virus-like particle vaccine in young women: A randomized double-blind placebo-controlled multicentre phase II efficacy trial. *Lancet Oncology* 6(5):271–278.

WHO (World Health Organization). 2001. *Macroeconomics and Health: Investing in Health for Economic Development: Report of the Commission on Macroeconomics and Health.* Geneva, Switzerland: WHO.

WHO. 2002. *Cervical Cancer Screening in Developing Countries: Report of a WHO Consultation.* Geneva, Switzerland, WHO.

WHO. 2005. *Report on the Consultation on Human Papillomavirus Vaccines (DRAFT).* Unpublished.

Zielinski GD, Snijders PJF, Rozendaal L, Voorhorst FJ, Van der Linden HC, Runsink AP, De Schipper FA, Meijer CJLM. 2001. HPV presence precedes abnormal cytology in women developing cervical cancer and signals false negative smears. *British Journal of Cancer* 85(3):398–404.

7

Palliative Care

When people develop cancer, whether they are rich or poor, whether they live in a rich or poor country, and whether they have access to the best that curative medicine can offer or no access, a large proportion will suffer pain and other distressing physical and psychological symptoms. These symptoms worsen as cancer advances and death approaches. Because cancers in low- and middle-income countries (LMCs) are much more likely to go undetected until late stages and curative treatment may not be available even for early stage cancers, an even greater proportion of patients will likely experience severe symptoms than in high-income countries. The appropriate response for all such patients is palliative care to relieve pain and other symptoms and care for the person, whether he or she is on the road to recovery, has completed treatment, or is near the end of life.

The World Health Organization (WHO) definition of palliative care (Box 7-1) is comprehensive and embodies an ideal situation. Treatment of cancer and palliative care are complementary activities. Figure 7-1 illustrates the shift over time from life-prolonging treatment to palliative care. The shift signifies not only a change in the type of treatment, but a change in the intensity of treatment as the end of life nears.

The availability of primary cancer treatment and the cancer infrastructure are extremely variable in LMCs. In many low-income countries treatment may be almost nonexistent for the large majority. To the extent that cancer care is available, and particularly where governments are developing and implementing programs, they should, of course, include palliative care as an essential component. But palliative care is possible even where little

BOX 7-1
The World Health Organization Definition of Palliative Care

Palliative care is an approach that improves the quality of life of patients and their families facing the problems associated with life-threatening illness, through the prevention and relief of suffering by means of early identification and impeccable assessment and treatment of pain and other problems, physical, psychosocial, and spiritual. Palliative care:

- Provides relief from pain and other distressing symptoms;
- Affirms life and regards dying as a normal process;
- Intends neither to hasten or postpone death;
- Integrates the psychological and spiritual aspects of patient care;
- Offers a support system to help patients live as actively as possible until death;
- Offers a support system to help the family cope during the patient's illness and in their own bereavement;
- Uses a team approach to address the needs of patients and their families, including bereavement counseling, if indicated;
- Will enhance quality of life, and may also positively influence the course of illness;
- Is applicable early in the course of illness, in conjunction with other therapies that are intended to prolong life, such as chemotherapy or radiation therapy, and includes those investigations needed to better understand and manage distressing clinical complications.

SOURCE: WHO (2002).

else for cancer exists. It can become the organizing principle for expanding cancer services. In either case, some official recognition of the need for and the requirements of palliative care are almost certain to be essential for progress. Ideally, medical, nursing, and social work students (and other relevant health care workers) will receive training in palliative care and practitioners will incorporate palliative care into routine practice. The starting point in each country for each of these aspects is likely to be somewhat different, depending on existing services and circumstances.

The starting point for this chapter is an overview of palliative care in Africa, the continent with the least developed programs. Because pain control is so central to palliative care, much of the remainder of the chapter is devoted to understanding the role of pain control in palliative care for

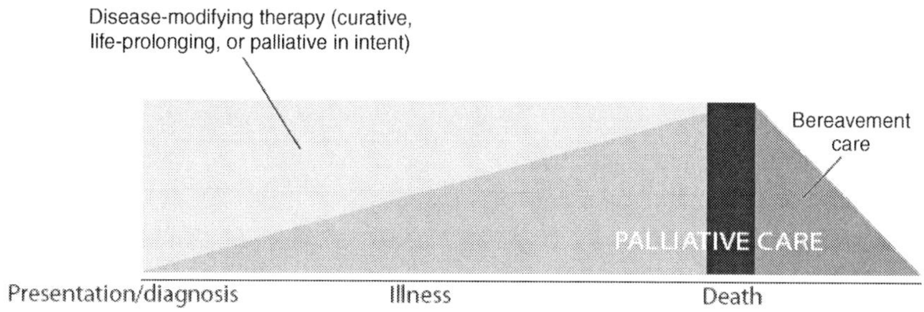

FIGURE 7-1 The need for palliative care throughout the course of serious illness. SOURCE: Reprinted, with permission, from WHO (2002). Copyright 2002 by WHO.

cancer, and to ways in which pain control can be expanded to form the core of expanded palliative care, which is taken up at the end of the chapter.

STATUS OF PALLIATIVE CARE IN AFRICA

The earliest developments in palliative care began about 25 years ago. Given the poverty, political turmoil, and myriad other challenges the African continent has had to face, it would be surprising if much effort had gone toward easing the suffering of those dying from cancer and other diseases. Progress has been slow and only a small fraction of those experiencing pain or other symptoms today receive palliative care. The general picture of a few hospices (organized services specifically for people approaching death in a matter of no more than months) and other foci of palliative care (e.g., places that provide care for symptoms at any time of illness, up to and including the end of life), and the more widespread absence of such care, has been generally acknowledged, but little detail has been attached to it. A recent survey by the Observatory on End-of-Life Care provides the first systematic look at palliative care in a large number of African countries.

Observatory on End-of-Life Care: Africa Assessment

During 2004–2005, representatives from the International Observatory on End-of-Life Care ("the Observatory") traveled around Africa meeting with contacts knowledgeable about palliative care (Personal communication, D. Clark, Director, International Observatory on End-of-Life Care, 2005). After surveying 47 countries, they developed a typology of 3 categories that captures the state of palliative care development in each country.

1. Capacity-building stage: no services operating yet, but evidence of individuals attending training programs or conferences; oral morphine largely unavailable.

2. Localized service provision: isolated palliative care and hospice services available in local areas; often heavily dependent on outside donors; no significant impact on broader national policy; oral morphine availability extremely limited.

3. Approaching integration: national recognition of the importance of palliative care (e.g., in policy documents); training readily available; reimbursement scheme for hospice/palliative care services in place; greater availability of morphine.

Of the 47 countries assessed, palliative care had no appreciable presence in 21 counties, 11 were at the "capacity-building" stage, 11 were at the stage of "localized service provision," and 4 were "approaching integration." The latter four are South Africa, Zimbabwe, Kenya, and Uganda (the most advanced, described below). The history of how services developed in each of these four is quite different, but each involves one or a few leaders without whom progress would not have occurred.

Countries may remain in stage 1 or 2 or they may progress. In countries where the situation remains unchanged for years, new or renewed leadership from within or assistance from the outside may be needed to generate movement. Progress can stop or be lost if the leaders have not been able to make headway, and this can lead to burnout and disillusionment.

The typology may be applicable outside of Africa, particularly in parts of the world where many countries are developing palliative care capacity. The Observatory will be assessing palliative care in the countries of Eastern and Central Europe and the Central Asian republics in the coming years, using this framework.

Palliative Care in Uganda: Hospice Uganda

Uganda has the most advanced hospice program in Africa that provides palliative care to patients nearing the end of life. Hospice Uganda began work out of a Kampala hospital with an old Land Rover, a grant to last 3 months, and a mandate to become the model home-based hospice for Africa for dying cancer and AIDS patients. It was started by Anne Merriman, a transplanted Irish palliative care specialist who had spent much of her career in Africa and Asia. Her experience at the Nairobi Hospice in Kenya—in 1990, only the third hospice in Africa—taught her that when trying to export the western hospice model to another continent, she needed ways that met the needs of poor Africans in their homes.

After systematically considering a number of countries interested in hosting the model project, Uganda was selected by the parent organization, Hospice Africa. The project has expanded from the original Kampala location, which has served about 4,000 patients living within 20 km of Kampala, to two rural sites. Mobile Hospice Mbarara commenced service in January 1998, using a similar model to the Kampala service. Little Hospice Hoima began one month later as a demonstration of an affordable service to reach the village level, and has treated a few hundred rural patients.

Hospice Uganda reaches farther than the three hospice programs. From the beginning, the aim was to train people from around the country to provide this care. As of February 2003, in Kampala, 20 courses to certify health professionals and 11 courses to certify volunteers had been held. More courses have been given in Mbarara, Hoima, and other districts. In total, nearly 1,000 professionals and 500 nonprofessionals have been trained. As a result, palliative care is being extended throughout the country.

In 1998, an advisory team to the Ministry of Health was formed, resulting in Uganda being the first government in Africa to list palliative care as an essential clinical service incorporated into a 5-year health plan (for 2000–2005). At this time, a senior physician and Chairman of the National Drug Authority was appointed as a senior advisor to Hospice Uganda. In 2000, the advisory team was replaced by a Palliative Care Country Team, which includes all the stakeholders, including the government, funders, and educators, as well as Hospice Uganda.

A barrier to pain relief in rural areas, in particular, was the legal requirement common to many countries that morphine be prescribed by a physician. This effectively barred most of the population from ever having access to effective pain control. Dr. Merriman insisted that oral morphine be available before starting palliative care. The government was persuaded to change the statute governing the prescribing of morphine. Guidelines were published by the Ministry of Health in 2001 to allow specialist palliative care nurses and clinical officers—trained and registered in Uganda—to prescribe morphine. Even the rural police are now aware that nurse practitioners carry morphine. Before Hospice Uganda arrived, these drugs were unavailable in the country.

Another requirement—that the diagnosis of terminal cancer or AIDS be made by a doctor—is recognized as a barrier because most people never see a doctor. In villages, the palliative care team will have to diagnose and treat without referrals, which requires training tailored to the particular area, but likely without much medical technology. As a result of these efforts, morphine is now available, paid for by the government, in about 15 of the 56 districts in the country.

The cost of treatment in Kampala and Mbarara is about $7 per week, including one home visit. About one-third of the cost is for medications (mainly liquid morphine, which is mixed locally, making it relatively inexpensive). If patients can come to the hospice center, the cost is less, about $4 per week. To the extent the service is integrated into existing systems, costs are kept low. Even with these low costs, the majority of patients cannot even afford the medicines. Hospice Uganda is funded largely by small contributions and more recently, a few larger grants. Much of the money goes to training and advocacy, but patient care is also largely subsidized.

The following are lessons learned:

- Using existing health facilities (government, private, and mission) as a base makes hospice care more affordable.
- For HIV/AIDS, grafting palliative care knowledge onto existing support teams is affordable and effective.
- Existing expertise in palliative care is very limited, so focused training is essential.
- Palliative care must be adapted to the cultural and economic needs and resources of patients and families. These vary from country to country, and from tribe to tribe within countries.
- Government support is essential, both for lowering legal barriers to the use of oral morphine and for support of the concept of palliative care.

Hospice Uganda has successfully begun a long process of assimilating palliative care into the lives of Africans in all types of places. Still, even in Uganda, only a few hundred of the estimated quarter million (out of the total population of 24 million) in pain at any one time currently receive adequate control of their symptoms.

Since 2001, Hospice Uganda has expanded its advocacy and training about innovative and low-cost ways to provide palliative care and morphine to other African countries. Hospice Uganda has introduced needs assessments in the catchment areas of the three hospice programs in the country, but these also serve as models. In 2002, WHO assisted five other countries in Africa with similar assessments as first steps toward establishing hospice programs, and this work continues. In 2006, the new African Palliative Care Association and partners sponsored a special workshop on opioid availability for palliative care for teams from six sub-Saharan African countries, using the template of the guidelines in WHO's *Achieving Balance in National Opioids Control Policy* (WHO, 2000) to develop action strategies to improve patient access to oral morphine. In addition, 12 African countries are receiving funding assistance from the President's Emergency Plan for AIDS Relief (PEPFAR), the U.S. bilateral program to assist 15 low-income countries with high rates of HIV infection and AIDS. One of PEPFAR's stated aims is to improve palliative care for people with AIDS. This could be a means for countries to build a palliative care program that would be equally appropriate for people dying from cancer and other diseases.

PAIN AND PALLIATIVE CARE

An essential part of cancer control is palliative care and pain management, which includes patient access to opioid drugs. According to WHO, "A palliative care programme cannot exist unless it is based on a rational national drug policy," and this includes "regulations that allow ready access of suffering patients to opioids" (WHO, 2002). One reason why pain control has been relatively slow to develop is that opioid pain medicines, while considered by international health authorities to be essential medicines, have been strictly regulated as narcotic drugs by government law enforcement and drug regulatory agencies to prevent diversion and abuse. Consequently, the cancer and palliative care community is faced with a unique challenge: how to develop cooperative relationships with government drug control and law enforcement agencies, leading to reform of overly restrictive opioid control policies at every level—international, national, and state or province.

The Impact of Pain

Unrelieved pain dramatically affects quality of life and sometimes the will to live. Patients with persistent pain rated as 5 or greater on a 10-point scale have clear and significant functional limitations that affect relationships, social activities, and ability to work and care for families (Daut et al., 1983). Increasing pain produces higher rates of depression and anxiety (Rosenfeld et al., 1996).

The suffering of an individual patient radiates throughout households, neighborhoods, and villages. Caregiver distress, anxiety, and depression are clearly associated with inadequate control of a family member's symptoms. In places where the burden of care falls on the family, the persistence of pain and the suffering of the individual erodes the quality of life of family members. Family caregivers often have to give up their schooling or employment to remain home to care for a family member. In developing countries, the loss of patient or caregiver income may dramatically affect the social status of the family. Families of people dying from cancer who provide care at home—the preferred place for many—must face unrelieved pain and suffering daily with little or no access to the palliative care interventions that could vastly improve the quality of life of all involved (Joranson, 2004; Murray et al., 2003).

Pain in Patients With Cancer

Several well-defined acute and chronic pain syndromes are associated with cancer and its treatment (Table 7-1) (Breitbart, 2003; Foley, 1878, 1994; Hewitt et al., 1997; Portenoy and Lesage, 1999). The prevalence of cancer pain syndromes differs between high- and low-income countries. In

TABLE 7-1 Cancer-Related Chronic Pain Syndromes

Tumor-Related Syndromes	
Bone pain	Multifocal or generalized bone pain Vertebral syndromes Back pain and epidural compression Pain syndromes of the bony pelvis and hip

Headache and facial pain	Intracerebral tumor
	Leptomeningeal metastases
	Base of skull metastases
	  Orbital syndrome
	  Parasellar syndrome
	  Middle cranial fossa syndrome
	  Jugular foramen syndrome
	  Occipital condyle syndrome
	  Clivus syndrome
	  Sphenoid sinus syndrome

Painful cranial neuralgias	Glossopharyngeal neuralgia Trigeminal neuralgia
Tumor involvement of the peripheral nervous system	Tumor-related peripheral neuropathy Cervical plexopathy Brachial plexopathy Paraneoplastic painful peripheral neuropathy
Pain syndromes of the viscera and miscellaneous tumor-related syndromes	Hepatic distention syndrome Midline retroperitoneal syndrome Chronic intestinal obstruction Peritoneal carcinomatosis Malignant perineal pain Malignant pelvic floor myalgia Ureteric obstruction
Cancer Therapy-Related Syndromes	
Postchemotherapy pain syndromes	Chronic painful peripheral neuropathy Avascular necrosis of femoral or humeral head Plexopathy associated with intra-arterial infusion Gynecomastia with hormonal therapy for prostate cancer
Chronic postsurgical pain syndromes	Postmastectomy pain syndrome Postradical neck dissection pain Postthoracotomy pain Postoperative frozen shoulder Phantom pain syndromes Stump pain Postsurgical pelvic floor myalgia
Chronic postradiation pain syndromes	Radiation-induced peripheral nerve tumor Radiation-induced brachial and lumbosacral plexopathies
Chronic radiation myelopathy	Chronic radiation enteritis and proctitis Burning perineum syndrome Osteoradionecrosis

SOURCE: Based on Foley (1979; 1994).

low-income countries, where patients often present late in the course of their illness, tumor-related chronic cancer pain syndromes are more common than treatment-related syndromes.

Prevalence of Pain in Patients with Cancer

Studies from around the world consistently report that 60 to 90 percent of patients with advanced cancer, and up to one-third of patients under active cancer treatment, experience moderate to severe pain, across all age groups, among men and women, and among ambulatory and hospitalized patients (Foley, 1979, 1999; Daut and Cleeland, 1982; Cleeland et al., 1988a; Cleeland et al., 1996; Stjernsward and Clark, 2003). Most studies are from Europe and North America, but results are similar in the few studies reported from developing countries, including India, Thailand, Vietnam, the Philippines, and China.

The intensity, degree of pain relief, and effect of pain on quality of life in patients vary according to the type and stage of cancer, treatment, and personal characteristics. Pain syndromes are common. Key studies have found:

- 90 percent of ambulatory lung or colon cancer patients in the United States experienced pain more than one-quarter of the time; for 50 percent, pain interfered with general activity or work. Pain lasted a median of 4 weeks at moderate intensity (Portenoy et al., 1992).
- 60 percent of outpatients in an oncology clinic in the Netherlands were in pain, with 20 percent reporting moderate to severe pain (Schuit et al., 1998).
- 56 percent of patients followed by the U.S. Eastern Cooperative Oncology Group reported moderate to severe pain half of the time, and for 36 percent, it interfered with daily functioning (Cleeland et al., 1994).
- 69 percent of cancer patients in France reported pain sufficient to interfere with their function (Larue et al., 1995).
- Anxiety, depression, and history of previous substance abuse negatively influence the experience of cancer pain (Kelsen et al., 1995).

Most cancer pain is directly related to the tumor itself, including 85 percent of patients referred to an inpatient cancer pain consultation service, and 65 percent of patients seen in an outpatient cancer center pain clinic in the 1970s in the United States (Foley, 1979). Bone pain is the most common tumor-associated pain, followed by tumor infiltration of nerves, and infiltration and obstruction of internal organs. Tumors that commonly metastasize to bone, such as breast or prostate cancer, result in a higher prevalence of pain (80 percent) than do lymphomas and leukemias (Foley, 1979). The prevalence and severity of pain increase with disease progression; fewer than 15 percent of patients with nonmetastatic disease report pain. Tumors near neurologic structures are more likely to cause pain. Cancer treatment causes pain in approximately 15 to 25 percent of patients receiving chemotherapy, surgery, or radiotherapy.

Burden of Pain in the Final Stages of Cancer

Pain-Days: A Metric for Moderate to Severe Pain

No standard metric describes the pain burden for people at the end of life. Measures used to quantify the effects of disease—disability-adjusted life-years (DALYs), years of life lost, quality-adjusted life-years (QALYs)—are less appropriate for the severe pain associated with dying. A transparent and direct measure, called *pain-days*, has been proposed (Foley et al., 2006), defined as the total number of person-days of moderate or severe pain requiring treatment with opioid drugs for adequate relief.

To the extent it is known, the patterns of pain from specific cancers at given stages are similar everywhere: a lung cancer patient dying in the United States and one dying in sub-Saharan Africa have similar pain, if untreated. But different cancers produce different symptoms (from the disease and from the treatment), so the mix of cancers in a country strongly influences the overall pain pattern. The mix is highly variable: The common cancers of many poor countries (e.g., of the liver, stomach, and esophagus) are less common in wealthy countries.

The two elements that determine the number of cancer pain-days in a population are (1) the numbers of people dying painful deaths and (2) the average prevalence and duration of severe pain in those individuals.

Numbers of Deaths from Cancer

About 2.1 million deaths from cancer occur annually in LMCs worldwide, and both the mortality rates and numbers are increasing. In contrast to wealthier countries, in developing countries about 80 percent of cancers are detected very late, when palliation is most needed (Stjernsward and Clark, 2003).

Prevalence and Duration of Severe Pain in Those Dying from Cancer

The extent of severe pain among people dying of cancer is poorly documented. Expert opinion suggests about 80 percent of people dying from cancer experience moderate or severe pain during their final days, and the average duration of severe pain is 90 days (Foley et al., 2006). This varies by type of cancer and the course of the particular cancer. Each patient is different and each situation requires assessment by a knowledgeable person to determine the degree of pain relief needed. The main point is that most people with cancer would benefit greatly from pain relief, and for most, the need will be greatest during the final days, weeks, or months.

INTERVENTIONS FOR PAIN RELIEF

The goal of pain treatment is not to cure disease, but to improve quality of life: to allow the patient to function as effectively as possible for as long as possible, and to die with as little pain as possible. Pain can occur at any stage of cancer, but is most severe near the end of life, when the strongest drugs—opioids—are needed. Interventions used for pain relief include drug treatment; radiotherapy; and anesthetic, neurosurgical, psychological, and behavioral approaches, each of which is appropriate for certain patients and situations. Analgesic drugs are the mainstay of treatment, however.

For patients with moderate to severe pain, opioids such as morphine that are *full agonists*, meaning that they bind completely to pain-transmitting receptors, are indispensable and should be easily available in adequate doses to all cancer patients who need them, wherever they are.

WHO Cancer Pain Relief Guidelines: The Three-Step Analgesic Ladder

The WHO Cancer Unit created a Cancer Pain Relief Program, including guidelines for the treatment of cancer pain (WHO, 1990, 1996). Its "Three-Step Analgesic Ladder" (the ladder) (Figure 7-2) embodies the concept that analgesic drug therapy is the mainstay of treatment for the majority of patients with cancer pain, and that a strong opioid (morphine) is an absolute necessity to control severe pain (Table 7-2). The ladder, which is accepted internationally, is equally appropriate for patients with HIV/AIDS (O'Neill et al., 2003).

The steps in the ladder match increasing pain severity with the appropriate drug treatment. New patients can enter at any step according to the severity of their pain. Step 1 is for mild pain and treatment with non-opioid drugs which, although they are widely available, can be expensive. A patient with mild pain from bone metastases could be helped by paracetamol, aspirin, or one of the non-steroidal anti-inflammatory drugs (NSAIDs). In a patient with mild pain from a peripheral neuropathy, the combination of a non-opioid with a tricyclic antidepressant (e.g., amitriptyline) or an anticonvulsant (e.g., gabapentin) would be appropriate.

Step 2 describes patients with moderate pain or those who fail to achieve adequate relief after a trial of a non-opioid analgesic. They are candidates for a combination of a non-opioid (e.g., aspirin or acetaminophen) with

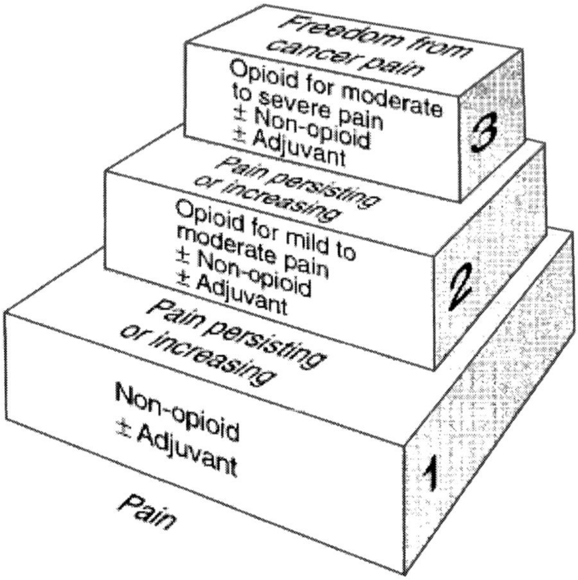

FIGURE 7-2 The Three-Step Analgesic Ladder.
SOURCE: Reprinted, with permission, from WHO (1996). Copyright 1996 by WHO.

an opioid (e.g., codeine) and also partial agonists such as propoxyphene, buprenorphine, or tramadol.

Step 3 is for patients with moderate to severe pain who require a pure opioid agonist for relief, such as morphine, hydromorphone, methadone, fentanyl, oxycodone, and levorphanol. Morphine is effective and can be less expensive than other strong opioids; however, several opioids should be available for rotation because efficacy and side effects differ between drugs and individuals. There are no recommended standard or maximum doses for opioid drugs—starting doses of oral morphine may be as little as 5 mg and therapeutic doses for severe pain may go up to more than 1,000 mg every 4 hours. The correct dose is the dose that relieves the pain. Non-opioid analgesics are often used in combination to improve efficacy and to spare opioid side effects.

Adjuvant drugs should be available at every step of the ladder to treat side effects of analgesics or provide additive analgesia (Table 7-2). Drugs in the following categories are essential to full use of the ladder: antiemetics, laxatives, antidiarrheal agents, antidepressants, antipsychotics, anticonvulsants, corticosteroids, anxiolytics, and psychostimulants.

The practical application of the ladder is summarized in five phrases: by mouth, by the clock, by the ladder, for the individual, and by attention

TABLE 7-2 Basic Drug List for Cancer and AIDS Pain Relief: Analgesics and Adjuvant Drugs

Category	Basic Drugs	Alternatives
Analgesics		
Non-opioids	acetylsalicylic acid (ASA; aspirin) paracetamol ibuprofen indomethacin	choline magnesium trisalicylate diflunisal naproxen diclofenac celecoxib rofecoxib
Opioids for mild to moderate pain	codeine	dihydrocodeine hydrocodone tramadol
Opioids for moderate to severe pain	morphine	methadone hydromorphone oxycodone pethidine buprenophine fentanyl
Opioid antagonists	naloxone	nalorphine
Adjuvant Drugs for Analgesia and Symptom Control		
Antiemetics	prochlorperazine	metaclopramide ondansetron
Laxatives	senna sodium docusate mineral oil lactulose magnesium hydroxide	bisacodyl bran dantron sorbitol
Antidiarrheal agents	loperamide diphenoxylate HCl/atropine sulfate	paregoric
Antidepressants (adjuvant analgesics)	amitriptyline	imipramine paroxetine
Antipsychotic	haloperidol	
Anticonvulsants (adjuvant analgesics)	gabapentin carbamazepine	valproic acid
Corticosteroids	prednisone dexamethasone	prednisolone
Anxiolytics	diazepam lorazepam midazolam	clonazepam
Psychostimulants	methylphenidate	pemoline

SOURCE: Foley et al. (2003).

to detail. Drugs given orally are the core treatment; other routes, including sublingual, transdermal, rectal, or subcutaneous may be needed for some patients. Analgesics should be given around the clock at fixed intervals to provide continuous relief. The dose should be titrated against the patient's pain, increasing gradually until pain is relieved or side effects are not tolerated. Effective doses should be administered on a regular schedule that maintains pain relief. Rescue doses for intermittent breakthrough pain should be readily available and administered as needed.

Effectiveness of Opioids in Pain Relief

Current recommendations for morphine use date from the mid-1980s, when WHO developed the ladder. Morphine has a much longer history, however (Wiffen, 2003). It was first extracted from opium in 1803. The properties of opium itself—a resin derived from the sap of the poppy—had been known for centuries, and noted in Pliny's Historia Naturalis in 77 A.D. In the 1950s, *Brompton's cocktail*, a mixture of morphine, chloroform, cocaine, and sometimes alcohol, was in vogue in England.

Although morphine's oral efficacy was doubted many years ago, the effectiveness of oral morphine in relieving pain today is unquestioned. The U.S. Agency for Healthcare Research and Quality sponsored an exhaustive review entitled *Management of Cancer Pain* (Goudas et al., 2001), which *assumed* the efficacy of morphine, despite the absence of large clinical trials testing morphine against no treatment or placebo. It concentrated instead on the *relative efficacy* of analgesics currently used for cancer pain. The evidence rests heavily on seminal studies of the 1960s and 1970s, when a group of investigators conducted a series of clinical trials comparing the analgesic potency of various opioid analgesics for cancer pain. Placebos were used in some studies, providing the only such comparisons of morphine versus no treatment. Most recent clinical trials have compared newer opioid formulations with morphine and other analgesics.

A Cochrane Collaboration systematic review, *Oral Morphine for Cancer Pain* (Wiffen, 2003), concludes:

> This literature review, and many years of use, show that oral morphine is an effective analgesic in patients who suffer pain associated with cancer. It remains the gold standard for moderate or severe pain.

The Cochrane review also affirmed that pain relief could be achieved in most patients by titrating the dose, and that, although sustained-release forms may be more convenient, they are not more effective than the standard immediate-release form of morphine (the least expensive formulation). They noted also that "a small number of patients . . . do not benefit from morphine or . . . may develop intolerable side effects."

Effectiveness of the Three-Step Analgesic Ladder

Field testing—confirmed by broad clinical experience—has demonstrated that 70–90 percent of cancer patients can achieve pain control if the ladder is used appropriately (Goudas et al., 2001). The evidence comes largely from developed countries, including studies using the Brief Pain Inventory (Bernabei et al., 1998), but experience has begun to accumulate in developing countries suggesting similar effectiveness (Cleeland et al., 1988b). Although the ladder has not been validated in formal AIDS studies, recent clinical reports have described its successful application to pain management in AIDS (Anand et al., 1994; Kimball and McCormick, 1996; McCormack et al., 1993; Newshan and Lefkowitz, 2001; Newshan and Wainapel, 1993; Schofferman and Brody, 1990).

Trials validating the specific choice of agents and their sequence within the ladder are limited (Mercadante, 1999), and few studies have examined relative efficacy of different drugs for specific types of pain (Eisenberg et al., 1994). There are commonly held beliefs, for example, that NSAIDs are particularly beneficial for bone pain, and that opioids are of little benefit for neuropathic pain. However, a meta-analysis of NSAIDs for metastatic bone pain suggests that they are no more effective than opioids (Eisenberg et al., 1994). Furthermore, a growing body of clinical trials has documented the effectiveness of opioids for neuropathic pain when titrated to effect (Foley, 2003).

Despite some gaps in knowledge, the ladder—with its associated drugs—is an effective tool for managing pain associated with cancer, from early to late stages. In an ideal world, a physician or other authorized and trained health workers would prescribe appropriately throughout the course of illness. Around the world, however, most patients are likely to self-medicate pain with weak or ineffective analgesics and traditional medicines they buy over the counter, sometimes leading to complications. In the real world, many people with cancer never reach the formal health care system, and if they do, they have late-stage disease and severe pain that requires oral morphine, which is largely unavailable in the health care systems of LMCs as well as some more developed countries.

ADEQUACY OF AND BARRIERS TO PAIN CONTROL IN LMCS

The adequacy of pain control in populations is not easily measured. A useful and available surrogate is the per capita consumption of morphine (Joranson, 1993), a figure based on mandatory annual reports by national governments to the International Narcotics Control Board (INCB). Of the 27 million kilograms of morphine used legally in 2002, 78 percent went to six countries—Australia, Canada, France, Germany, the United Kingdom, and the United States. The rest was consumed by the other 142 countries that reported. Morphine is largely unavailable in Africa, the eastern Mediterranean, and Southeast Asia (Table 7-3 and Figure 7-3).

Legal Controls on Opioid Drugs

The Single Convention on Narcotic Drugs of 1961, amended by the 1972 Protocol (United Nations, 1961), is an international treaty that aims both to prevent the illicit production of, trafficking in, and nonmedical use of narcotic drugs and also to ensure their availability for medical and scientific needs. The INCB, established in 1968 by the Single Convention, is the independent, quasi-judicial organization that implements the Single Convention.

The Single Convention requires that all governments (even nonsignatories) estimate annually the amounts of opioids needed for medical and scientific purposes and report annually on imports, exports, and distribution to the retail level (consumption). It also sets out the following principles on which countries can base their own policies and regulations:

- Individuals must be authorized to dispense opioids by virtue of their professional license or be specially licensed to do so.
- Opioids may only be transferred between authorized parties.
- Opioids may be dispensed only with a medical prescription.
- Security and records are required.

Many governments impose tighter restrictions that constitute significant barriers to patient access, such as burdensome licensing and prescription procedures, heavy penalties for mistakes, and limiting the amount or the number of days or the diagnoses for which an opioid prescription can be written (International Narcotics Control Board, 1989; WHO, 1996).

Cost-Effectiveness of Pain Medications

Foley and colleagues (Foley et al., 2006) analyzed the costs and cost-effectiveness of pain medications, including oral morphine, in three LMC countries: Uganda, Romania, and Chile. Based on this analysis, the cost of oral morphine ranged from $216 to $420 (Table 7-4) per year of pain-free life gained in the three sample countries. The next question is whether the pain relief that could be achieved would be worth the cost. We know that pain-free days are valued highly by patients. A day lived with the certainty of experiencing severe pain is of very low value, perhaps even lower than death itself (Furlong et al., 2001; Le Gales et al., 2002). Bryce and colleagues (2004) found that people said they were willing to give up several months of healthy life for access to good end-of-life care. Patients in low-income

TABLE 7-3 Morphine Consumption by Country According to Income Level, per Capita, 2004

Morphine mg/capita	Low	Lower Middle	Upper Middle	High
≤0.01	Burkina Faso Burundi Cambodia Central African Republic Congo, Dem. Rep. Cote d'Ivoire Guinea Mozambique Pakistan Sao Tome and Principe Sierra Leone Yemen, Rep.	Cameroon	Estonia	
>0.01–0.1	Benin Bhutan Mali Myanmar Nepal Rwanda Senegal Uzbekistan Vietnam Zambia	Algeria Bolivia Cape Verde Egypt, Arab Rep. Guatemala Indonesia Marshall Islands	Libya	
>0.1–1.0	Chad Guinea-Bissau Kenya Mongolia Tanzania Uganda Zimbabwe	Azerbaijan Belarus Bosnia and Herzegovina China Colombia Dominican Republic Ecuador El Salvador Iran, Islamic Rep. Jordan Kazakhstan Micronesia, Fed. Sts. Moldova Morocco Nicaragua Paraguay Peru Philippines Sri Lanka	Botswana Dominica Grenada Mauritius Mexico Oman Palau Panama Russian Federation St. Vincent and the Grenadines Turkey Venezuela, RB	Bahrain Brunei Darussalam Greece Kuwait Qatar Saudi Arabia United Arab Emirates

continued

TABLE 7-3 Continued

Morphine mg/capita	Low	Lower Middle	Upper Middle	High
>0.1–1.0 (continued)		Suriname Swaziland Syrian Arab Republic Thailand Tonga Turkmenistan Vanuatu		
>1.0–10.0		Brazil Bulgaria Georgia Jamaica Macedonia, FYR Namibia Serbia and Montenegro Tunisia Ukraine	Argentina Barbados Chile Costa Rica Czech Republic Hungary Latvia Lebanon Lithuania Malaysia Poland Romania Seychelles Slovak Republic South Africa Uruguay	Andorra Bahamas Cyprus Finland French Polynesia Hong Kong Israel Italy Japan Korea, Rep. Macao Malta Netherlands Antilles New Caledonia Portugal Singapore Slovenia
>10.0–20.0				Belgium Germany Ireland Netherlands Spain United Kingdom
>20.0				Australia Austria Canada Denmark France Iceland New Zealand Norway Sweden Switzerland United States

SOURCE: Pain and Policy Studies Group, University of Wisconsin/WHO Collaborating Center (2006).

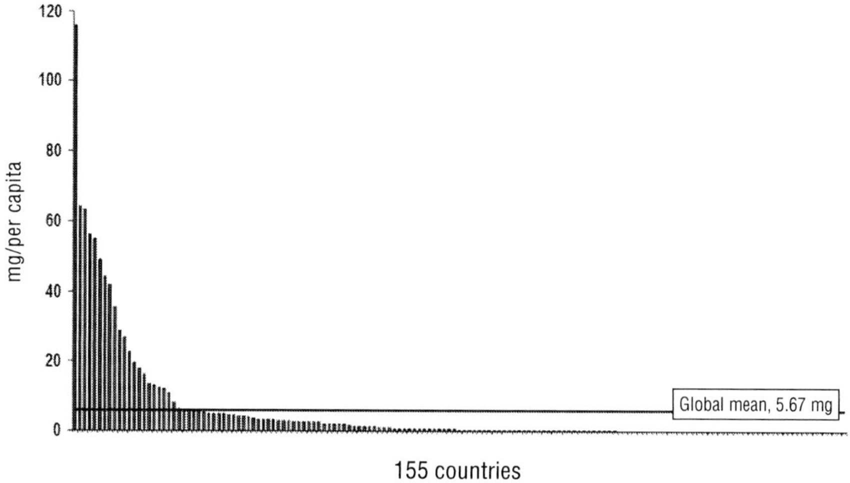

FIGURE 7-3 Global morphine consumption for 155 countries (mg/per capita, 2004).
SOURCE: Pain and Policy Studies Group, University of Wisconsin/WHO Collaborating Center (2006).

countries place as great or even greater value on pain relief as patients in high-income countries (Cleeland et al., 1988; Murray et al., 2003).

IMPROVING PALLIATIVE CARE IN LMCS

Only a handful of LMCs have thus far made significant progress in palliative care, and each case is unique. Although there is no recipe for either initiating or upgrading palliative care services in countries with little or no

TABLE 7-4 Cost Analysis Results (all costs in $US, 2002)

	Uganda	Chile	Romania
Total incremental annual cost of oral morphine (US$ millions)	$4.2 m	$1.0 m	$2.2m
Incremental annual cost per capita	$0.18	$0.06	$0.10
Incremental number of pain-days per year avoided with oral morphine	3.6 m	0.9 m	1.9 m
Incremental cost per person-day of pain avoided	$1.17	$1.17	$1.17
Incremental cost per year of pain-free life added	$420	$420	$420

SOURCE: Reprinted, with permission, from Foley et al. (2006). Copyright 2006 by the World Bank.

capacity, common elements suggest some ways forward. At the heart of change invariably is a small core of motivated, dedicated, and charismatic leaders who champion palliative care and hospice services. Often, these are health care professionals who have been burdened with the care of patients dying in unrelieved pain. Progress usually depends on links to expertise and partners from inside and outside the country to assist with a variety of unfamiliar tasks. These include expertise in setting up nongovernmental organizations, creating an inclusive platform for advocacy, and training and mentoring enough people to reach the critical mass needed to begin providing services. Technical, financial, and motivational assistance to local leaders can make these tasks manageable. These same the local leaders also become involved in the advocacy work necessary to obtain opioid pain medications and to address the barriers to patient access.

Improving Pain Control as the Entry Point in Improving Palliative Care

In the many countries that lack adequate pain control and palliative care, the basic reasons tend to be similar: low priority of pain relief and palliative care in the national health care system, lack of knowledge about how to treat pain on the part of health care practitioners, patient fears and misunderstanding of the medications (including opioid analgesics), and regulatory barriers to opioid analgesics. WHO's position (which is widely accepted) is that a palliative care program cannot exist without patient access to opioid drugs. Creating access where it does not exist invariably requires policy activities at national and local levels within a country, as well as international interactions, e.g., with the INCB. It involves not only the health care sector, but regulators, law enforcement, and others. The centrality of drug availability has made it a cornerstone for the development of palliative care in LMCs. The University of Wisconsin Pain and Policy Studies Group (PPSG) on Policy and Communications in Cancer Care, or WHOCC (a WHO Collaborating Center), is a leading international resource for providing assistance to national efforts to expand access to opioid drugs as a means of improving palliative care. The PPSG has tried different approaches to moving pain control forward in different parts of the world by providing tools and training for professionals in the public and private sectors and fostering collaboration among different sectors within countries.

A major thrust of PPSG's work has been, in collaboration with WHO and the Open Society Institute, regional workshops, of which four have been held: in Quito for six Latin American countries (in 2000), in Gabarone for five sub-Saharan African countries (2002), in Budapest for six central and Eastern European countries (in 2002), and in Entebbe (in 2006) for six sub-Saharan countries. More recently (October 2006), PPSG hosted leaders in palliative care from 8 LMCs in Wisconsin for one week of training and discussion. An aim of each of these meetings has been the development of an action plan for each participating country to improve the availability of opioid medications for relief of pain and suffering of cancer and AIDS patients at the end of life.

A weakness of the regional workshops had been lack of resources for follow-up by PPSG and for taking forward the plans developed on the part of the participants. This was possible in only limited cases (e.g., Romania, described in detail below). A change with the October 2006 effort is that each participant is also being supported for a part of his or her time on return to work, and the PPSG will be involved with each one.

PROGRESS IN PAIN CONTROL IN ROMANIA: A CASE EXAMPLE

A team from Romania participated in the Budapest regional workshop and emerged as ready to pursue change more immediately than any other country team. This section recounts their situation and progress.

Prerevolution narcotics policies dating back more than 35 years frequently prevented physicians in Romania from providing pain relief to cancer and AIDS patients even at the end of life. Romania's annual medical consumption of morphine, at 2.2 mg per capita (2001 data), was well below the global mean and among the lowest in Eastern Europe. After the workshop in Budapest in 2002 (see above), Romania was selected among the participating countries for a follow-up national project. The situation was that palliative care was severely impeded by regulatory barriers, leaders in palliative care wanted to work with the government to address the barriers, and the Ministry of Health appointed a Palliative Care Commission to study the law and regulations and recommend changes, demonstrating that a key ingredient—political will—was present.

The Opioid Regulatory Situation

Just a few years ago, the regulations for prescribing opioids in Romania were so complicated, restrictive, and burdensome that it was sometimes impossible for outpatients to receive oral morphine. The least restrictive option was a single 3-day prescription, even for a dying cancer patient. For certain exceptions, including incurable cancer (but not HIV/AIDS), with governmental permission, an application could be made for "long-term prescribing" for a 3-month period with each prescription lasting a maximum of 10 to 15 days. Many forms, some requiring special stamps, had to move from the hospice physician to the district oncology hospital, to the district health department, and finally to the patient's family physician, who would write a triplicate prescription for the pharmacy, where all the paperwork came together. Modern cancer pain management was basically precluded.

Process of Change

From 2003 to 2005, the Ministry of Health and its Palliative Care Commission examined and prepared a revision of the national narcotics law and regulations, with review and comment by the PPSG at the University of Wisconsin at Madison (Ryan, 2005). A new law eliminating the regulatory barriers was adopted by the Romanian Parliament in November 2005. Implementing regulations consistent with the new law have been adopted. The study and drafting process took place during a visit from a five-member Romanian team to the PPSG in late 2004.

Under the new law and regulations, the previous special authorization procedure is no longer necessary for opioids to be prescribed. Physicians now have, for the first time, independent ability to prescribe an amount for 30 days with no limit on dose. Patient eligibility based on diagnosis has been removed (Mosoiu et al., 2006).

The example being set by Romania could be a model for Central and Eastern Europe and the Former Soviet Union countries that lack policy models for improving opioid availability. However, the situation is unique in each country and change will still require country-by-country approaches and outside assistance as the situation requires.

The WHOCC and Development of Pain Control and Palliative Care in India[1]

For decades, the only morphine available in India was injectable, used for postoperative pain. Enactment of a strict national narcotics law in 1985 caused legal morphine consumption reported by the Government of India to decline even further, from a high of 573 kilograms to 18 kilograms in 1997, among the lowest per-capita consumption in the world. The reporting of morphine consumption has since ceased. Ironically, much of the world's morphine supply originates in legal poppy cultivation in India, but only a trickle was used domestically. It was during the period of declining consumption that international efforts to promote pain control and palliative care programs began to reach India. The first program, Shanti Avedna Ashram, was established in 1986. In 1992, pain relief and the availability of morphine were designated priorities in the National Cancer Control Programme and WHO provided substantial education in palliative care.

The Ministry of Health convened a series of national workshops from 1992 to 1994 in cooperation with the WHOCC to find out why morphine

[1]Based on Joranson et al. (2002); Rajagopal and Venkateswaran (2003); and Rajagopal et al. (2001).

was so difficult to obtain. The following experience, recounted by a former Narcotics Commissioner of India, is instructive:

> . . . [Hospital name] is a referral hospital for cancer management. The annual requirement of morphine is approximately 10,000 tablets of 20 mg. But the Institute has not been able to procure a single tablet till date, primarily due to the stringent state laws and multiplicity of licenses. After a lot of effort, the Institute had been able to obtain the licenses in 1994 and had approached [a manufacturer] for a supply of tablets. At the relevant time [the manufacturer] did not have the tablets in stock and by the time the tablets could be arranged, the licenses had expired. The doctors at the Institute and the associated pain clinic have stopped prescribing morphine tablets because they would not be available (Joranson et al., 2002).

The situation was so extreme that in 1999, the INCB called on the Government of India to take measures to make morphine available for medical uses (Joranson et al., 2002).

In 1994, an initiative begun by the WHOCC, the Indian Association of Palliative Care, and the Pain and Palliative Care Society systematically studied the reasons for the lack of morphine. The 1985 national law passed to diminish narcotic trafficking and abuse included stringent punishments for narcotics infractions, which increased doctors' reluctance to prescribe morphine and pharmacists' reluctance to stock it. At the state level, palliative care programs had to obtain multiple licenses from two different departments to obtain opioids and to move morphine between different states in India. The result was gridlock.

In 1997, the WHOCC developed a proposal to reduce the number of licenses and extend their period of validity, among other measures. The Revenue Secretary in New Delhi accepted the recommendations and in 1998, sent instructions to all state governments to adopt a model simplified licensing rule developed from the proposal. This request had little initial effect, so the WHOCC and the WHO Demonstration Project at the Pain and Palliative Care Society in Calicut held workshops with officials and cancer and palliative care stakeholders in several states to encourage the needed changes. Gradually, rules have begun to change. By 2002, 7 of 28 states or territories had adopted the model rule, but only in the state of Kerala (population 32 million) has it been implemented successfully, so that community-based palliative care programs can be licensed to order morphine and thus can provide uninterrupted access to it.

Four factors have led to the success in Kerala:

1. The state government simplified the licensing process and agreed that oral morphine could be available to palliative care centers with at least one doctor having at least one month of practical experience in palliative care;

2. The national Drugs Controller exempted palliative care programs from needing a drug license, thereby eliminating the need for a pharmacist and the associated costs;

3. A hospital pharmacy in the state became a local manufacturer and distributor of inexpensive oral morphine tablets, obtaining its supply of morphine powder from the national factory; and

4. A palliative care network has been established, consisting of about 50 small programs, each having a physician licensed to obtain and dispense morphine. Statewide coverage has increased to about 20 percent of those needing palliative care.

Another New Approach in India

While the success in Kerala is remarkable, the overall picture in the rest of India is not. Those who have led in Kerala, through "Pallium India," a nongovernmental organization, and the WHOCC are beginning to test a new strategy to extend palliative care with oral morphine to other parts of India where cancer hospitals lack palliative care and oral morphine. The plan builds on the fact that palliative care in India (as elsewhere) started and is growing mainly as a result of local interest and leadership, rather than through policy directives from the national government (although the fact that the government has pronounced palliative care a priority enables further development). The new approach is aimed at cancer institutions with little or no palliative care and is based on the "WHO triangle," which asserts that the three basic ingredients of success are policy, education and training, and drug availability. The approach seeks to integrate the following into cancer institutions: (1) a policy to provide palliative care; (2) staff training about pain control and morphine; and (3) assurance of a continuous supply of oral morphine.

The availability of funds will allow the project to establish palliative care in three cancer centers over a period of 2 years. To begin with, all cancer centers in the country were informed of the project and given the opportunity to apply. The response was more enthusiastic than expected, with 27 cancer institutions applying. Three centers were selected in the states of Manipur, Mizoram, and Uttar Pradesh. The program has two phases: phase 1 involves training two professionals from each center and phase 2 involves education of local health care professionals and the public when the trained professionals return home. Phase 1 has been completed and the teams have returned to their cancer centers. By prior agreement (a Memorandum of Understanding), the home cancer center will be obligated to do the following:

- Initiate a palliative care service within 3 months.

• Include the cost of immediate-release morphine in their annual drug budget, take steps to ensure its uninterrupted availability, and ensure its rational use with proper documentation. Pallium India and the WHOCC will assist the centers with these tasks.

• Contribute the time of the trainees during the training period, and ensure that the trained personnel will be able to devote at least half of their working time to palliative care.

• Provide the funds to continue palliative care and morphine availability when the project terminates at the end of 2 years.

• Evaluate outcomes by submitting statistics on patient numbers, morphine prescriptions, and dispensing, according to agreed-on specifications.

Pallium India and the WHOCC will support and assist the trainees back in their home centers through periodic follow-up and e-mail consultations.

Phase 2 involves education of local health care professionals, the public, and institution administrators in each locality. The program will be directed primarily at professionals in the institution, but would be available to other professionals in the area, medical students, the public, and administrators. The acceptance of the community is essential to successful establishment of palliative care. Each 1- to 2-day workshop would take place as soon as possible after the return of the trained professionals, but not later than 6 months.

Experience in Kerala has been that once a proper palliative care program has been developed and its benefits become apparent, it can be sustained by community support. Cancer pain being emotive, support from the community is usually forthcoming. Over the long term, a visible palliative care service in one location should result in more such facilities developing elsewhere. Evaluation by the organizers will, of course, be carried out during and after the program. The external funding cost of the 2-year program for three institutions is estimated at about $40,000, provided by the U.S. National Cancer Institute. This does not include costs incurred by the institutions participating.

DISCUSSION AND RECOMMENDATIONS

Palliative care is an essential component of cancer control that is lacking or vastly underrepresented in LMCs. Because cancers tend to be recognized only at advanced stages in LMCs (and curative treatment may not be available or at least accessible), palliative care is particularly important in these countries. Among the elements of palliative care, pain control is the most essential. Severe pain is common at the end stages of many cancers, degrading quality of life for the patient and family. Palliative care cannot be adequate without pain control, which requires the use of opioid analgesics such as morphine. The legal and societal barriers to providing oral morphine to cancer patients (and others) at the community level, where it is needed, are formidable in many or most LMCs (and many high-income countries), even though the actual cost of the intervention is modest. Successes in establishing palliative care with pain control in a few places—such as Romania, India, and Uganda—demonstrate that change is possible, with considerable effort. Building on these experiences as models, it may be possible to accelerate the pace in other countries. The knowledge of how to do this now exists and should be applied more widely.

RECOMMENDATION 7-1. Governments should collaborate with national organizations and leaders to identify and remove barriers to ensure that opioid pain medications, as well as other essential palliative care medications, are available under appropriate control. *The INCB and WHO should provide enhanced guidance and support, and assist governments with this task.*

RECOMMENDATION 7-2. Palliative care, not limited to pain control, should be provided in the community to the extent possible. *This may require developing new models, including training of personnel and innovations in types of personnel who can deliver both psychosocial services and symptom relief interventions.*

REFERENCES

Anand A, Carmosino L, Glatt AE. 1994. Evaluation of recalcitrant pain in HIV-infected hospitalized patients. *Journal of Acquired Immune Deficiency Syndromes* 7(1):52–56.

Bernabei R, Gambassi G, Lapane K, Landi F, Gatsonis C, Dunlop R, Lipsitz L, Steel K, Mor V. 1998. Management of pain in elderly patients with cancer. *Journal of the American Medical Association* 279(23):1877–1882.

Breitbart W. 2003. Pain. In: O'Neill JF, Selwyn P, Schietinger H, eds., *A Clinical Guide to Supportive and Palliative Care for HIV/AIDS*. Washington, DC: Health Resources and Services Administration. Pp. 85–122.

Bryce CL, Loewenstein GARMSJ, Wax RS, Angus DC. 2004. Quality of death: Assessing the importance placed on end-of-life treatment in the intensive-care unit. *Medical Care* 42(5):423–431.

Cleeland CS, Gonin R, Hatfield AK, Edmonson JH, Blum RH, Stewart JA, Pandya KJ. 1994. Pain and its treatment in outpatients with metastatic cancer. *New England Journal of Medicine* 330(9):592–596.

Cleeland CS, Ladinsky JL, Serlin RC, Thuy NC. 1988. Multidimensional measurement of cancer pain: Comparisons of U.S. and Vietnamese patients. *Journal of Pain & Symptom Management* 3(1):23–27.

Cleeland CS, Nakamura Y, Mendoza TR, Edwards KR, Douglas J, Serlin RC. 1996. Dimensions of the impact of cancer pain in a four country sample: New information from multidimensional scaling. *Pain* 67(2–3):267–273.

Daut RL, Cleeland CS. 1982. The prevalence and severity of pain in cancer. *Cancer* 50(9):1913–1918.

Daut RL, Cleeland CS, Flanery RC. 1983. Development of the Wisconsin Brief Pain Questionnaire to assess pain in cancer and other diseases. *Pain* 17(2):197–210.

Eisenberg E, Berkey CS, Carr DB, Mosteller F, Chalmers TC. 1994. Efficacy and safety of nonsteroidal antiinflammatory drugs for cancer pain: A meta-analysis. *Journal of Clinical Oncology* 12(12):2756–2765.

Foley KM. 1979. Pain syndromes in patients with cancer. In: Foley KM, Bonica JJ, Ventafridda V, eds. *Advances in Pain Research and Therapy.* New York: Raven Press.

Foley KM. 1994. Cancer pain syndromes. In: Stanley TH, Ashburn MA, eds. *Anesthesiology in Pain Management.* Amsterdam: Kluwer Academic Publisher. Pp. 287–303.

Foley KM. 1999. Pain assessment and cancer pain syndromes. In: Doyle D, Hank G, MacDonald N, eds. *Oxford Textbook of Palliative Medicine.* 2nd ed. New York: Oxford University Press.

Foley KM. 2003. Opioids and chronic neuropathic pain. *New England Journal of Medicine* 348(13):1279–1281.

Foley KM, Wagner JL, Joranson DE, Gelband H. 2006. Pain control for people with cancer and AIDS. In: Jamison DT, Breman JG, Measham AR, Alleyne G, Claeson M, Evans DB, Jha P, Mills A, Musgrove P, eds. *Disease Control Priorities in Developing Countries.* 2nd ed. New York: Oxford University Press. Pp. 981–993.

Furlong WJ, Feeny DH, Torrance GW, Barr RD. 2001. The Health Utilities Index (HUI) system for assessing health-related quality of life in clinical studies. *Annals of Medicine* 33(5):375–384.

Goudas L, Carr DB, Bloch R. 2001. *Management of Cancer Pain. Evidence Report/Technology Assessment No. 35. AHRQ Publication No. 02-E002.* Rockville, MD: Agency for Healthcare Research and Quality.

Hewitt DJ, McDonald M, Portenoy RK, Rosenfeld B, Passik S, Breitbart W. 1997. Pain syndromes and etiologies in ambulatory AIDS patients. *Pain* 70(2–3):117–123.

International Narcotics Control Board. 1989. *Demand for and Supply of Opiates for Medical and Scientific Needs.* New York: United Nations.

Joranson DE. 1993. Availability of opioids for cancer pain: Recent trends, assessment of system barriers. New World Health Organization guidelines, and the risk of diversion. *Journal of Pain and Symptom Management* 8(6):353–360.

Joranson DE. 2004. *Regulations for Prescribing Opioids in Europe and Romania.* Bucharest, Romania.

Joranson DE, Rajagopal MR, Gilson AM. 2002. Improving access to opioid analgesics for palliative care in India. *Journal of Pain & Symptom Management* 24(2):152–159.

Kelsen DP, Portenoy RK, Thaler HT, Niedzwiecki D, Passik SD, Tao Y, Banks W, Brennan MF, Foley KM. 1995. Pain and depression in patients with newly diagnosed pancreas cancer. *Journal of Clinical Oncology* 13(3):748–755.

Kimball LR, McCormick WC. 1996. The pharmacologic management of pain and discomfort in persons with AIDS near the end of life: Use of opioid analgesia in the hospice setting. *Journal of Pain & Symptom Management* 11(2):88–94.

Larue F, Colleau SM, Brasseur L, Cleeland CS. 1995. Multicentre study of cancer pain and its treatment in France. *British Medical Journal* 310(6986):1034–1037.

Le Gales C, Buron C, Costet N, Rosman S, Slama PR. 2002. Development of a preference-weighted health status classification system in France: The Health Utilities Index 3. *Health Care Management Science* 5(1):41–51.

McCormack JP, Li R, Zarowny D, Singer J. 1993. Inadequate treatment of pain in ambulatory HIV patients. *Clinical Journal of Pain* 9(4):279–283.

Mercadante S. 1999. World Health Organization guidelines: Problem areas in cancer pain management. *Cancer Control* 6(2):191–197.

Mosoiu D, Ryan KM, Joranson DE, Garthwaite JP. 2006. Reform of drug control policy for palliative care in Romania. *Lancet Online* DOI:10.1016/S0140-6736(06)68482-1.

Murray SA, Grant E, Grant A, Kendall M. 2003. Dying from cancer in developed and developing countries: Lessons from two qualitative interview studies of patients and their carers. *British Medical Journal* 326(7385):368–371.

Newshan G, Lefkowitz M. 2001. Transdermal fentanyl for chronic pain in AIDS: A pilot study. *Journal of Pain & Symptom Management* 21(1):69–77.

Newshan GT, Wainapel SF. 1993. Pain characteristics and their management in persons with AIDS. *Journal of the Association of Nurses in AIDS Care* 4(2):53–59.

O'Neill JF, Selwyn PA, Schietinger H. 2003. *A Clinical Guide to Supportive and Palliative Care for HIV/AIDS.* Washington, DC: Health Resources and Services Administration.

Pain and Policy Studies Group. 2006. Morphine consumption figures [unpublished].

Portenoy RK, Lesage P. 1999. Management of cancer pain. *Lancet* 353(9165):1695–1700.

Portenoy RK, Miransky J, Thaler HT, Hornung J, Bianchi C, Cibas-Kong I, Feldhamer E, Lewis F, Matamoros I, Sugar MZ, Olivieri AP, Kemeny NE, Foley KM. 1992. Pain in ambulatory patients with lung or colon cancer: Prevalence, characteristics, and effect. *Cancer* 70(6):1616–1624.

Rajagopal MR, Joranson DE, Gilson AM. 2001. Medical use, misuse, and diversion of opioids in India. *Lancet* 358(9276):139–143.

Rajagopal MR, Venkateswaran C. 2003. Palliative care in India: Successes and limitations. *Journal of Pain & Palliative Care Pharmacotherapy* 17(3–4):121–128.

Rosenfeld B, Breitbart W, McDonald MV, Passik SD, Thaler H, Portenoy RK. 1996. Pain in ambulatory AIDS patients. Impact of pain on psychological functioning and quality of life. *Pain* 68(2–3):323–328.

Ryan K. 2005. Progress to remove regulatory barriers to palliative care in Romania. *Palliative Care Newsletter* 1(4).

Schofferman J, Brody R. 1990. Pain in far advanced AIDS. In: Foley KM, Bonica JJ, Ventafridda V, eds. *Advances in Pain Research and Therapy.* New York: Raven Press.

Schuit KW, Sleijfer DT, Meijler WJ, Otter R, Schakenraad J, Van den Bergh FCM, Meyboom-De Jong B. 1998. Symptoms and functional status of patients with disseminated cancer visiting outpatient departments. *Journal of Pain & Symptom Management* 16(5): 290–297.

Stjernsward J, Clark D. 2003. Palliative medicine—a global perspective. In: Doyle D, Hanks GWC, Cherny N, Calman K, eds. *Oxford Textbook of Palliative Medicine.* 3nd ed. New York: Oxford University Press.

United Nations. 1961. *Single Convention on Narcotic Drugs.* [Online] Available: http://www.incb.org/e/conv/1961/ [accessed 7/12/04].

WHO (World Health Organization). 1990. *Cancer Pain Relief and Palliative Care, Technical Report Series 804.* Geneva, Switzerland: WHO.

WHO. 1996. *Cancer Pain Relief.* 2nd ed. Geneva, Switzerland: WHO.

WHO. 2000. *Achieving Balance in National Opioids Control Policy: Guidelines for Assessment.* Geneva, Switzerland: WHO.

WHO. 2002. *National Cancer Control Programmes: Policies and Managerial Guidelines.* 2nd ed. Geneva, Switzerland: WHO.

WHO Regional Office for Europe. 2002. *Assuring Availability of Opioid Analgesics for Palliative Care: Report of a WHO Workshop Held in Budapest, Hungary; 25–27 February 2002.* Copenhagen, Denmark: WHO Regional Office for Europe.

Wiffen PJ. 2003. Pain and palliative care in The Cochrane Library: Issue number 4 for 2002. *Journal of Pain & Palliative Care Pharmacotherapy* 17(2):95–98.

8

Cancer Centers in Low- and Middle-Income Countries

Cancer centers are the focal points for cancer research and treatment advances in high-income countries. Cancer treatment takes place throughout health care systems, however, where sufficient oncology expertise exists. In the United States, for example, an estimated 80 percent of newly diagnosed cancer patients are treated in local hospitals rather than specialized cancer centers (Hewitt and Simone, 1999). In middle-income countries and some low-income countries, cancer centers have been established for cancer diagnosis and treatment and for palliative care, both in the public and private sectors. In general, most of the oncology expertise in LMCs resides in these centers.

Major cancer centers in the United States and other high-income countries take part in other aspects of cancer control, in particular programs in prevention, public education, surveillance, and research. Cancer centers in low- and middle-income countries (LMCs) tend to be less involved in other aspects of cancer control, and therein lies an opportunity. Where resources are limited, cancer centers can play an especially important role in the development of cancer control programs, as catalysts for cancer control nationally, and as points of contact for the global community. This chapter describes LMC cancer centers and their roles, discusses aspects of establishing or expanding the scope of cancer centers with at least some government support and recognition, suggests and emphasizes ways in which international efforts can help LMC centers and thus LMC cancer control, and identifies the functions that these centers might carry out. The recommendation arising from this review is that every country should aim to have at least one publicly supported "cancer center of excellence" as a cancer focus that encourages the broad objectives of cancer control and that provides exemplary patient care, appropriate to the local circumstances. This is not to suggest that a single model applies everywhere or that, as in high-income countries, a goal should not be to expand treatment to the local level, within the health care system more generally. Here, too, the notion of "resource-level appropriateness" applies. A center of excellence in Timbuktu need not look like one in Buenos Aires, Paris, or New York.

DEFINITION OF A CANCER CENTER

The term "cancer center" has no fixed definition. The United States has a well-developed network of cancer centers with official designation from the National Cancer Institute (NCI), however, and some of the language used to describe them is useful in discussing the goals and functions of cancer centers envisioned in this report for LMCs. The specifics of LMC cancer centers might differ, but the underlying goals are similar.

The NCI-designated cancer centers are the centerpiece of the U.S. effort to reduce morbidity and mortality from cancer. This includes not only providing state-of-the-art treatment, but research for the production of new knowledge about the basic nature of cancer, and about new and more effective approaches to prevention, diagnosis, and therapy. NCI describes officially recognized cancer centers as follows:

> The cancer centers are . . . the principal deliverers of medical advances to patients and their families and the chief educators of health care professionals and the public. An excellent cancer center is a local, regional, and national resource, having an impact that goes well beyond its own walls into the communities it serves directly and, by the generalizable knowledge it creates, into the world at large. . . . It is expected, for example, that centers will give greater emphasis to the particular challenges presented by special populations. The disproportionate burden of cancer in minority and other underserved groups is poorly understood and badly in need of attention from the research community. . . . Cancer centers . . . are expected to inform the public about their ongoing activities in these areas through public outreach and education (National Cancer Institute, 2006a).

Cancer centers are actual, physical places, although they may differ in how they are organized. In the United States and other countries, many cancer centers are single institutions (one building or one campus) that specialize, first and foremost, in the diagnosis and treatment of cancer. In other cases, the cancer center may be a cancer unit within a larger hospital, such as a university medical hospital that treats the full range of health conditions. In still other cases, the cancer "center" is actually a consortium of hospitals or institutions that cooperate in an integrated cancer program.

Except for government-financed medical care, such as Medicare, in the United States the financial federal contribution to officially designated cancer centers is largely NCI support of research and other activities. Patient services and, to some extent, education and outreach, are funded by other means, including patients themselves and their insurers, philanthropic donations, and support from state or local government.

CANCER CENTERS IN LMCS

By virtue of their sole focus on cancer, cancer centers in LMCs have common ground with cancer centers in the United States and other high-income countries. However, they may differ in emphasis, in structure, and in the specific components of the cancer program they carry out. They may emphasize basic research compared with patient care, outreach, and other functions, for example. In the United States, the patient care components are assumed to be well developed as part of the health care system itself. Thus, research on the full spectrum of cancer control primarily distinguishes NCI-designated cancer centers from the many hospitals and other sites where cancer patients are treated. While some of the more developed middle-income countries may have an existing health care infrastructure that provides adequate cancer diagnosis and treatment, this is not generally the case. Therefore, the development of cancer management (even if limited in scope) will be a primary goal of cancer centers in LMCs.

As in high-income countries, cancer centers in LMCs also act as focal points for cancer control nationally and as points of contact internationally. Both of these functions are vital. Being a recognizable international point of contact can bring substantial benefits, discussed later in this chapter. The reasons for being a national focal point may seem obvious. Cancer centers pioneer new treatments, establish the state of the art in treatment and other aspects of cancer control, and act as a reference center for the country. Either formally or informally, leaders in regions where cancer control is poorly developed may also act as reference centers, training centers, or perform other leadership roles. The King Hussein Cancer Center in Amman, Jordan, with the support of the NCI, has begun to fill this role in the Middle East region (NCI, 2006b).

Establishment and Core Functions of LMC Cancer Centers

The pattern of financing cancer centers in LMCs may be different from that in high-income countries. Ideally, the national government will support at least some functions, and the cancer center will be officially recognized or designated as a national cancer center. In most LMCs, where a large proportion of people do not have health insurance and cancer care is expensive relative to income, the majority may find it impossible to pay for cancer services on their own. Without covering the costs of treatment, and possibly additional expenses incurred by patients and their families (e.g., travel, subsistence of family members accompanying patients), a cancer center may be essentially inaccessible, even for those nearby. A mixture of public (national and international) and private (including philanthropic) funding may be needed to allow access to a wide range of patients.

This report recommends that every country aim to establish at least one officially designated or recognized cancer center that incorporates as many of the core functions (listed below) as possible. This could be designated as a "center of excellence." Where multiple cancer centers exist already, one (or more, if appropriate) could be selected as a center of excellence, with the addition of resources as needed to carry out the core functions. As in the United States and elsewhere, the cancer center may be a single free-standing institution, may be part of a larger complex (university or hospital), or may consist of a consortium of institutions and experts in close collaboration, but identified primarily with the cancer center. This critical mass of expertise and resources is needed to establish the cancer center presence locally and internationally. ("Critical mass" has not yet been defined for low-resource settings, and is a task that should be undertaken by an international collaborative group, possibly as part of the resource-level-appropriate definitions.)

It is encouraging that some cancer centers in LMCs have taken on broader roles in cancer control, even without official recognition (see Box 8-1). Cancer institutes such as these, where they exist, may be good candidates to take on national or regional responsibility, with official recognition.

We suggest that the core functions that cancer centers in LMCs should strive to offer include:

- **Patient care**, including the services of medical oncology, radiotherapy, surgery, supportive services (imaging, pathology), psychosocial services, and palliative care
- **Training** in all functions available at the cancer center, as appropriate to the needs and resources of the country (or smaller area, if more than one cancer center of excellence exists in the country)
- **Research**, focusing on clinical questions of particular local importance (including research on "resource-level-appropriate" questions)
- **Cancer detection and prevention programs**, locally and throughout the country, that are tailored to resource levels
- **Community outreach**, including education, prevention programs, and community-based palliative care with pain management using oral morphine

BOX 8-1
Some Leading Cancer Centers In LMCS

Cancer Institute at Chennai, India

The Cancer Institute in Chennai (formerly Madras) carries out a broad agenda of cancer control in South India, where it is the only major cancer center. The Cancer Institute was founded in 1954 by the Women's Indian Association (WIA, which is the abbreviation by which the Center is known) Cancer Relief Fund by India's first woman medical graduate. WIA began and remains a voluntary institution with no official acknowledgment of the government (Sharma, 2004).

As is the case with cancer centers worldwide, the initial focus was treating patients with cancer, which is still the mainstay. About 100,000 patients are treated each year, regardless of ability to pay. Most patients are poor and pay little or nothing for state-of-the-art care, including surgery, chemotherapy, and radiotherapy for potentially life-prolonging treatment; they also receive palliative care at little or no cost.

What distinguishes WIA is its activities beyond patient care. A College of Oncologic Sciences was established in 1984, the first in India to offer specialty training in surgical and medical oncology and medical physics. Graduates of the college are now found in cancer centers all over India. Training in cancer research is now also offered (Sharma, 2004).

Early on, WIA adopted cancer prevention and early detection as part of its mission, developed outreach programs for rural areas, developed a population-based cancer registry, and began carrying out a program of basic and applied research on cancer of local importance (cancers of the cervix, breast, and oral cavity and pediatric leukemias).

The prevention program consists of a network of initiatives for the public and professionals. Rural training centers train village health nurses and other health workers in cervical cancer screening, breast examinations, and early detection of oral cancer (Shanta, 2000).

WIA has been active at a policy level, as well. It was instrumental in exempting cancer drugs from import duty and in launching a national scheme to fund a series of regional cancer centers (Sharma, 2004).

WIA has been recognized internationally for its work, which has attracted collaborations and forged strong ties to the global cancer community. It partnered with the World Health Organization (WHO) in 1969 to establish the first international cancer control program in a developing country. Current collaborators and research supporters include the International Network for Cancer Treatment and Research, the World Bank, WHO, and the University of Oxford (Shanta, 2000).

Ocean Road Cancer Institute, Dar es Salaam, Tanzania

Sub-Saharan Africa has few cancer centers outside of South Africa.

continued

BOX 8-1 Continued

The most prominent is the Ocean Road Cancer Institute (ORCI) in Dar es Salaam, Tanzania, one of the world's poorest countries. ORCI was established by the government in 1996 and is still the only dedicated cancer center in the country. Cancer is still not a health priority, but the existence and influence of ORCI has begun to change that (Ngoma, 2003).

From its origins in the radiotherapy department of Muhimbili University teaching hospital, ORCI offers the full range of cancer management for adults and children—surgery (through Muhimbili hospital), chemotherapy, radiotherapy, palliative care—as well as cervical and breast cancer screening. About 2,000 new patients are seen each year and recently, about 5,000 women have been screened for cervical cancer annually. Services are paid for by the government with no charge to patients.

ORCI also acts as the focal point for the Tanzanian National Cancer Control Program. Goals and activities include research, training, prevention programs, improving cancer treatment facilities around the country, and networking nationally and internationally. Recent research collaborations have involved cervical cancer screening using visual inspection, with the International Network for Cancer Treatment and Research (INCTR) and International Agency for Research in Cancer, and treatment of Burkitt's lymphoma, also with INCTR.

ORCI is, in fact, a magnet for international collaboration. INCTR's only African office operates from ORCI. In early 2006, IAEA announced that ORCI will be the site of the first PACT "Centre of Excellence" (IAEA, 2006). These developments would have been unlikely in Tanzania without the modest nucleus provided by ORCI, and the steady progress it has made during its initial years.

Instituto Nacional de Enfermedades Neoplasicas, Lima, Peru

The Instituto Nacional de Enfermedades Neoplasicas (National Institute for Neoplastic Illnesses, INEN) was established by the Peruvian government

- **Defining resource-level-appropriate standards of care** and providing this information to relevant practitioners and institutions throughout the country (see Chapter 4)
- **Surveillance and monitoring** of relevant risk factors and cancer-specific data, consistent with national data collection programs (see Chapter 3)
- **Communications and information technology** leadership by early adoption of low-cost advanced technology for a number of purposes, linking inside the country and internationally

in 1939 as a center for cancer treatment. It has grown in size and scope over the years and is still the only major cancer institute in the country. INEN is part of the Ministry of Health and has national responsibility for cancer prevention, detection, treatment, and education. The Maes Heller Research Institute has a wide range of programs in basic and clinical research. INEN also functions as a hub for satellite centers that it has organized in other parts of the country (Pinillos, 1990). Early detection and prevention—including antismoking campaigns—have long been high on the INEN agenda. Community support is important to INEN, with several hundred volunteers working regularly at the center.

In 1952, INEN was the first Peruvian institution to establish formal postgraduate training programs for medical specialties. Most of the current surgical and medical oncology staff received their training through INEN, as well as additional postgraduate study abroad. INEN is recognized internationally as the focal point for cancer control in Peru, among relatively few such centers in Latin America.

The institute is currently the leader in developing a new National Cancer Control Plan and program for Peru, a process that INEN initiated in 2002 (Coalición Multisectorial Peru Contra el Cáncer, 2006). It is collaborating with a large number of Peruvian partners as well as the American Cancer Society, U.S. National Cancer Institute, Pan American Health Organization, and International Union Against Cancer. Support from the American Cancer Society has been made available not only to develop the plan, but to help defray staff costs of the program for the first 2 years of start-up. A major task during the early phase is to secure the future of the program by raising internal funds. This arrangement of support and the centralization of the work in a major cancer center is the first such effort of its kind in Latin America (Personal communication, E. Huerta, Cancer Preventorium, Washington Cancer Center, 2006).

International Partnerships and Communication for LMC Cancer Centers

One of the observations of this report is that the international health community—cancer centers, the many academic global health programs, and the international development community—have established relatively few activities related to cancer in LMCs. The reasons for this are complex, involving the perceived and real burdens of cancer in comparison with other conditions (especially infectious "tropical diseases" and HIV/AIDS). Another factor appears to be a lack of perceived opportunity for identifying specific projects or types of projects that would further cancer control in important ways. If the international community is going to become more engaged in the coming years, these issues must be addressed. Once interest is piqued, however, it will be important for international partners to recognize institutions and individuals in LMCs with whom they can establish connections. We see an important function of the cancer center to be an easily identifiable, officially recognized gateway for international collaboration. From the beginning of cancer center establishment (or enhancement of existing centers), the international community should be involved. This does not mean that all outside collaboration should be with a single cancer center. The cancer center is likely to be the first point of contact, however, and could identify other institutions and individuals within the country, for example. This "moth phenomenon" is already apparent, where countries with cancer centers of some prominence attract international attention in preference to countries with no obvious point of contact.

Information and communications technologies and applications, including the development of specialized content, continue to proliferate and improve at relatively low cost and can be important sources of international support, as described below. The circumstances of each cancer center, including who its partners are, will determine exactly which ones are adopted—both the technologies and the applications. Connectivity is still a problem in places, but improving globally. Whatever the constraints, high-quality information and communication technology can be available and will be important components at any site. One caveat, however, is that the information actually needed in LMCs may be scarce or may not be accessible easily (e.g., resource-level-appropriate guidelines for most cancers). Health research of direct relevance to LMCs, and to cancer in particular, is rare. Research conducted locally may be published in developing country journals, few of which are indexed by Medline or other major databases, so they may not appear in literature searches (Edejer, 2000). Language is another barrier: Most of the published literature and other material on the Internet is in English. Some of this can be addressed by programs that develop and provide content as well as technology, but this is still limiting. Nonetheless, the field moves quickly and can be made more relevant as time goes on.

A few examples of successful tools and programs for developing country health care that could be useful to cancer centers include those described below.

SatelLife

SatelLife was founded with the purpose of putting technology, in particular space technology, to use for the benefit of people in developing countries. Since the early 1990s, it has accomplished this with both technology and content for the health care community (SatelLife, 2006). HealthNet "knowledge networks" were created in Eritrea, Ethiopia, Kenya, Uganda, Zimbabwe, and Nepal. The organizations are now locally owned and managed, but supported by SatelLife to provide a variety of services, including free or low-cost email, computer literacy training, health data collection, and information resources. Global information services are accessed in 120 countries.

A few years ago, SatelLife began expanding the use of handheld computers (personal digital assistants, or PDAs) to collect and transmit health information in Africa. A collaborative project with the American Red Cross and the Acumen Fund used PDAs to undertake surveys of measles vaccination in Ghana and Kenya. In Ghana, 2,400 parents were surveyed at vaccination centers in 3 days, and in Kenya, the 28 Kenyan Red Cross volunteers surveyed 2,000 parents. The results were ready for analysis immediately. A traditional paper and ink survey would have yielded only 1/10 the number of reports, and would have taken weeks or months to process. The information is of strategic value for planning further immunization campaigns in both countries (American Red Cross, 2002). PDAs are also useful as portable information resources. SatelLife, in collaboration with Skyscape, has provided PDAs with treatment guidelines, essential drug lists, and medical textbooks to doctors and medical students in Uganda (American Red Cross, 2002).

World Health Organization: Health InterNetwork Access to Research Initiative

Health InterNetwork Access to Research Initiative (HINARI) is a program organized by WHO that provides online access to the full text of 2,900 major biomedical and related journals to local, nonprofit institutions in developing countries. The service is free or low cost, depending on the economic status of the country. Currently, about 1,400 institutions (including cancer centers) in 104 countries (out of 113 eligible) have registered for HINARI. During 2004, users at these institutions downloaded nearly 2 million articles (WHO, 2006).

WiRED International Programs

WiRED International (for World Internet Resources for Education and Development) is a nonprofit organization that provides medical and health care information, education, and communications resources to communities in low-income areas and postconflict countries (WiRED International, 2006). Projects have been developed in 11 countries in Latin America, Eastern and Central Europe, the Middle East, and Africa. Of particular interest to the discussion of cancer centers are Medical Information Centers (MICs) for medical schools and teaching hospitals, and telemedicine centers to link health professionals in different parts of the world.

The MICs are computer-based information systems using both local information storage (large fixed disk drives and CD-ROMs) and Internet connectivity to proprietary sites (e.g., WHO's HINARI database). As comprehensive print libraries are increasingly impractical and computer-based libraries are made more practical and user-friendly, they are beginning to fill the information void in many locations. WiRED has installed MICs in Honduras, Kenya, Kosovo, Iraq, Montenegro, Nicaragua, and Serbia, with installations at multiple sites in most countries.

Video conferencing with high-quality cameras has been developed for a variety of activities, including face-to-face meetings in seminars, lectures, and workshops, and for clinical assessment and consultation. An April 2006 video conference between physicians at Baghdad's Medical City Center and physicians at Children's Hospital in Washington, DC, was devoted to evaluating the cases of several Iraqi children. During the same month, video conferences were conducted between Rizgari Hospital in Erbil, Iraq and Massachusetts General Hospital and California Pacific Medical Center. Linkages among different hospitals in Iraq are also part of the program.

WiRED also has another set of programs dealing with health information for the general public, as well as some specialized uses. A "Video Visit" program was set up in 2000 for Albanian children being treated for cancer in Italy to see and hear their families in Tirana, Albania over live video.

St. Jude Children's Research Hospital International Outreach Program: Cure4Kids

Cure4Kids is an Internet-based distance learning program provided free to physicians, nurses, scientists, and health care workers who treat children with catastrophic illnesses (St. Jude Children's Research Hospital, 2006). The Internet tools include:

- Online education about catastrophic childhood illnesses
- Collaborative work spaces for document sharing and online meetings
- Access to consultation and mentoring by St. Jude faculty
- Technology and training for better management of patient information

More than 8,400 Cure4Kids users in 155 countries were registered as of 2005 (St. Jude Children's Research Hospital, 2006). Its 200 online seminars about catastrophic childhood illnesses, primarily cancer, are available in seven languages. (See Chapter 6 for more on St. Jude's programs.)

Programme of Action for Cancer Therapy: A Path to Cancer Centers of Excellence

The International Atomic Energy Agency (IAEA) has recently taken the lead in efforts to help expand cancer control services in resource-poor countries through a new initiative, the Programme of Action for Cancer Therapy (PACT). Since 1981, IAEA has supported radiotherapy services in its member countries, having spent more than $50 million through the year 2000. Radiotherapy projects were initiated at the request of IAEA Member States under technical cooperation agreements. The projects ranged from setting up a country's first radiotherapy center to upgrading facilities. All projects included the radiotherapy equipment and, as needed, training in clinical use of the machinery, dosimetry, safety, and maintenance (Levin et al., 2001). As befitted IAEA's institutional mission, IAEA did not provide for other cancer treatment modalities, nor deal with cancer control more broadly.

PACT, although an IAEA initiative, has much broader objectives. It is intended to go beyond radiotherapy by partnering with a range of organizations to establish comprehensive, multidisciplinary cancer control capacity, including training in prevention, early detection, palliative care, and potentially curative treatment in IAEA Member States. PACT was endorsed by the IAEA Board of Governors in June 2004, with a 10-year horizon and the following expectations (IAEA, 2004), assuming partnerships and funding are solidified:

At the end of the programme, it is expected that PACT's engagement with Member States and with other organizations in the public and private sectors will have met the needs of Member States because it will have served to:

- Strengthen national programmes for cancer control in developing countries.
- Enable institutions in health sectors to design and support the implementation of policies and projects for the sound application of radiation therapy.
- Establish radiotherapy centers in each developing country appropriate for its needs, taking into account economic and demographic factors, and in the context of an appropriate national strategy for cancer control.
- Establish centers of excellence for radiation therapy that will serve as centers of training in all regions served by PACT.

- Review the status of radiation protection, safety, and security arrangements at national and local levels, and, as needed, put in place the technical, legal, and regulatory capacities appropriate to take best advantage of radiation therapy.
- Promote strategic partnerships on cancer therapy between countries and their national research, education, and regulatory systems at the subregional and regional levels; between national and international organizations; and between the public and private sectors.

These are ambitious goals. IAEA has a history of collaboration with a variety of other organizations, both governmental and nongovernmental, but the scale intended under PACT is vastly greater than has been the case to date. The success of the program will depend on building robust partnerships that bring funding and technical expertise to the enterprise. PACT's intended partners include Member States (developed and developing), other United Nations (U.N.) and non-U.N. institutions including those operating at regional and subregional levels, WHO in particular and its regional offices, the International Agency for Research in Cancer (IARC), charitable trusts, foundations, and others in the public and private sectors.

IAEA announced in February 2006 (on World Cancer Day) that the first PACT Center of Excellence will be established in Dar es Salaam, Tanzania. Tanzania has one of the few publicly funded cancer centers in sub-Saharan Africa outside of South Africa. This will be the first major IAEA project that goes beyond radiotherapy toward helping the country advance its National Cancer Strategy and Action Plan. IAEA will focus on radiotherapy for treatment and palliation, while other PACT partners will assist with cancer surveillance, prevention, and early detection as well as strengthening civil society and community support for cancer control.

Promoting Cancer Center Twinning for LMCs

Institutional "twinning" is conceptually simple and appealing as a way to support the establishment and functioning of cancer centers in LMCs by partnering with established cancer centers or units in more developed countries. Twinning represents a long-term commitment of the partners, involving a range of individuals on both sides, with agreement on the expectations of all parties. The relationships should be mutually beneficial and not be seen as a one-way transfer from a high-income to a lower income partner. The concept of resource-level-appropriate care should apply, and equally important, cultural and societal characteristics and norms on both sides must be understood and respected.

The best developed examples of twinning in cancer are limited to pediatric cancer centers or units, which are described in detail in Chapter 6. The major program in the United States is St. Jude Children's Research Hospital International Outreach Program. The program began in 1991 with middle-income-country partners in Latin America. There are now nine countries with one or more centers, and another five countries in other parts of the world.

An example originating in Europe is a twinning program begun in 1986 between a pediatric cancer unit in Monza, Italy (the Hemato-Oncology Center of Milan-Bicocca University, Saint Gerardo Hospital) and the Manuel de Jesus Rivera-La Mascota Hospital (referred to as "La Mascota") in Nicaragua. The program's success led to greater involvement by Monza, which established the Monza International School for Pediatric Hemato-Oncology (MISPHO), mainly to assist more countries in Latin America through training, workshops, and other collaborative functions. This, in turn, led to the formation of a network of Latin American countries, and additional twinning projects between other Italian pediatric cancer units and units in Bolivia, Cuba, Paraguay, and the Dominican Republic (Masera et al., 2004).

Both the St. Jude and Monza programs have resulted in documented improved survival of treated cancer patients. The two most important factors leading to this improvement are use of standard, optimized treatment protocols and a strong emphasis on creating conditions that allow patients to complete, and not abandon, their treatment.

World Heart Federation Twin Centres Programme: Twinning for Cardiology

An example of twinning outside of cancer is the World Heart Federation's (WHF's) "Twin Centres Programme," the aim of which is "to enhance the quality and capacity of cardiology centres in less advantaged countries or regions" through formal links with leading centers or institutions with high-quality cardiology programs, including prevention, clinical cardiology, research, and training. The program can be used to strengthen existing links and to encourage new ones (World Heart Federation, 2006). The role of the WHF is twofold: to catalyze twinning between institutions and to provide a range of exchange fellowships and traineeships.

A central feature of this initiative is the fellowship program, considered an integral part of the development of a twinning arrangement. Fellowships allow young cardiologists and cardiovascular scientists from the lower income country to get training at the partner institution. Awardees must agree to return to their home institution after the training.

Observations and Lessons Learned Regarding Twinning Arrangements

From the pediatric cancer programs, the most important observation is that twinning arrangements have succeeded in treating children with cancer in low-income countries in an appropriate and sustainable way. The programs also serve as demonstrations that such programs can work and that some cancers can be cured. The impacts of twinning programs (and cancer centers more generally) are limited to their resources and reach, of course. As stated by MISPHO leaders:

> The micro-approach promoted by twinning programs in the context of the "childhood cancer family" is both a symbolic intervention in the direction of globalization with a human face and a concrete contribution towards saving the lives of a minority of the children with cancer . . . (Masera et al., 2004).

Certain characteristics of the institutional relationships in twinning arrangements and of the centers themselves are considered important by those involved. These include (Masera et al., 2004):

- Long-term commitment
- Attracting additional (less comprehensive) relationships with other organizations to strengthen the overall effort
- A reciprocal respect for the autonomy, culture, and local traditions between partners
- An active but noninvasive role of supervision and scientific advice from the higher income partner
- A comprehensive disease-oriented approach to program development, including training professionals, assuring the availability of essential drugs and diagnostic tools, and strengthening physical facilities
- Alliance among health professionals, families, and volunteers to support the center and its patients
- Development of financial support through a diversified donor pool without excessive reliance on a single source (in particular, not assuming that all financial support will come from the higher income partner); local fundraising, at whatever level possible, is important
- Assured salary support for at least a core of center personnel
- Attention to quality of care, with standards and monitoring, from the inception
- Promotion of collaborative research projects of local relevance, with LMC scientists in the lead

Cancer Centers and Other Chronic Diseases

One potential drawback of promoting cancer centers to lead in the full range of cancer control activities is the isolation of cancer from other noncommunicable diseases. This concern is timely given WHO's recent reorganization and major report on chronic disease prevention, which emphasizes the commonalities among the major noncommunicable diseases, including cancer. WHO recommends that every country develop a chronic disease policy "that sets out the vision for prevention and control of the major chronic diseases and provides the basis for action in the next 5–10 years" (Epping-Jordan et al., 2005). The 2005 World Health Assembly Resolution on Cancer Prevention and Control calls for universal national cancer control plans and programs (World Health Assembly, 2005). This suggests a need for coordination, while recognizing that cancer control has unique requirements apart from those of other chronic diseases.

The WHO chronic disease emphasis is focused largely on prevention and not the other aspects of control. The most significant shared risk factor, by far, is tobacco. Tobacco control continues to gain momentum internationally as an independent issue with its own initiatives, stimulated by the Framework Convention on Tobacco Control. The cancer control community (in particular, the International Union Against Cancer, also known as UICC) has been a strong force for tobacco control and this will undoubtedly continue, unaffected by cancer centers taking the lead in cancer control. To a lesser extent (but still important), the promotion of healthy diets and weight control are beneficial for cancer as well as other chronic diseases.

Palliative care is the aspect of cancer patient care that is of greatest relevance for the range of chronic diseases. Historically, palliative care developed in high-income countries specifically for cancer patients and even now, that is the main focus. Rather than the other major noncommunicable diseases, people with AIDS are benefiting from palliative care structures (mainly hospice programs) put in place for cancer. Developing palliative care more broadly—at least initially, concentrating on end-of-life care—is a challenge for all countries (WHO, 2005). Although cancer centers with cancer control responsibilities should organize palliative care, the care itself should be delivered to a large extent as home care, in the community through local health workers. So, although it is unlikely that many non-cancer patients will receive palliative care at cancer centers, all patients should benefit from programs in the community, organized through the health care system and serving all people in need, regardless of diagnosis.

DISCUSSION

Cancer centers are recognized around the world first and foremost as institutions specializing in cancer diagnosis and treatment. The concentration of clinical expertise and the large number of patients with cancers of all types and stages make cancer centers an obvious place for cancer research to flourish, as well. This is, in fact, the natural evolution that has taken place in high-income countries and some LMCs. A natural extension of cancer center functions is in prevention programs, which require outreach to the community to educate the public about the value and availability of screening and to inform them about other prevention approaches. In LMCs, where resources are scarce, the cancer center may take on even greater importance than is the case in high-income countries. Many low-income countries, mainly in Africa, have no recognized cancer centers (Personal communication, T. Ngoma, Ocean Road Cancer Institute, Dar es Salaam, Tanzania, March 2006). Most, if not all, middle-income countries do have cancer centers, although most appear to be limited to cancer diagnosis and treatment; if they offer screening, it is for people referred to or requesting the service (i.e., opportunistic screening) and not part of an organized screening program for the broader population. This is the norm in Latin America, at least (Eisenchlas, 2006).

Where recognized public-sector cancer centers do not exist or are very few (which is the case in at least a number of low-income countries), it is likely that there are also very few physicians and other health care personnel trained in oncology in the country. To create the conditions under which a multidisciplinary team can assemble to provide appropriate care in the public sector (as well as take on the other challenges discussed in this chapter), the idea of the cancer center is most appealing. The critical mass of cancer professionals includes physicians, nurses, social workers, and the variety of necessary technicians for patient care and training new personnel, at a minimum. This critical mass is needed to attract and retain excellent staff and to take advantage of economies of scale and of scope. Going a step farther, cancer centers in LMCs—where cancer expertise and resources are concentrated—are the logical centers of gravity for national cancer control programs involving both clinical services to patients as well as public awareness, prevention, surveillance, research, and other functions in the cancer plan and program. It will be necessary for each country to first take stock of their existing capacities, including the human and material resources needed for cancer control and then decide how to move forward. This is the approach currently being developed in Peru, for example (see Box 8-1).

It is recognized that creating cancer centers of excellence either from scratch or by augmenting existing cancer centers might also have negative consequences. By definition, they will concentrate already scarce resources for cancer, and in most cases, require additional funding, which might be diverted from other health priorities. Access inevitably will be limited, at least geographically, benefiting some more than others. Thus health care equity will not be served, although the intent is that the cancer center will develop outreach programs and become a reference center for other cancer centers. However, these developments may take years or decades to achieve, depending on resource availability and on the management and accomplishments of the keystone center. There is always a danger that the cancer center will be seen as a political prize to be awarded other than on the basis of merit—both the choice of which site will become a center of excellence and the choice of high-level administrators. On balance, we believe the positives outweigh the negatives, but this cannot be guaranteed everywhere.

SUMMARY AND RECOMMENDATIONS

The goal of creating and supporting centers of excellence for cancer control in many countries over the next decade is ambitious but achievable. The scope of the task is not easily definable, however, because there is no inventory of cancer centers and their current capabilities. In Latin America, where every country has cancer centers—some have many—almost all are centers for diagnosis and treatment only, with no broader cancer control functions (Eisenchlas, 2006).

Countries should not have to undertake these efforts on their own. The number of international programs—including PACT, described earlier—demonstrates that there is support from the global community to expand cancer centers. The amount and nature of this support over the coming decade is not predictable at present; it will depend, among other things, on the success of PACT in attracting partner organizations. To some extent, it will also depend on the demand by LMCs, which must demonstrate commitment to these projects. No other global effort comparable to PACT exists, although arrangements among individual countries are always possible.

In addition to support for the creation or expansion of public cancer centers through PACT or other sources, global partners—one or more—can greatly enhance the development of cancer control capabilities. In cancer, twinning relationships have been largely unexplored outside of pediatric cancer units, but these serve as useful examples. One way of promoting twinning would be for a convener or organizer to establish one or more models (e.g., for different levels of involvement) for institutions to follow, and to facilitate matching institutions. Fellowships, such as those offered by WHF, could also be useful incentives for new twinning programs. Various organizations could play this role, including the U.S. National Cancer Institute (and other high-income-country research and funding organizations).

RECOMMENDATION 8-1. Countries should consider establishing a government-supported cancer "center of excellence" that provides resource-level-appropriate services to the public and acts as a reference point for national cancer control. *This could be a new center or designation of an existing one.*

RECOMMENDATION 8-2. International partners should assist in developing and improving cancer centers in LMCs through twinning arrangements and other means. *The recently formed PACT, established by the IAEA, could—in collaboration with a range of partners—take on this role. Financial contributions from national governments (research funding institutions and bilateral aid agencies) could be channeled into this effort as a means of progressively increasing the global donor community's investments in cancer control in LMCs in ways likely to have the biggest impact.*

REFERENCES

American Red Cross. 2002. *SATELLIFE Wins Swedish Health Award for IT Program in Africa.* [Online]. Available: http://www.redcross.org/news/in/measles/021022satelife.html [accessed May 3, 2006].

Coalicion Multisectorial Peru Contra el Cancer. 2006. *Documento De Consenso.* Lima, Peru: Ministerio de Salud.

Edejer TT. 2000. Disseminating health information in developing countries: The role of the Internet. *BMJ* 321(7264):797–800.

Eisenchlas J. 2006. *Cancer Prevention and Management in Latin America.* Commissioned by the Institute of Medicine. Unpublished.

Epping-Jordan JE, Galea G, Tukuitonga C, Beaglehole R. 2005. Preventing chronic diseases: Taking stepwise action. *Lancet* 366(9497):1667–1771.

IAEA (International Atomic Energy Agency). 2004. *Programme of Action for Cancer Therapy: Report by the Director General to the Board of Governors.* Vienna, Austria: IAEA.

IAEA. 2006, February. *IAEA Responds to Cancer Crisis in Tanzania.* [Online]. Available: http://www.iaea.org/NewsCenter/PressReleases/2006/prn200603.html [accessed May 8, 2006].

Levin V, Meghzifene A, Izewska J, Tatsuzaki H. 2001. Improving cancer care: Increased need for radiotherapy in developing countries. *IAEA Bulletin* 43(2):25–32.

Masera G, Baez F, Biondi A, Cavalli F, Chiesa R, Conter V, Fossati-Bellani F, Marinoni M, Sala A, Valsecchi MG, Tognini G. 2004. Bridging the childhood cancer mortality gap between economically developed and low-income countries: Lessons from the MISPHO experience. In: Tannenberger S, Cavalli F, Pannuti F, eds. *Cancer in Developing Countries: The Great Challenge for Oncology in the 21st Century.* Munich, Germany: W. Zuckschwerdt Verlag GmbH. Pp. 42–60.

National Cancer Institute. 2006a. *Cancer Centers: Policies and Guidelines Relating to the Cancer-Center Support Grant; Part I: Description of the Program and Its Policies.* [Online]. Available: http://www3.cancer.gov/cancercenters/ccsg_comp_pt1_5.html#5essential [accessed April 28, 2006].

National Cancer Institute. 2006b. *NCI International Portfolio: Addressing the Global Challenge of Cancer.* Bethesda, MD: National Institutes of Health.

Ngoma T. 2003. Partner profile: Ocean Road Cancer Institute. [Online]. *INCTR Newsletter* 3(3). Available: http://www.inctr.org/publications/2003_v03_n03_w09.shtml.

Pinillos L. 1990. Instituto Nacional de Enfermedades Neoplasicas: Past and present. *Seminars in Surgical Oncology* 6(4):203–206.

SatelLife. 2006. *The Global Health Information Network.* [Online]. Available: http://www.healthnet.org/ [accessed May 3, 2006].

Shanta V. 2000. Partner profile: Cancer Institute (WIA), Chennai, India. [Online]. *INCTR Newsletter* 1(1). [Online]. Available: http://www.inctr.org/publications/2000_v01_n01_a07.shtml [accessed January 25, 2006].

Sharma DC. 2004. Cancer Institute at Chennai: A model for resource-poor countries. *Lancet Oncology* 5(4):204.

St. Jude Children's Research Hospital. 2005. *International Outreach Program—I.O.P. Annual Report 2005.* Memphis, TN: St. Jude Children's Research Hospital.

St. Jude Children's Research Hospital. 2006. *Cure4Kids.* [Online]. Available: http://www.stjude.org/international-outreach/0,2564,455_3209_5203,00.html [accessed November 1, 2006].

WHO (World Health Organization). 2005. *Preventing Chronic Diseases: A Vital Investment.* Geneva, Switzerland: WHO.

WHO. 2006. *HINARI: Health InterNetwork Access to Research Initiative.* [Online]. Available: http://www.who.int/hinari/en/ [accessed May 3, 2006].

WiRED International. 2006. *WiRED International.* [Online]. Available: http://www.wiredinternational.org/ [accessed May 3, 2006].

World Health Assembly. 2005. *Cancer Prevention and Control.* WHA58.22.

World Heart Federation. 2006. *Twin Centres.* [Online]. Available: http://www.worldheart.org/texts/capacity-twin-centres.htm [accessed May 3, 2006].

9

Advocacy for Cancer Control

Cancer advocacy groups—defined broadly as cancer societies, survivor advocates, and other groups of volunteers outside of government, all by definition nongovernmental organizations, or NGOs—are well established in most developed countries. They have been a potent influence in high-income countries in raising awareness about the cancer burden and directing public and private efforts and resources into cancer control. In most low- and middle-income countries (LMCs), where cancer is a low priority, advocacy is also largely undeveloped. As we have argued in this report, cancer control deserves higher priority based on its large and increasing burden of disease. Advocacy has a role to play in bringing the public's concerns about cancer to decision makers.

In most developed countries, cancer advocacy begins with national cancer societies, often formed by physicians, other health care professionals, and business leaders (e.g., the forerunner of the American Cancer Society was founded in 1913). Advocacy by the interested public develops later, usually around specific issues. These groups compete for funds and influence, but often develop formal and informal alliances. Cancer advocacy groups in developed countries have proven to be powerful forces for the advancement of cancer control and provide a considerable amount of leadership in the establishment of national cancer priorities.

Independence from government is essential to advocate for something the government is reluctant to do, which means not being dependent financially on government. This is true even if, as occurs in many countries, NGO cancer societies undertake joint projects with government or undertake specific contracts. This principle has been affirmed over and over in the history of tobacco advocacy, where governments are often in receipt of funds from the tobacco industry, and in some countries this extends to individual politicians and even office bearers. Although the tobacco situation is unique, the principle of independence applies to any advocacy group, be it for support for breast cancer patients or for cervical cancer screening programs. Ideally, advocates should be free to use the media, mass volunteer influence, and all other mechanisms of persuasion to achieve their objectives.

It is not possible nor desirable to "control" the advocacy movement, as its very nature is a societal response to a variety of situations often, initially at least, driven by emotion. Success, however, does depend on advocating things that are achievable. A set of priorities and actions must be developed that are feasible economically and politically, and acceptable to society. This, in turn, requires analytical and planning expertise that may not exist among the advocates. Training to develop these skills should be a natural role for successful advocacy organizations in high-income countries.

The International Union Against Cancer is the undisputed leading international umbrella organization for cancer advocacy. Its work is described next. Among national cancer societies, the American Cancer Society (ACS) is the most active in promoting cancer advocacy in LMCs. The ACS work is described later in the chapter. What follows is a brief review of cancer advocacy in LMCs, followed by some basic principles and ideas by which the global community could help LMCs in this area.

AN UMBRELLA FOR ADVOCACY: THE INTERNATIONAL UNION AGAINST CANCER

The International Union Against Cancer, also known as UICC, is the most prominent and inclusive international body dedicated to cancer control. It is a membership organization with a small administrative head office, with controlling committees made up of volunteers. The most visible UICC activity is the World Cancer Congress, held every 2 years in a major city, the most recent in Washington, DC, in 2006. Several thousand participants from all sectors attend these meetings, the great majority from high-income countries, but with increasing representation from LMCs and attention to developing effective cancer control in those countries.

UICC has 270 member organizations in 80 countries. Many of these organizations are typical nongovernment, volunteer-based cancer societies, but many are also government-funded (often national) cancer institutes and research institutions. For example, Fiji and Estonia list only NGO members; Egypt and El Salvador list only government-funded cancer institutes. Many countries have only one member. This mix is beneficial for UICC, but government-funded institutes are not usually considered to be true advocacy bodies because they are not independent of government.

Most UICC funding comes from member organization subscriptions that are prorated based on member income. About 20 of the larger national cancer bodies (e.g., the American Cancer Society, the Australian Cancer Society, and Cancer Research UK) pay substantially more than the hundreds of smaller, less well-endowed organizations, but still a very small fraction of their total income. The UICC annual income is a modest $5 million (out of well over $500 million total budgets for the three organizations named above) (International Union Against Cancer, 2006).

Major UICC Activities

UICC has four "strategic directions," including prevention and early detection, tobacco control, knowledge transfer, and capacity building. Each area is led by a "strategic leader," a globally recognized expert.

In "Prevention and Early Detection," UICC promotes public education and the training of health care professionals to understand and act on opportunities. Activities include reviewing available cancer data to identify priorities and to develop training and other programs to address the priority areas; strengthening local capacity through training in epidemiology, cancer registration, and needs analysis; promoting cost-effective, sustainable prevention and early detection strategies, and promoting national policy changes to reinforce the strategies; and establishing networks of professionals and experts at various levels to interact in mutually beneficial ways.

In "Tobacco Control," UICC continues to support the ratification and adoption of the Framework Convention on Tobacco Control (FCTC), and is taking the next steps by working the strong NGO network to help countries adopt the measures specified in the FCTC. LMCs are a high priority. A tool in tobacco control is UICC's electronic information source, "GLOBALink," for tobacco control professionals worldwide. Tools, listservs, web hosting, petitions, and news are all available to members. Other goals in tobacco control include increasing the information base and identifying research needs; establishing standards for best practices in tobacco control; encouraging and facilitating collaboration among UICC members; developing consensus positions on key issues; and representing cancer organizations in interactions with international governmental bodies.

The goal of "Knowledge Transfer" is to narrow the gap between what is known and what is applied in cancer control. Activities include facilitating research and training fellowships for health care and advocacy professionals and volunteers; maintaining a global network of cancer experts; providing forums for information exchange; publishing a range of journals, manuals, and other material for health care professionals; and promoting specific activities that advance the cancer control agenda.

In "Capacity Building," UICC works with organizations within member countries through a wide variety of programs to increase the capacity in countries to further cancer control through advocacy. Specific activities involve providing training for advocacy leaders to develop skills to effectively influence cancer policy makers; improving fundraising capacity; teaching knowledge and skills to allow advocates to participate effectively in national cancer control planning; developing strategic alliances with other organizations and groups to create synergies; and developing resources for all the educational activities, both online and in other formats. A major recent effort has been in developing resources for NGOs to be involved in, or to spearhead, national cancer control planning (International Union Against Cancer, 2006).

THE AMERICAN CANCER SOCIETY

ACS has taken a leading role in global cancer advocacy by promoting cancer advocacy in countries with emerging cancer societies. Their major activities in this area are mentioned below (American Cancer Society, 2006).

American Cancer Society University

The centerpiece of the ACS global effort is training international cancer control leaders through the "American Cancer Society University (ACSU)" in all aspects of running a community-based cancer control organization or program. The ACSU program begins with a week-long course, which is held a few times each year in different parts of the world, followed by support of participants in home countries. Key aspects of the training include:

- Building an organization and defining its mission
- Developing a successful cancer control message and getting the message out
- Identifying and working with the various collaborators necessary for cancer control
- Raising funds to support the organization and its advocacy messages
- Promoting cancer control needs assessment and planning
- Recruiting and involving volunteers
- Assessing the status and importance of existing cancer services, including prevention and treatment

When participants return home, ACS provides "seed grants" to help them launch new initiatives. They have been used, for example, for the following activities:

- Establishing a tobacco and cancer study unit in Ethiopia
- Creating and training a network of tobacco and cancer control advocates in India
- Starting a prostate cancer awareness program in Jamaica
- Producing a tobacco- and cancer-related, youth-focused mini magazine in Nigeria
- Translating cancer and smoking information into Romanian
- Holding a workshop on building and effectively running a cancer organization in Vietnam
- Recruiting and training volunteers to serve as educators in Bolivia

After participating in activities, ACSU participants are brought back together in regional meetings to share their experiences, including reporting on activities funded by the seed grants. More than 250 people from about 60 LMCs have completed the ACSU training.

International Partners Program

The International Partners Program (IPP) creates collaborations between ACS units in the United States and cancer organizations in LMCs to build advocacy appropriate to the setting in specific areas, and to strengthen and support the organizations on both sides of the partnership. Programs in tobacco control, cancer prevention and early detection, cancer information, and fundraising are all part of the IPP agenda. In addition to the capacity building benefit to the lower income partner, those associated with the ACS units (volunteers and others) learn about conditions in other countries, which could have direct benefits in serving immigrants to the United States. The linkages also create bridges to establish additional programs in cancer control.

The two most successful partnerships currently are between the ACS South Atlantic Division and Bolivia, and the ACS California Division and the Philippines. In Bolivia, the emphasis is on improving cancer awareness among women. In the Philippines, the focus has been promoting universal immunization against the hepatitis B virus to prevent liver cancer.

International Grant Programs

ACS offers grants in tobacco control in LMCs, for which ACS acts on its own and collaborates with the UICC, Cancer Research UK, The Canadian Tobacco Control Research Initiative, and others. The work of individual campaigners and advocacy groups is supported by several different grant programs.

ACS supports the development of tobacco control infrastructure in

LMCs by supporting groups that hold meetings and workshops for local advocates, work with governments, produce information for the public, and other activities. Programs are active in Guatemala, India, China, and the Latin American region. In addition to these specific partnerships and programs, ACS is active around the world in tobacco control in many other ways.

CURRENT STATUS OF CANCER ADVOCACY IN LMCS

No worldwide inventory of cancer advocacy groups exists outside of the UICC members. Undoubtedly, many small ones lie beyond the reach of organized information systems. Of the 270 UICC members in 80 countries, nearly all can be categorized as NGOs or government cancer institutes.

Information to categorize specifically the ways in which these NGOs arose is not available. Based on observation, however, a major driving force—perhaps *the* driving force—has been the need to improve palliative care. Once started, however, most of the organizations have broadened their focus to encompass treatment and in due course, the full spectrum of cancer control activities. The NGOs in LMCs are all small resource organizations. Their cancer institutes almost invariably have poor resources. There are rare exceptions, such as the Cancer Institute in Lima, Peru, that was built by funds derived from tobacco taxes.

Apart from the drive arising from the desire for palliative care, a number of NGOs were started through government initiative, and office bearers include relatives of government officials. The next most common type of organization is the support group, mostly for breast cancer. In low-income countries, a number of these have been started by expatriate cancer survivors currently living in the country.

Determining how effective these organizations are in the field is simply not possible. Some organizations distribute pamphlets, often using text derived from materials from developed countries. Others do not publicize their activities. Few are likely to have substantial reach within their communities and for most, finances are invariably fragile (Gray, 2005).

Selected Advocacy Efforts in LMCs

Europa Donna

Europa Donna (ED) is the dominant breast cancer advocacy group in Europe, consisting of national organizations from 39 countries. The original core and impetus came from Western Europe, but the membership currently includes about a dozen mostly middle-income countries from Eastern and Central Europe and the former Soviet republics. The most recent member is the state of Georgia. Bulgaria joined in 2004 and has initiated activities (Box 9-1). The organization was formed in the early 1990s, based on the recognition of the success of breast cancer advocacy in the United States. The 10 goals (Box 9-2) involve influencing women, health care professionals, health care systems, and government (European Breast Cancer Coalition, 2006).

Each ED member country has its own National Forum and interacts with its own national government, as well as through the Europe-wide network to influence the broader political structures in Europe. National Fora include patients, female health professionals, breast cancer-related organizations and institutions, and women supporting the fight against breast cancer. Education, information, and lobbying are the three major activities. Lobbying takes place nationally in member countries and throughout Europe.

Lobbying at the European level began in 2000. A milestone was the launch of the European Parliamentary Group on Breast Cancer in 2001 and the passage of a breast cancer resolution by the European Parliament in 2003. Most of the LMCs are not members of the European Union, so they may not benefit directly from European Parliamentary action.

BOX 9-1
Europa Donna Bulgaria

Europa Donna (ED) Bulgaria was established in 2004. In cooperation with cancer patient organizations and others, it has developed a variety of programs focusing on direct contact with cancer patients, producing and distributing cancer-related information, working with health care institutions, and participating in the European patients' forum. ED organized a forum on problems in oncology, where specialists emphasized the importance of prevention and timely diagnosis. Information sessions included visits to an oncology hospital, a self-education center to enable people to consult with competent specialists, and an art therapy club to help women express their feelings about the disease through drawing.

ED has been working toward developing European standards for patients' rights, screening and early diagnosis, availability of up-to-date treatment for all, and social adaptation. On a visit to Bulgaria in 2004, the President of ED met the Vice-Minister of Health to discuss breast cancer problems, drug policies, and a national screening program.

SOURCE: European Breast Cancer Coalition (2006).

BOX 9-2
Europa Donna's 10 Goals

1. To promote the dissemination and exchange of factual, up-to-date information on breast cancer throughout Europe
2. To promote breast cancer awareness
3. To emphasize the need for appropriate screening and early detection
4. To campaign for the provision of optimum treatment
5. To ensure provision of quality supportive care throughout and after treatment
6. To advocate appropriate training for health professionals
7. To acknowledge good practice and promote its development
8. To demand regular quality assessment of medical equipment
9. To ensure that all women understand fully any proposed treatment options, including entry into clinical trials and their right to a second opinion
10. To promote the advancement of breast cancer research

SOURCE: European Breast Cancer Coalition (2006).

Reach to Recovery International

Reach to Recovery International (RRI), a UICC program, is a network of voluntary breast cancer support groups around the world. The underlying premise is "that of one woman who has lived through breast cancer giving of her time and experience to help another woman confronting the same challenge." The original, and still main, purpose of RRI is psychosocial support for women with breast cancer, but the group is also involved in broader advocacy.

At the start of 2006, the network included 84 groups in 50 countries. Some groups are mature, but the majority are relatively new, from Africa, Asia, Eastern Europe, and Latin America. The network helps volunteers to start new groups, helps to establish support services, and enhances existing groups' skills in communication and advocacy. RRI also works to promote services to meet the needs of women with breast cancer. Groups just getting started may work with an established group in a "twinning" program.

The RRI network offers peer support training, the chance to attend regional and international conferences, and the RRI newsletter, *bloom*. RRI meetings at the international level are held every 2 years, and an Asia–Pacific conference is held in the years in between. Train-the-trainer workshops are offered to develop skills in volunteer training and management.

Malaysian Breast Cancer Council

The concept of the Malaysian Breast Cancer Council (MBCC) was developed at the conclusion of the First Asia-Pacific Reach to Recovery International Breast Cancer Support Conference, which was held in Malaysia in 2002. MBCC consists of Reach to Recovery groups (peer support groups of women with breast cancer), in coalition with cancer societies, hospices, national societies of health care professionals in cancer care, and agencies with special interest in breast cancer and women's issues. MBCC was formed to:

- Influence policies regarding breast cancer
- Create a sociocultural change in attitude toward breast cancer
- Facilitate communication and break down barriers on breast cancer issues
- Prevent duplication of services and activities
- Maximize resources to help enable effective support services

Breast cancer survivors and health care professionals work in partnership in this advocacy endeavor. The advantages of this partnership are:

- Improved doctor–patient communication and relationships, including the beginnings of shared decision making
- Advocates who have had breast cancer and are supporting the rights of cancer patients not only in providing information to the public, but also in encouraging health care professionals to make the treatment environment more patient friendly
- With increased mutual respect, increased referrals by health care providers of patients to Reach to Recovery groups for psychosocial support
- Giving Reach to Recovery groups, cancer societies, and societies of health care professionals in cancer care the common ground to resolve differences and work together toward common goals for women with breast cancer and cancer in general

Issues raised with Malaysian government officials and the public relate to:

- Availability of sources to provide information on access to cancer care and treatment
- The importance of seeking evidence-based screening, diagnostic services, and treatment

- Equity of services in cancer treatment for all women
- Rising cost of cancer treatment drugs
- Tobacco control measures

A major activity of the MBCC network is monitoring cancer-related information being delivered to the public by companies and other organizations, and taking action to publicly correct misinformation. Topics range from misleading advertising to breast cancer screening by a range of (costly) technologies other than mammography. Member organizations write letters to the media, contact government officials, and take other measures to set the record straight.

Informing women about early detection of breast cancer is another priority. In addition to distributing brochures, MBCC organizes public events to spread the message. "Outrageously Pink Night" consisted of a street party aimed at young people. People in pink took to the streets for dancing. At the same time, the Minister of Women, Family and Community Development, who was guest of honor, distributed goody bags with gifts and information on early detection of breast cancer.

In August 2004, 20 women living with breast cancer participated in a Patients' Forum. The Parliamentary Secretary from the Ministry of Health and several medical specialists were also present. Issues discussed included treatment needs of women with breast cancer, the escalating cost of chemotherapy drugs, and the acute shortage of specialized cancer treatment services in Malaysia. These issues are being addressed jointly by the Ministry of Health and MBCC committee members.

ROLE OF THE GLOBAL ADVOCACY COMMUNITY IN PROMOTING CANCER ADVOCACY IN LMCS

Advocacy groups may arise within a country with little outside influence, but in most LMCs, that has not happened. Just as governments and professionals in LMCs can make much greater progress in developing cancer programs with technical assistance and resources from high-income countries, so can the fledgling advocacy movement benefit from the inputs of the international advocacy community. The first target has to be a core of people in individual countries who understand that cancer is a growing problem for them, and second, that things they do can elevate the status of cancer control through advocacy efforts.

Because of the way advocacy develops—around issues that directly affect the advocates and their communities—going international may not be a natural priority for most groups. Everywhere, regardless of the services available and the attention paid to cancer, there is always more to be done locally by advocates without expanding beyond national borders. Some mature groups with significant resources have offered assistance to developing countries (including ACS, discussed above). Outreach in tobacco control has been extensive, and the breast cancer advocacy community also has become active. In addition to the global Reach to Recovery program under UICC auspices (see below), individual groups, such as the U.S.-based Susan G. Komen Breast Cancer Foundation, reach out to advocates in developing countries to offer tools that can be used to help develop their movements at home. What is less common, and clearly more difficult, is to help to build advocacy where no leaders have yet emerged.

There can be no doubt that the experience of high-income-country cancer societies and other organizations can help develop advocacy in low-income countries. However, it is essential to recognize the different situations that exist and help tailor advocacy to what is appropriate. Setting out some basic questions is relatively simple:

- What are the common cancers?
- Which of these are avoidable by effective prevention strategies?
- What else is missing on the spectrum of cancer care?
- Is cancer education a useful role for the cancer society?
- What services does government provide?
- Is research an appropriate target for the particular society?
- What are the available resources?

International advocacy groups can play a number of roles:

- **To advise on the practicalities of cancer control choices, and to provide training workshops on relevant topics in the host country.**

Advocacy groups that organize around specific issues—breast cancer and palliative care are the two most frequent—have chosen their priorities. Cancer societies that have more all-encompassing aims, however, need to select priorities and organize plans of action, key tasks that international partners could assist, either through UICC or as society-to-society partnerships. Here it may be appropriate to establish the principle that such training is best conducted in the concerned LMC, where a suitable and representative audience can be garnered.

- **A two-way exchange of staff with the object of benefiting both.**

Just as "twinning" of cancer treatment institutions is of benefit, twinning of cancer societies or international NGOs (e.g., Rotary International) could be used to develop long-term relationships to benefit both sides.

- **Providing funding for expanded advocacy in LMCs.**

Funding is a major constraint to the expansion of advocacy in LMCs. Cancer organizations from high-income countries provide some funding for low-income-country activities, but the amount is relatively small. This issue needs to be addressed, but new sources of funding are also needed.

Advocacy for Tobacco Control: An Example

The history of international tobacco advocacy begins in the 1970s with UICC and the International Union of Tuberculosis and Lung Disease. This involved a concerted program of training workshops based on a model published by UICC initially in 1976 (Gray and Daube, 1976). More than 100 such workshops were run over three decades with major input from the U.S.-based Advocacy Institute and the American Cancer Society. From this activity grew a coherent international group of advocates that now runs a triennial world conference attended by several thousand active participants. These individuals belong to a variety of national and international organizations coming to tobacco control from a variety of perspectives. Global tobacco control policy is, with the exception of a few difficult issues, generally agreed on, although individual groups have particular priorities. This movement is largely responsible for the Framework Convention on Tobacco Control (see Chapter 5).

However, international conferences, although essential, do not take action. The action items are left to those working in their home environment. Viewed internationally, the tobacco control movement sorely lacks funding to assist LMCs. Trained, internationally oriented advocates exist in significant numbers, but funding and a formal global program are missing.

Is tobacco control advocacy different from lobbying for other cancer control causes? In one way, it is. The evidence indicting tobacco in disease had been known for 20 years before the UICC tobacco program began and was accepted by most wealthy governments, but the evidence and possible solutions had not been considered in LMCs, where smoking rates were still relatively low in most places. Health officials welcomed such interventions as they were usually well informed and frustrated by their situation. However, it may also be significant that most tobacco prevention interventions are cost free or low cost in comparison to tax income from tobacco, and lobbying for tax increases has a logic of special appeal to governments. Treatment for tobacco-related cancers was not one of the targets this program was advocating as it was both relatively unsuccessful and in very limited supply in LMCs.

Tobacco advocacy provides a concrete example of a successful international movement that arose from small beginnings more than three decades ago. The expertise of support groups and the experience showing they can widen their horizons to become comprehensive cancer control advocates is encouraging.

SUMMARY AND RECOMMENDATION

Advocacy for cancer control is just beginning in LMCs, and has yet to take root in many. The history of cancer advocacy is very recent even in high-income countries, yet its impact has been great. Where the public has spoken out, governments and health care professionals have listened, at least in the United States and Europe. One should not underestimate the challenges of developing advocacy in LMCs, but the potential benefits in terms of more appropriate resources and attention to cancer make investing in advocacy very attractive. The global advocacy community has a role to play in assisting those in LMCs with information and strategies, while respecting the local political and social structures. As is the case with other aspects of cancer control, much of this work must take place person to person and country by country.

> **RECOMMENDATION 9-1. Established cancer advocacy organizations, mainly in high-income countries, should actively support and assist the growth of cancer advocacy in LMCs.** *Specific activities would include setting up advocacy networks within countries, within regions and internationally; identifying successful approaches to cancer advocacy and replicating or adapting them for use in other settings; and providing hands-on training and technical assistance.*

REFERENCES

American Cancer Society. 2006. *American Cancer Society.* [Online]. Available: http://www.cancer.org/docroot/home/index.asp [accessed July 3, 2006].

European Breast Cancer Coalition. 2006. *Europa Donna.* [Online]. Available: http://www.cancerworld.org/CancerWorld/home.aspx?id_sito=5&id_stato=1 [accessed July 3, 2006].

Gray N. 2005. *The Role of Advocacy in Cancer Control in Low- and Middle-Income Countries.* Paper commissioned by the Institute of Medicine.

Gray N, Daube M. 1976. *Guidelines for Smoking Control.* Geneva, Switzerland: UICC.

International Union Against Cancer. 2006. *Making a World of Difference.* [Online]. Available: http://uicc.org/index.php?id=516 [accessed July 3, 2006].

10

Expanding the Role of the Global Community in Cancer Control

This report makes the case—not for the first time—that recognition of the burden that cancer imposes and some level of response are feasible in every country. It also identifies feasible opportunities of particular importance in the countries where resources have constrained the response to cancer. Another critical element is support—both in resources and in expertise—from the "global community." Until now, international support has been forthcoming almost exclusively from cancer-focused organizations, but not from the broader based health and development sector, such as foreign aid from individual countries (through agencies such as the U.S. Agency for International Development, or USAID), the World Bank, and major nonprofit organizations, which provide substantial support for health infrastructure and for infectious diseases in low- and middle-income countries (LMCs). Another largely untapped resource is the U.S. and international academic community, particularly given a large increase in interest in global health and the establishment and growth of university global health programs. The support of all of these groups strongly influences the health agendas of the recipient countries. A lack of focus on cancer from these external parties easily translates to a lack of focus of LMCs themselves on cancer.

This chapter reviews the programs and activities of major sectors of the international community in relation to cancer control in LMCs and discusses further needs and opportunities. The role of advocacy, including by the global community, is covered separately in Chapter 9.

THE "GLOBAL COMMUNITY" IN GLOBAL CANCER CONTROL

A few major organizations support cancer control internationally: United Nations (U.N.) organizations, mainly the World Health Organization (WHO) and its research affiliate, the International Agency for Research on Cancer (IARC), and the health program of the International Atomic Energy Agency (IAEA); government cancer institutions, such as the National Cancer Institute (NCI) of the U.S. National Institutes of Health (NIH), the International Network for Cancer Treatment and Research; cancer societies and advocacy groups, such as the American Cancer Society and the international umbrella organization for cancer societies and advocacy, the International Union Against Cancer (UICC). All these groups play high-level, visible roles in raising awareness about the magnitude of the cancer problem, and in promoting cancer control.

Beneath the layer of major organizations and major programs is a much broader array of organizations and professionals with narrower roles, confined either to a country or area, or to a particular aspect of cancer control research or practice. No global inventory of these efforts exists. Efforts include, for example, the Open Society Institute and the Diana Fund, which are major supporters of expanding hospice and palliative care programs in Eastern and Central Europe, Africa, and elsewhere. Individual cancer centers in Europe and the United States have entered into "twinning" relationships with centers in low-resource settings, providing technical assistance, training, research support, and financial support, over the long term. Professional societies, notably the American Society of Clinical Oncology (ASCO) and the European Society for Medical Oncology (ESMO), provide training, fellowships, and other types of assistance to colleagues and institutions in LMCs. Some multinational pharmaceutical companies have programs to make oncology drugs available to cancer centers in low-resource countries where patients or governments otherwise would not be able to afford them. Foundations also fund research projects and service delivery. The Gates Foundation has been the main supporter of cervical cancer prevention research in low-resource settings.

UN AGENCIES: WHO, IARC, AND IAEA

The United Nations and its agencies relate directly to national governments. Governments look to WHO for guidance on health priorities, policy, and planning and for technical assistance. IAEA also acts through agreements with governments. It has pursued an active role in establishing and upgrading radiotherapy facilities and providing for their safe and effective operations.

World Health Organization Cancer Control Activities

WHO is the most prominent voice in global health. WHO has maintained at best a modest cancer control program for the past 30 years. As part of a reorganization in 2006, the program became part of the Department of Chronic Diseases and Health Promotion. Cancer control is also a part of other WHO programs, including those focused on tobacco control, reproductive health, occupational health, childhood immunizations, and essential medicines.

The high-level policy of WHO is carried out largely at the Geneva, Switzerland, headquarters. Work performed in countries is carried out mainly through the six WHO regional offices and the offices maintained in every member country.

The WHO cancer control program has concentrated on the following areas:

- Promoting and strengthening national cancer control programs
- Building international networks and partnerships for cancer control
- Promoting organized, evidence-based interventions for early detection of cervical and breast cancers
- Developing guidelines on disease and program management
- Advocating for a rational approach to effective treatments for potentially curable cancers
- Supporting low-cost approaches to pain relief and palliative care

The work of the cancer control program contributed strongly to adoption by the 58th World Health Assembly of a resolution on cancer prevention and control in May 2005, a milestone for the field (see Chapter 1). The resolution is designed to reinforce comprehensive cancer policies and strategies among all member states. It urges development and integration of comprehensive cancer control programs into current and future health care initiatives; the sharing of scientific research; and the development of appropriate information systems, including outcome and process indicators that support planning, monitoring, and evaluation of cancer prevention and control programs.

WHO's 2002 report, *National Cancer Control Programs: Policy and Managerial Guidelines* (World Health Organization, 2002), provides information on planning, implementing, managing, and evaluating cancer programs. It outlines the scientific basis for cancer prevention, early detection, cure, and care; discusses the appropriateness of particular technologies; and describes how to manage national programs tailored to different resource settings. (See Chapter 1 for a more complete discussion.)

The Cancer Control Programme has co-established or actively promoted the following programs and initiatives for cancer prevention:

- The Tobacco Free Initiative (TFI), established in July 1998 to focus international attention, resources, and action on the global tobacco epidemic. TFI provides global policy leadership, encourages mobilization at all levels of society, and promotes the WHO Framework Convention on Tobacco Control.
- WHO Framework Convention on Tobacco Control (FCTC), ratified in November 2004 and the first public health treaty negotiated under the auspices of WHO. FCTC includes provisions that set international standards on tobacco price and taxes, advertising, labeling, illegal trade, and secondhand smoke. The Treaty became law for the signatories in February 2005.
- Global Strategy on Diet, Physical Activity and Health, endorsed by the May 2004 World Health Assembly, to improve public health through healthy eating and physical activity.
- WHO Initiative for Vaccine Research, including vaccines against some of the infections that can cause cancer, such as hepatitis B and C and human papillomavirus, as well as schistosomiasis and other helminths.
- The INTERSUN Program, established in 1992 by WHO and a number of international partners, to improve protection against ultraviolet radiation and prevent its effects, including skin cancer.
- Global Strategy on Occupational Health for All: The Way to Health at Work, supporting healthier workplaces, including reduction in exposure to carcinogens.
- "A Community Health Approach to Palliative Care for HIV and Cancer Patients in Africa," a joint project including five countries[1] to improve the quality of life of HIV/AIDS and cancer patients in sub-Saharan Africa.

WHO Regional Offices

WHO divides the world into six regions: Africa, the Americas, Southeast Asia, Europe, Eastern Mediterranean, and Eastern Pacific. One country in each region houses the permanent regional office. The staff of regional offices work directly with their designated countries. In addition, each country has its own resident WHO representative and delegation of varying size. Regional staffs include a chronic disease advisor, who may or may not be a cancer specialist (although no current advisors are cancer specialists).

[1]Botswana, Ethiopia, Tanzania, Uganda, and Zimbabwe.

International Agency for Research on Cancer

IARC, established in May 1965 as a WHO agency, is a research organization located in Lyon, France. Its mission is to "coordinate and conduct research on the causes of human cancer, the mechanisms of carcinogenesis, and to develop scientific strategies for cancer control." IARC's work focuses on epidemiology, environmental carcinogenesis, and research training. IARC does not conduct clinical trials or conduct research on other aspects of cancer patient care, nor is it directly involved in the implementation of control measures or legislation aimed at controlling carcinogens. Most of IARC's efforts have been in and about high-income countries, but they have maintained an interest and some specific initiatives directed at LMCs in each major area of emphasis.

IARC has four main objectives (International Agency for Research on Cancer, 2006):

- **Monitoring global cancer occurrence:** IARC gathers data on incidence, mortality, and survival for hundreds of countries. The data are available electronically and in published reports. Most prominently, the 8th edition of its report, *Cancer Incidence in Five Continents*, includes information on more than 200 countries. IARC also estimates cancer incidence and mortality for every country in the world in its GLOBOCAN electronic database.
- **Identifying the causes of cancer:** Through committees, IARC assesses the carcinogenicity to humans of various agents, mixtures, and exposures. More than 800 agents have been reviewed since 1972 and published through the *IARC Monographs Programme on the Evaluation of Carcinogenic Risks to Humans*.
- **Exploring the mechanisms of carcinogenesis:** IARC laboratory research concentrates on the interaction of carcinogens with DNA, with particular emphasis on identifying carcinogen-induced, endogenous, and inherited mutations. The aim is to identify potential points of intervention to prevent progression to clinical disease.
- **Developing scientific strategies for cancer control:** The goals of IARC's programs are primary prevention and early detection of cancer. A recent example is the evaluation of low-technology screening methods for cervical, breast, and oral cancers in developing countries.

IARC maintains a number of databases related to its core functions. These include descriptive epidemiology, carcinogens, and molecular epidemiology.

Training Programs

IARC coordinates an annual 3-week summer school program of 1-week modules designed to stimulate cancer research by improving scientific knowledge and developing skills. Course selection preference is given to professionals from resource-poor countries to strengthen their research institutions and build local capacity. Researchers and support staff from groups or institutions involved in cancer monitoring, evaluation of care practices, prevention activities, or etiological research are eligible to attend IARC training programs. Subjects of the modules may include cancer registration, epidemiologic methods and research, and interpretation of cancer statistics.

Fellowships

More than 500 cancer research fellowships have been awarded to junior scientists since 1966. Recently, the program was broadened to award postdoctoral fellowships to junior scientists from LMCs to work directly with one of the research groups at IARC headquarters.

Visiting Scientist Awards are also offered for experienced investigators from universities or research institutions to spend up to one year at IARC working with one of the research groups on a topic related to the Agency's objectives.

International Atomic Energy Agency (UN)

IAEA may seem an unlikely home for a cancer control program for resource-poor countries, but it takes its mandate directly from the 1956 statute creating the "Atoms for Peace" agency: "The Agency shall seek to accelerate and enlarge the contribution of atomic energy to peace, health and prosperity throughout the world" (IAEA, 1956). IAEA began in 1980 to provide radiotherapy equipment and train staff in its use in LMCs. IAEA has provided more than $145 million in cancer-related assistance to developing countries (IAEA, 2006). In 2004, the Programme of Action for Cancer Therapy (PACT) was established as a comprehensive cancer control assistance program, with IAEA leading collaborations with a wide range of partners (IAEA, 2004) (see Chapter 8 for a discussion of PACT's potential role in supporting cancer centers in LMCs). This perspective represents a significant evolution of strategic thinking and investment on the part of IAEA, beyond radiotherapy. In the past IAEA has established a number of radiotherapy-only centers. In some places, these have formed a nucleus for developing more comprehensive treatment, but in other places they have remained solely radiotherapy centers.

Historically, IAEA Member States asked for assistance with radiotherapy through "technical cooperation" projects, which ranged from setting up a country's first radiotherapy center to upgrading facilities. All projects included providing equipment as well as training in clinical use of the machinery, dosimetry, safety, and maintenance, following internationally accepted guidelines for safety (Levin et al., 2001).

Where the request from a Member State was for a first radiotherapy center, a comprehensive feasibility study was carried out by IAEA and involving the relevant Ministry of Health and the medical community. Staff training, equipment, and expertise needs were estimated and a layout of the buildings was produced. The framework for feasibility studies is laid out in IAEA technical documents that cover various aspects of the use and safe operation of radiotherapy units. Since 1995, radiotherapy has been initiated in several resource-poor countries, such as Ethiopia, Ghana, Namibia, Uganda, Mongolia, Zambia, and Yemen, and expanded or upgraded in numerous others.

Projects in Eastern Europe, for example, have focused on upgrading technology and improving the skills of radiotherapy professionals, both of which had deteriorated during the period of regional economic decline following the collapse of the Soviet Union. Two regional projects, with cost sharing by recipient governments, upgraded facilities in Albania, Armenia, Bosnia and Herzegovina, Croatia, Macedonia, Georgia, and Moldova. Several hundred radiotherapy professionals from these countries were supported for participation in basic and continuing professional development courses. These projects continue and others have been initiated to address the still-serious inadequacies in low- and middle-income countries in Africa, Latin America, Asia, and Eastern Europe (Levin et al., 2001).

Radiotherapy Resource Inventories

In 1959 IAEA began compiling a registry of radiation therapy facilities in clinical settings, with a final update published in 1976. The inventory was restarted in 1995 as the Directory of Radiotherapy Centres (DIRAC) and is now available on the Internet (http://www-naweb.iaea.org/nahu/dirac/default.shtm). DIRAC is updated as IAEA receives information from the various countries.

OTHER SOURCES OF GLOBAL SUPPORT FOR CANCER CONTROL

National Research Agencies: The Example of the U.S. National Cancer Institute

NCI is the main source of U.S. government support for international cancer research and training. Most of the international interaction is with other high-income countries, but NCI has a substantial portfolio of work in

LMCs. NCI works cooperatively with the Fogarty International Center of NIH and with extramural institutions through bilateral agreements, grants, and contracts. NCI international expenditures are primarily devoted to foreign grants and contracts, bilateral scientist exchanges and training under the NIH Visiting Program, workshops, and international dissemination of cancer information.

Most recently, in 2006, NCI has made a major commitment to partner with IAEA and the PACT Alliance (see above and Chapter 8) to improve cancer control in LMCs. NCI will support a pilot of the expanded PACT, which will involve providing a team of cancer control experts from the United States (Clanton, 2006).

Two of the most prominent activities supported by NCI in LMCs are the Middle East Cancer Consortium (MECC; see below) and the International Network for Cancer Treatment and Research (INCTR; see below). The other area of emphasis in multiple countries is cancer registration. Training is carried out through the scientist exchange programs and other educational opportunities, and research through a large number of individual research projects involving LMCs. NCI also contributes support to many large and small workshops and meetings around the world.

Scientist Exchange and Other Training Programs

In FY 2005, more than 1,000 foreign scientists spent time at NCI, about one-third of them from LMCs. NCI also supports scientists from developing countries for training in U.S. laboratories outside of NCI, and in overseas laboratories in developed countries.

The Oncology Research Faculty Development Program helps young but established scientists from developing countries prepare for careers as investigators and for leadership positions in cancer research in their home country. The cost is shared by NCI and the sponsoring laboratory. Participants from LMCs are also given support to attend an annual NCI course on cancer prevention and control offered by the NCI Division of Cancer Prevention.

NCI Research

NCI supports a wide range of research in all aspects of cancer control and in many LMCs. A few examples include:

- A community-based, randomized-control evaluation of low-cost methods for early detection of breast and cervical cancers in women at the Tata Memorial Hospital, in Mumbai, India, including clinical breast examination without mammography, self-examination, and visual inspection of the cervix by trained female health workers

- Research on esophageal cancer in China, where incidence of the disease is highest in the world, including two nutritional intervention trials, in collaboration with the Chinese Academy of Medical Sciences
- A collaborative study between NCI and investigators in Ukraine and Belarus to study the long-term health consequences of the Chernobyl nuclear accident
- A binational study with Brazil on Epstein-Barr virus-associated lymphoma, particularly Burkitt's lymphoma, in Brazil

Cancer Registration in Developing Countries

NCI assists with training and sponsors participation of personnel from developing countries at courses on cancer registration conducted by IARC in Lyon, France, and the School of Public Health at Emory University in Atlanta, Georgia. In cooperation with the Middle East Cancer Consortium, cancer registry training programs have been held around the Middle East. In recent years, training programs also have been held regionally around the world, drawing participants from many countries.

The Middle East Cancer Consortium

MECC was founded in 1996 as a partnership between the United States and the Ministries of Health of Cyprus, Egypt, Israel, Jordan, the Palestinian Authority, and most recently, Turkey. The MECC objective is to reduce the incidence and impact of cancer in the Middle East through collaborative research. Since its inception, MECC's major activities have been the Cancer Registry Project and the Small Grants Programme. Cancer communication is another priority.

The Cancer Registry Project supports population-based cancer registries within member countries, and develops linkages among them. The first monograph about cancer incidence in the region, based on the new registries, was published in 2006 (Freedman et al., 2006). The consortium also supports training, basic research, enhancement of public health and patient care, quality control, and international communications.

The Small Grants Programme is for clinicians and scientists to conduct research. All research projects, which are funded based on a merit review, require collaboration between more than one MECC country.

International Network for Cancer Treatment and Research

INCTR is a not-for-profit, nongovernmental organization dedicated to cancer control in the developing countries of Asia, Africa, and Latin America. It was founded in 1998 by UICC and the Institut Pasteur in Belgium, and is supported by NCI as well as by membership fees, project-related grants and contracts, and corporate sponsorships. INCTR headquarters are at the Institut Pasteur, with branches and offices in the United States, France, England, Brazil, Egypt, Tanzania, India, and Nepal.

Mission and Strategy

INCTR's mission is to build capacity for cancer treatment and research in countries with limited resources through long-term collaborative projects focused on local or regional problems. Projects are designed to bring immediate benefits to patients or to prevent cancer in the population while providing professional education and training as well as opportunities for cancer research. INCTR promotes collaborations between wealthy countries and countries with limited resources, and encourages the formation of cooperative groups, consortia, networks, and partnerships with corporate, professional, academic, and governmental and nongovernmental organizations. Partners include IARC (for cervical cancer screening), NCI (for education and training), King Faisal Research Center in Saudi Arabia (for translational research), and Eli Lilly and Novartis (for clinical trials workshops and data management).

Projects are developed with the advice and participation of various INCTR committees and strategy groups as well as independent scientific advisors and the Special Panel of the INCTR Advisory Board, which is made up of distinguished oncologists and pathologists from developing countries.

INCTR Collaborating Units, Associate Members, Branches, and Offices

Projects are conducted in participating institutions or their departments, referred to as INCTR collaborating units, which are involved with cancer research, treatment, and education in the developing world. Projects, whether related primarily to research or to training and education, are conducted jointly, often in concert with other organizations or INCTR member institutions. They may entail the preparation of protocols, guidebooks, or training manuals; the transfer of technology; or the development of policy.

INCTR Associate Members include individuals, corporations, institutions, and organizations (e.g., professional societies and associations) from developed and developing nations. Branches are legally independent nonprofit entities at the national or regional level, working to raise and disburse funds in support of the INCTR mission. Branches interact with cancer centers or units, professional organizations, or elements of national or regional governments, and coordinate ongoing INCTR programs and projects within the country or region. Each branch has an administrative structure and may employ medical, scientific, and support staff. Current INCTR branches include:

- Alliance Mondiale Contre le Cancer (France)
- INCTR Egypt
- INCTR USA
- INCTR Brazil
- Nepalese Network for Cancer Treatment and Research

INCTR offices, which are extensions of INCTR, Brussels, conduct activities similar to branches and may evolve into branches. Offices currently exist in Tanzania, United Kingdom, and India.

Education Program

INCTR runs workshops, training courses, and symposia, as well as a Visiting Expert Program in which cancer specialists in a variety of disciplines spend days to weeks in institutions in developing countries. Training is conducted in-country where possible by Visiting Experts, or in INCTR-accredited centers in nearby countries of similar socioeconomic status. An attempt is made to focus training activities on specific countries, which currently include Iraq, Jordan, Afghanistan, and several African countries.

The Education Program has a strong focus on clinical trials and data management, oncology nursing, pediatric oncology, and hematological neoplasms. Past meetings have included:

- Workshop on Chemotherapy Administration and Palliative Care for Oncology Nurses (Yaoundé, Cameroon, March 2003)
- Pediatric Oncology Update (with Shaukat Khanum Memorial Cancer Hospital & Research Centre, Dubai, October 4–6, 2003)
- Lymphoma Workshop (Cairo, Egypt, October 16–18, 2003)
- Cancer Nursing Training (Cairo, Egypt, October 16–18, 2003)
- Pediatric Oncology Update (with the Chinese Pediatric Oncology Society, Chongqing, November 20–23, 2003)
- Clinical Trials Workshop (São Paolo, Brazil, September 2004)
- Multidisciplinary Workshop (for social workers, psychologists, and others involved in the support of patients with cancer, São Paolo, Brazil, September 2004)

Palliative Care Program

INCTR has begun work in palliative care in Nepal. INCTR has sent medical and nursing palliative care experts to Nepal and identified four institutions where patients can receive palliative care. Training has been organized for local staff members, and patients are now being cared for in these units. A home hospice program is also being established. INCTR plans to use this as a demonstration program and to train personnel. Similar work is planned for other countries in Asia and Africa.

Translational Research

The Translational Research Program is based at the King Fahad National Children's Cancer Centre within the King Faisal Specialist Hospital and Research Centre in Riyadh, Saudi Arabia. This program is focused on improving understanding of pathogenesis, improving diagnosis, and defining prognostic factors, particularly in acute lymphoblastic leukemia (ALL).

Other Activities

INCTR has helped to establish three cooperative groups to carry out epidemiological research and clinical trials in developing countries. They are described below.

The Leukemia Study Group of India This group is focusing initially on ALL, conducting clinical trials with the aim of improving survival rates through a better understanding of epidemiology, clinical features, and biological characteristics. The major cancer centers organizing the effort will serve as regional centers for education and training for peripheral centers and hospitals.

The Middle East Children's Cancer Association MECCA has members from 13 Middle Eastern countries who have agreed to work together in improving the prevention, early detection, and treatment of children with cancer. The group will focus initially on ALL.

The Retinoblastoma Group of Mexico This group has representatives from most regions in Mexico and is in the process of establishing a registry for retinoblastoma and common treatment protocols.

DEVELOPMENT ASSISTANCE FOR NONCOMMUNICABLE DISEASES, 1995–2002

In the only analysis of its type, Michaud (2004) examined the share of development assistance going toward noncommunicable diseases (referred to in this report as chronic diseases), including cancer. The chronic disease portion of the global burden of disease by region in 2001 was a point of reference. Worldwide, chronic diseases accounted for 46 percent of the global burden of disease and communicable diseases, 42 percent (the balance of disease burden is due to injuries). In developing regions chronic diseases accounted for about 40 percent of the total burden of disease, in contrast to developed countries, where the corresponding figure was nearly 80 percent. Heterogeneity is also significant among developing regions: Communicable diseases still predominate in sub-Saharan Africa and part of the Eastern Mediterranean region. Everywhere else—Latin America and the Caribbean, parts of the Eastern Mediterranean, Southeast Asia, and the Western Pacific, representing 3.8 billion people—chronic diseases have surpassed noncommunicable diseases.

Data Sources

The review included the major sources of data on funding provided by bilateral and multilateral agencies to developing country health sectors. For bilateral development agencies, the Organization for Economic Cooperation and Development (OECD) creditor reporting system (CRS) is the most comprehensive source of comparable data. The database lists all projects funded by donor and recipient country, with a short description of the project and the total funding. Chronic disease projects were identified through the project descriptions. The only multilateral agencies for which projects related to chronic diseases could be identified were WHO and the World Bank. To improve comparability and minimize year-to-year fluctuations, the funding levels (commitments in the case of WHO and disbursements for all others) are reported as 3-year rolling averages.

The overall result is likely an underestimate of the actual amount. For some projects, the descriptions were not specific enough, and other projects (e.g., infrastructure projects) could have a wide range of effects, including improved chronic disease control. Finally, other sources of funding, such as IAEA, are not included.

Results

Bilateral Agencies

In 2002, the latest year in the analysis, official development assistance from bilateral agencies totaled $2.9 billion. A total of $3.2 million—0.1 percent—was allocated to the prevention and control of chronic diseases. The 8-year total from 1995 to 2002 was $35.5 million. The 3-year rolling averages increased from $3.4 million in the early period (1995 to 1997) to $5.5 million for 1998 to 2000, and decreased to $4.4 million for 2000 to 2002. Of the total allocated to chronic diseases from1995 through 2002, 6 percent was allocated to cancer, 35 percent to mental disorders, 8 percent to tobacco control, and the remaining 50 percent for other NCDs. The specific projects identifiable as cancer related (including tobacco control) are listed in Table 10-1.

On the donor side, the United Kingdom and Sweden contributed 43 percent of the 8-year total ($8.7 million and $6.7 million, respectively). Trends over the period for individual donor countries were mixed. Australia and Sweden increased funding the most. Finland and the Netherlands substantially decreased their commitments. For all other countries, there was little change (Table 10-2).

The Eastern Mediterranean region and Europe received the most bilateral funding for chronic diseases ($6.4 million and $5.7 million, respectively, 1995–2002). Southeast Asia received the least ($1.4 million) (Table 10-3).

Multilateral Agencies

In 2002, WHO allocated 3.6 percent of its total budget ($44 million) to chronic diseases (Table 10-4). About one-third went to mental health, 30 percent to tobacco control, and 37 percent to unspecified chronic disease projects. The chronic disease share of total regional expenditures was lowest in sub-Saharan Africa (1.6 percent) and highest in Southeast Asia (6.6 percent). The specifics of global and interregional activities (apart from tobacco control and mental health) were available for about half the total $7.6 million. Approximately $1.1 million went for risk factor prevention and risk factor surveillance for diet, nutrition and physical activity, and cardiovascular risk management. A total of $2.4 million was allocated to cardiovascular diseases, diabetes, cancer, chronic respiratory conditions, and aging.

WHO expenditures for noncommunicable diseases (NCDs) nearly tripled between 1998–1999 and 2002, increasing from $16 million to $43.6 million per year, with most of the increase in funding for tobacco control and mental health. For all other chronic diseases, the increase was from $9.4 million to $14.3 million per year.

World Bank loans for chronic diseases between 1997 and 2002 totaled $109.5 million, with the 3-year average increasing from $7 million (1997–1999) to $20–21 million between 1998 and 2002. Nearly all of these loans went to Eastern Europe (the Russian Federation, Albania, Armenia, Latvia, Croatia, Lithuania, Romania, and Azerbaijan) as part of larger health-sector loans, mostly for cardiovascular disease prevention and the control of smoking and alcohol abuse.

In late 2005, the World Bank began to reexamine its investments in chronic diseases. A new work program will examine the economic and health burden of the major chronic diseases in the Bank's client countries,

TABLE 10-1 Bilateral Development Assistance Projects for Cancer 1995–2002

Year	Donor	Recipient	Short Description	US$ (000)
1995	Canada	Americas unspecified	Cervical cancer research	2
		Unspecified	Tobacco policy research initiative	809
		Vietnam	Tobacco control political mapping	20
	Sweden	Africa unspecified	Workshop on tobacco control	1
1996	Canada	Unspecified	Tobacco control research initiative	306
1997	Belgium	Kenya	Cervical cancer and sexually-transmitted diseases (STDs)	136
	Sweden	South Africa	Tobacco control	10
1998	Australia	Unspecified	WHO Tobacco or Health program	75
	Canada	Unspecified	Tobacco policy research	492
		Turkey	Tobacco control strategies	151
		Vietnam	Tobacco control political mapping	5
1999	Belgium	Kenya	Cervical cancer and STDs	65
	Canada	India	International initiative for tobacco policy research	24
		Unspecified	International initiative for tobacco policy research	134
		Unspecified	Tobacco and ecohealth workshop	1
	Italy	India	Epidemiologic study of hepatic neoplasia risk	22
		Tunisia	Technical assistance to Habib Hospital and Cancer Institute of Tunisia	624
	United Kingdom	Unspecified	Cervical cancer prevention	337
2000	Australia	Unspecified	Health education for tobacco control	86
	Italy	Tunisia	Technical assistance to Habib Hospital and Cancer Institute of Tunisia	554
2001	Australia	Unspecified	Tobacco control capacity-building workshop	51
	Belgium	Kenya	Cervical cancer and STDs	30
	Canada	Unspecified	International initiative for tobacco policy research	171
		South Africa	International initiative for tobacco policy research	6
	Finland	Nepal	Health education: diseases and disability due to tobacco	24
	Sweden	Unspecified	Tobacco policy cooperation	96
2002	Sweden	Vietnam	Tobacco control	325
	United Kingdom	Unspecified	Cervical cancer prevention	173
1995–2002 Total Cancer-Related Projects				*4,730*
1995–2002 Total All Chronic Disease Projects				*35,452*

SOURCE: Reprinted, with permission, from Michaud (2004). Copyright 2004 by Catherine M. Michaud, Harvard Initiative for Global Health.

TABLE 10-2 Bilateral Commitments 1995–2002 for Noncommunicable Diseases by Country, US$ 000s

Donor Country	1995–2002 Commitment
United Kingdom	8,663
Sweden	6,748
Finland	3,746
Australia	3,519
Netherlands	3,361
Canada	3,272
Italy	2,808
Spain	1,056
Belgium	722
Norway	630
United States	302
Austria	212
Denmark	173
Ireland	92
New Zealand	65
Switzerland	48
France	35
Total	*35,452*

SOURCE: Reprinted, with permission, from Michaud (2004). Copyright 2004 by Catherine M. Michaud, Harvard Initiative for Global Health.

TABLE 10-3 Bilateral Commitments 1995–2002 for Noncommunicable Diseases by Recipient Region, US$ 000s

WHO Region	1995–2002 Commitment
Africa	2,904
Americas	2,088
Eastern Mediterranean	6,416
Europe	5,662
Southeast Asia	1,403
Western Pacific	3,104
Unallocated to region	3,832
Total	*25,409*

SOURCE: Reprinted, with permission, from Michaud (2004). Copyright 2004 by Catherine M. Michaud, Harvard Initiative for Global Health.

the rationale for public interventions and the roles of government in the control of chronic disease, and the Bank's comparative advantage in assisting clients in chronic disease control. It will define a strategy to address the priorities across multiple sectors to lay the basis for improved policy advice to clients, as well as more efficient allocation and use of existing resources

TABLE 10-4 WHO Budget by Region and Major Chronic Disease Component, 2002, US$ 000

WHO Region	Total Budget	Total for NCDs (% total)	NCD Subcategories: Unspecified NCDs[a] (% NCD total)	Mental Health (% NCD total)	Tobacco (% NCD total)
Africa	309,539	4,927 (1.6)	2,131 (43)	1,306 (27)	1,490 (30)
Eastern Mediterranean	104,415	2,234 (2.1)	1,257 (56)	416 (19)	562 (25)
Western Pacific	63,037	2,784 (3.3)	919 (33)	1,327 (48)	537 (19)
Southeast Asia	110,679	7,313 (6.6)	3,118 (43)	2,339 (32)	1,856 (25)
Americas	46,590	2,242 (4.8)	1,148 (51)	508 (23)	587 (26)
Europe	68,198	3,194 (4.7)	656 (21)	865 (27)	1,673 (52)
Regional total	*702,459*	*22,694 (3.2)*	*9,229 (41)*	*6,760 (30)*	*6,705 (29)*
Global and interregional total	*534,964*	*21,542 (4.0)*	*7,612 (35)*	*7,491 (35)*	*6,439 (30)*
Overall total	***1,237,423***	***44,236 (3.6)***	***16,841 (38)***	***14,251 (32)***	***13,144 (30)***

[a]Cancer is included in this category.

SOURCE: Reprinted, with permission, from Michaud (2004). Copyright 2004 by Catherine M. Michaud, Harvard Initiative for Global Health.

for impact on chronic diseases (Personal communication, O. Adeyi, Coordinator, Public Health Programs, Human Development Network, World Bank, October 13, 2005).

Conclusion

The allocation of funds for chronic diseases in recent years bears little relation to the importance of these diseases in terms of burden of disease. The traditional communicable disease targets still dominate health-sector funding.

THE UNTAPPED POTENTIAL OF THE ACADEMIC COMMUNITY

Major universities across the United States and elsewhere have become increasingly interested and involved in global concerns, especially in health in developing countries. Many have established formal global health programs, the primary goal of which is teaching students. However, some portion of their effort is also directed at carrying out research or other activities in developing countries. Both faculty and students may participate in the overseas portion of these programs.

University global health programs are an untapped resource for cancer control. The point is already made that progress in cancer control involving collaborations between low- and high-resource countries will require services and research at ground level. The example of institutional "twinning" has involved cancer centers per se, not global health programs, and the expertise required is largely clinical, including clinical research. However, many major universities house cancer centers as well as global health programs. One could envision a collaboration with a core clinical component that also takes on other projects. Examples might be helping to develop cancer registries along with IARC, working on community education and outreach about cancer, and exploring the legal and policy aspects of opioid drug availability (e.g., in collaboration with the WHO Coordinating Center for Policy and Communications in Cancer Care). This type of commitment could contribute in a meaningful way to improving cancer control in the partner country and provide opportunities for faculty and students in a variety of disciplines. The challenge is, at least in part, letting those in decision-making roles in global health programs know what opportunities exist or could be created in cancer control. The formation of a university consortium on global health could aid this process (see next section).

University Consortium on Global Health

Representatives of 17 major North American universities with active commitments to global health, and several academic associations, met in April 2005 at Boston University to explore the potential value of coming together in a consortium to support and expand global health programs and promote "global health literacy." A main purpose of the consortium—should it be developed formally—would be to create the means for a collective voice for global health that could communicate with greater strength than individual members. It would also be a place for exchange of ideas among members and for input from outside the academic community. We propose that an explicit goal be to explore the range of opportunities that could be open to university global health programs, with the aim of broadening the areas in which work is taking place. The consortium idea appears to have a good chance of taking hold, with next steps being planned (Keusch, 2006).

SUMMARY AND RECOMMENDATIONS

Global health and development organizations and institutions are highly influential in helping LMCs develop, funding, and carry out their health agendas. Historically, the priorities have been overwhelmingly the infectious diseases that kill children and increasingly adults (mainly AIDS and tuberculosis). Cancer, although not the leading health problem in these countries, imposes a significant and growing burden, but has been overlooked by most of the global development and academic communities. The exceptions are those that are exclusively cancer focused, which do concern themselves to varying degrees with cancer in LMCs. Still, only a tiny share of global health resources has been devoted to cancer.

There are signs that the balance has begun to change, with recognition by WHO and others that chronic, noncommunicable diseases must be addressed at the same time as infectious diseases. However, the danger is that the common risk factors for other chronic diseases will continue to dominate activities, leaving cancer (which shares fewer risk factors) behind. Cancer must have its own identity and recognition if the compelling opportunities across the spectrum of cancer control, highlighted in this report, are going to be acted upon.

RECOMMENDATION 10-1. *International Organizations*
WHO should maintain a strong capacity for cancer control analysis and guidance to assist the many countries that rely on them for health-related information and policy advice. *Capacity is needed both at WHO headquarters and in the regional offices.*

RECOMMENDATION 10-2. *Development Assistance*
The bilateral aid agencies, including the U.S. Agency for International Development, should consider adding aspects of cancer control to their discussion agendas with LMCs, *and adding funding for specific projects that fit into national cancer control plans and programs.*

RECOMMENDATION 10-3. *National Institutions*
The U.S. National Cancer Institute and other established cancer research and funding organizations both in the United States (e.g., the Centers for Disease Control and Prevention) and in other countries should help to establish and facilitate relationships between U.S. cancer centers and centers in LMCs *and encourage U.S. researchers, through grant programs, to undertake collaborative research of relevance to LMCs.*

RECOMMENDATION 10-4. *The Academic Community*
Universities with active global health programs should consider opportunities in cancer control, as well as the more traditional areas of focus. *If a university consortium is developed, one function should be to encourage and facilitate a broader agenda of topics, cancer control among them.*

REFERENCES

Clanton M. 2006. *Implementing the IAEA Program for Action in Cancer: The National Cancer Institute's Supporting Role*. Presented at the UIC World Cancer Congress 2006, Washington, DC. Unpublished.

Freedman LS, Edwards BK, Ries LAG, Young JL, eds. 2006. *Cancer Incidence in Four Member Countries (Cyprus, Egypt, Israel, and Jordan) of the Middle East Cancer Consortium (MECC) Compared With US SEER*. Bethesda, MD: National Cancer Institute.

IAEA (International Atomic Energy Agency). 1956. Statute of the International Atomic Energy Commission.

IAEA. 2004. *Strengthening the Agency's Activities Related to Nuclear Science, Technology and Applications: Resolution Adopted on 24 September 2004*. Vienna, Austria.

IAEA. 2005. *Where We Work*. [Online]. Available: http://www.iaea.org/pact/where_we_work/index.html [accessed December 1, 2005].

International Agency for Research on Cancer. 2006. *IARC's Mission: Cancer Research for Cancer Control*. [Online]. Available: http://www.iarc.fr/ENG/General/index.php [accessed January 23, 2006].

Keusch G. 2006 (July). Meeting of the University Consortium on Global Health, Executive Summary and Participant Comments, Boston University, April 26–27, 2005.

Levin V, Meghzifene A, Izewska J, Tatsuzaki H. 2001. Improving cancer care: Increased need for radiotherapy in developing countries. *IAEA Bulletin* 43(2):25–32.

Michaud CM. 2004. *Official Development Assistance for Noncommunicable Diseases, 1995–2002*. Background paper prepared for the WHO report "*Towards a WHO Long-Term Strategy for Prevention and Control of Leading Chronic Diseases*," submitted April 2004. Typescript.

World Health Organization. 2002. *National Cancer Control Programmes: Policies and Managerial Guidelines*. 2nd ed. Geneva, Switzerland: World Health Organization.

APPENDIX A

Cancer Control in Malaysia and Tanzania

Cancer Control In Malaysia[1]

Malaysia is a an upper middle-income nation of 24 million (2006), made up of peninsula Malaysia and East Malaysia, which occupies one-third of the island of Borneo (the remainder of Borneo is part of Indonesia). It gained independence in 1957. Less than half the population now live in the rural areas. The gross domestic product (GDP) per capita in 2005 was $1,210 (purchasing power parity). Only 2 percent of the population earns less than $1 per day. By 2002, the youth literacy rate was 98 percent for males and females, and most youth were staying in school past the compulsory 6 years (Central Intelligence Agency, 2006).

HEALTH INDICATORS

Malaysia has raised the health status of its population to a remarkable degree. It spends about 4 percent of GDP (2001) on health care.

- In 2004, life expectancy at birth was 69 years for males and 74 years for females (World Health Organization, 2006).

[1]This country profile is taken from a paper commissioned by the Institute of Medicine and prepared by Dr. Ednin Hamzah and colleagues in Petaling Jaya, Malaysia (Hamzah, 2005).

- Infant mortality was 10 per 1,000 live births in 2004 (by comparison the U.S. infant mortality rate was about 6 per 1,000 live births) (World Health Organization, 2006), down from 73 per 1,000 in 1960.
- The under-5 mortality rate has dropped from 105 per 1,000 in 1960 to 13 per 1,000 in 2004 (World Health Organization, 2006).
- For adults, the age-standardized mortality rate was 200 per 1,000 for males and 109 per 1,000 for females in 2004 (World Health Organization, 2006). In 1999, the leading causes of adult mortality in medically certified deaths were cardiovascular diseases, cancers, septicemia, motor vehicle accidents, and pneumonia.
- The maternal mortality rate in 2000 was 41 per 100,000 live births, down from 500 per 100,000 live births before independence (World Health Organization, 2006).

Undernutrition and malnutrition are now rare, and the prevalence of diet-related noncommunicable diseases (cardiovascular disease, diabetes) is increasing. These issues are recognized by the health authorities and are being addressed.

THE HEALTH CARE SYSTEM

The Ministry of Health (MOH) runs health care facilities. There is also an active private sector and a presence of traditional healers. The government health service provides practically free medical care for all, but facilities and personnel are overworked, and waiting lists can be very long. Private health services have no waiting lists, but are expensive. Patients in the private sector are covered by insurance, or care is provided by their employer, or they pay out of pocket. Only about 10 percent of the population has health insurance. A rapidly expanding private sector, coupled with unsatisfactory working conditions in the government services, has drained away skilled personnel from the public sector, which is chronically understaffed (Lim, 2002).

In the public sector, primary care (immunization, family planning, maternity care, communicable disease prevention, and accident and emergency services) is provided in a range of institutions. Secondary and tertiary care are available at the district and general hospitals, but with variable staffing and services offered. Complex tests (e.g., immunological studies, tumor markers) and complex radiological investigations (e.g., mammography, CT scans, and MRI scans) are available only in larger hospitals (Ministry of Health Malaysia, 2006).

Health clinics, staffed by health assistants, are easily accessible in every village and town, with the exception of the interior jungle of East Malaysia, where aboriginal tribes live. The MOH sends teams of health workers who travel to the interior by river to run the community health clinics. Traditional medicine is still relied on, particularly in rural areas.

Health Care Personnel

About equal numbers of physicians work in the public and private sectors—about 9,000 in each in 2003. The public sector is very short of specialists, so the MOH recruits in nearby countries, mostly from the Indian subcontinent. Public health nurses and medical assistants serve in the rural clinics, where doctors may not be available. The medical assistant is being phased out as the number of trained doctors continues to increase.

Pharmaceuticals

The MOH provides essential medicines (from a list) to the public free of charge or heavily subsidized. Most routine drugs for common illnesses are on the list, and whenever available the use of generic drugs is encouraged. Very expensive drugs are not listed, including oncologic drugs such as Herceptin. Some expensive oncologic drugs, such as Taxotere, are listed, but availability depends on the budget.

Morphine is strictly controlled. Private pharmacies do not stock morphine because they are afraid their stores will be broken into by addicts, so cancer patients are able to access morphine in hospitals only. Even so, the supply is limited and most hospitals will give patients no more than a 2-week supply at one time.

Mortality Statistics and Disease Surveillance

The Department of Vital Statistics produces mortality statistics, but their usefulness is limited because only about 40 percent of deaths are medically certified. Old age—defined as death in a person over 65 years old—is one of the most common causes of death (Department of Statistics Malaysia, 2006).

Only a few diseases, such as HIV/AIDS and tuberculosis, require mandatory reporting, and these are underreported as most doctors are not aware of reporting requirements. Reporting cancer cases is not mandatory. A National Cancer Registry was started in 2002, but its accuracy has been questioned. Few regional cancer registries exist; examples are the Penang Cancer Registry and the Sarawak Cancer Registry, which may not be very complete.

TABLE A-1 Leading Cancers in Men and Women in Malaysia, 2002

Men			Women		
Site	% All Cancers Reported	Age-Standardized Rate per 100,000 Adults	Site	% All Cancers Reported	Age-Standardized Rate per 100,000 Adults
Lung	13.9	25.9	Breast	30.4	52.8
Nasopharynx	8.0	11.4	Uterine cervix	12.0	21.5
Colon	7.8	13.9	Colon	5.6	11.2
Leukemias	7.2	9.3	Ovary	5.0	8.6
Rectum	6.4	11.7	Leukemias	4.4	6.9
Prostate	5.7	11.6	Lung	4.3	8.7

SOURCE: Ministry of Health Malaysia (2003).

CANCER CONTROL

Cancer Burden

About 26,000 people were diagnosed with cancer in 2002—12,000 men and 14,000 women. An estimated 10,600 cases were unregistered. Incidence rates in Malaysia fall between rates typical of low- and high-income countries. The leading cancers in adults are shown in Table A-1. The most frequent cancers in children were leukemias, lymphomas, and cancers of the brain, eye, connective tissue, and bones (Ministry of Health Malaysia, 2003).

In 1998 (the most recent year for which this information is available), of the medically certified deaths, 10 percent were due to cancer, making it the fourth leading cause of death. Of the 40,000 new cases of cancer reported in 2002, 12,000 were treated in oncology centers (which are few and unevenly distributed). Those treated outside of oncology centers would have been seen by a surgeon or physician. Because oncology is a relatively new field in Malaysia, surgeons may decide on their own that surgery alone is enough and the patient does not need radiotherapy or chemotherapy. In some of the more peripheral areas, chemotherapy is initiated by the surgeon after surgery without referral to an oncologist.

National Cancer Control Plan

In 2003, the Cancer and Tobacco Control Unit of the MOH held a workshop on the National Cancer Control Plan. Key aspects are efficient use of resources, appropriate use of technology, and active community participation, supporting an ambitious list of goals covering all aspects of cancer control. Policies have been developed in prevention, screening, early detection, adequate treatment, and palliative care. A plan to set up a national cancer institute in Malaysia has been developed, but is not currently feasible because of a lack of staffing. Implementation of the National Cancer Control Programme in Malaysia has been limited by funding and personnel (Lim, 2002).

STATUS OF CANCER CONTROL ACTIVITIES

Prevention and Early Detection Activities

The enormous significance of tobacco is well recognized by the Ministry of Health (see Chapter 5 for more on tobacco control in Malaysia). Hepatitis B vaccination to prevent liver cancer and other serious liver disease was added to the national schedule of immunization in Malaysia in the early 1990s, achieving 88 percent coverage in 2003 (Ministry of Health Malaysia, 2006). A healthy lifestyle campaign was launched in 1991, followed by several thematic campaigns, such as the early detection of cancer campaign (1996) and the healthy diet and nutrition campaign (1997) (Ministry of Health Malaysia, 2006).

No national population-based screening program for any cancer exists in Malaysia. Screening is opportunistic, with Pap smears and clinical breast examinations offered to women at wellness clinics and maternal and child health clinics. The Ministry of Women, Family and Community Development offers screening and early detection of breast and cervical cancers. In 2003, this Ministry gave a grant to the National Council of Women's Organisations (NCWO), a group of nongovernmental women's organizations, to carry out a Pap smear campaign and to teach breast self-examination to women in rural areas, a program that is now operating in almost all states in Malaysia.

In a 1996 survey, 26 percent of eligible women reported having undergone at least one Pap smear examination. In the same year, 47 percent of women reported having some form of breast examination, either breast self-examination, health worker examination, or mammography (4 percent of women) (Lim, 2002).

Diagnosis and Treatment

In Malaysia, as in other developing countries, cancers are typically diagnosed in late stages. The reasons include delay in access to public hospitals because of waiting lists, cultural beliefs, and misconceptions that lead people to prefer treatment by traditional healers. The National Cancer Registry does not collect data on stage of disease at diagnosis, hence the stage at diagnosis is known only from some hospital-based registries. In Hospital Kuala Lumpur (HKL), the main referral hospital for oncology in the country, 80 percent of patients with cervical cancer presented at Stages IIB to IV. In Sarawak, 26 percent presented at Stages I and IIA, with Stage III the most common stage (36 percent). Fifty to sixty percent of breast cancers are diagnosed in Stages III and IV at HKL (Hisham and Yip, 2004). In Sarawak, at least 70 percent of patients with cancers of the nasopharynx, breast, and cervix present in advanced stages.

Early detection is being encouraged through public education and through medical assistants and nurses who are being trained to identify the early signs and symptoms of common cancers. The impact of this program is not yet known (Lim, 2002).

Treatment Resources

In Malaysia the rich can afford the best treatment anywhere in the world, while the poor and underprivileged are forced to travel long distances to the nearest oncology center, do not have access to the necessary drugs because of lack of money, are given suboptimal care, and suffer in silence. The necessary cancer specialists—surgeons, radiologists, pathologists, radiation and medical oncologists, plastic surgeons oncology nurses, and counselors—are not present in most hospitals.

The country has only 21 cancer treatment centers, 6 of them in the public sector. Twelve centers are concentrated in or near the national capital of Kuala Lumpur while most places have none. The public-sector centers are overloaded, and waiting lists are long. In 2000, the Quality Assurance Committee in HKL reported that the waiting time for radiotherapy treatment in HKL was 5 to 8 weeks (Lim, 2002).

Palliative Care, Including Pain Control

Palliative care programs and hospice home care are being developed. More than 50 units of various sizes have been set up in government hospitals. Care of patients after discharge is carried out by medical personnel in the peripheral hospitals who have been trained in basic cancer care, with regular communication from the specialist units. Palliative care in the home is mainly the purview of nongovernmental organization (NGO) hospices, of which there were 20 in 2005. Two hospices operate 8-bed inpatient units. Palliative care in Malaysia is still very much end-of-life care. The perception that it represents only supportive terminal care and a loss of hope of curative treatment means that relatively few cancer patients are referred for palliative care.

Many cancer patients experience pain, but few professionals are trained in pain control. Strong (morphine and fentanyl) and weak (codeine and tramadol) opioids are available, but their use remains low. Per-capita morphine consumption in 2001 was 0.88 mg/capita, compared with the global mean of 5.44 mg/capita, which is itself very low (Pain and Policy Studies Group, 2003).

Misconceptions about morphine—the drug of choice, according to the World Health Organization, and the least expensive choice—abound not only with the public, but also with health care workers. Conversely, transdermal fentanyl is heavily promoted despite its high cost and lack of recommendation for use in the acute setting. Pethidine is still popular with doctors in chronic cancer pain management despite its known dangers. Unfortunately, the choice of pharmaceuticals is often based more on promotion than on clinical guidelines.

There is room for improvement in palliative care services. Several local medical schools, postgraduate courses in family medicine, and nursing colleges have introduced palliative care into their teaching programs. Workshops and seminars are held, and palliative care teams in hospitals are being developed. However, few doctors are interested in pursuing palliative care.

CANCER HEALTH CARE PROVIDERS

Oncologists

Malaysia had 35 oncologists in 2005, almost all of them clinical oncologists who practiced both radiation and medical oncology. None were specialized radiation oncologists. Only 12 of these 35 oncologists were in the public sector, and about half of the total practiced in and around Kuala Lumpur. As a partial solution to the maldistribution and shortage, doctors in peripheral hospitals may refer patients to the oncology unit in HKL, and if chemotherapy is required, the oncologist will send the drugs to the referring doctor to administer. If radiotherapy is required, the MOH may buy the services of a private oncology unit if there is one in the area. In addition, oncologists at HKL run clinics in the peripheral general hospitals once a month. The problem with the shortage of oncologists is in the public sector, where the "brain drain" is not to other countries, but to the private sector, where doctors can earn 5 to 10 times a public-sector salary.

Historically, physicians were trained in oncology overseas, mainly in the United Kingdom. They were sent by the MOH on a scholarship, after which they had to return to Malaysia. Opportunities for training in the United Kingdom have become more difficult in recent years, however. In addition, those who have gone abroad for medical training are unlikely to return to Malaysia to practice.

In 2003, the National University of Malaysia, in conjunction with the MOH, started a 4-year Master of Clinical Oncology Program with the goal of producing oncologists for the country. Because it is so new, no trained oncologists have yet emerged from this program.

Oncology Nurses and Other Specialists

The University of Malaya and HKL conduct oncology nursing courses, where nurses learn to administer chemotherapy and to counsel patients. A shortage of oncology nurses exists, however, because trained nurses leave the service.

There is also a shortage of radiographers to assist with radiotherapy, although the University of Malaya runs a diploma course in radiography. Medical physicists are also in short supply, with usually only one per radiotherapy unit. Degree programs in medical physics are offered by a few universities (Ministry of Higher Education Malaysia, 2006).

CANCER REGISTRATION AND MORTALITY

The Malaysian National Cancer Registry (NCR) was started in 2002, and although there are deficiencies, the data are probably the most accurate cancer data available. The registry covers only Peninsula Malaysia, and not East Malaysia. A few regional cancer registries also exist, but these are not considered reliable. The value of hospital-based registries depends on the quality of medical records, including the degree of computerization, which is not high in most places. The NCR registers an estimated 85–90 percent of diagnosed cancers, and the validity of the data is comparable to those of established registries (Ministry of Health Malaysia, 2003). The first report of the NCR appeared in 2003.

The Penang Cancer Registry, established in 1993, has also published incidence data. Case registration there is based primarily on voluntary notifications received from medical professionals in Penang, an island in the northwest region of Malaysia with a population of about 1.2 million (Yusoff et al., 2003).

Malaysia still has a problem with accurate certification of deaths. Because of traditional and religious beliefs that an autopsy is a desecration of the body, postmortem rates are very low even in hospitals where the cause of death is not known. As seen from the causes of non-medically certified deaths, the most common cause of death is old age. Traditionally, the tribal races in Malaysia prefer to die at home, and hence there are more deaths at home than in the hospital. Deaths at home are certified by the police or village headman.

PATIENT ADVOCACY

More than a dozen NGOs are involved in cancer support and advocacy in Malaysia. Some have established treatment centers, while others work to support public education and early detection. Almost all offer supportive and counseling services, and almost all operate in urban areas, although some organize early detection campaigns in rural areas. One NGO, the Cancer Research Initiatives Foundation, is purely a cancer research organization. Advocacy is also an activity of a few of these organizations, although the organizations do not seem to work together. They all raise money and some are supported by the government.

A CANCER PATIENT'S JOURNEY IN MALAYSIA

Madam C, 73 Years Old

Madam C lived with her husband in a low-cost flat in Kuala Lumpur. She had two daughters and three sons. Madam C presented with Dukes D (advanced) carcinoma of the rectum in September 2003. She had a surgical resection of her tumor followed by radiotherapy. Chemotherapy was commenced, but she failed to complete the course. All services were provided in a private facility. In June 2004, she returned with lung and lymph node metastases. She was aware of her diagnosis but not her prognosis, though it was obvious that she slowly became aware.

Following her disease progression, she moved into her eldest daughter's house, which was more comfortable. Another daughter who lived a few hundred kilometers away also moved in to help. Her husband, unable to accept his wife's condition, sought the assistance of an alternative practitioner. His treatment consisted of making deep incisions in her back and neck and filling the cavity with herbs. He charged RM 200 (about $50) for each appointment and saw her three times a week.

She continued to deteriorate and in November 2004 was referred by her oncologist for palliative care. She presented as a woman in pain at multiple sites with a grossly swollen face, lymphedema of her left arm, skin metastases over her chest, and extensive cellulitis over the areas where incisions were made on her back. A combination of morphine and haloperidol was started as a subcutaneous infusion as she also had some vomiting. She was given antibiotics and steroids. The family was also convinced to cease the use of alternative treatment. Within a week, she had improved considerably. She was pain free and had regained some function. Over the next 4 months, however, her condition worsened.

In the initial stages of Madam C's illness, her husband had been dominant. As the illness progressed, the decision-making authority shifted to the patient's daughter and the patient herself. Although the patient and family generally were prepared for the eventual outcome, the amount of palliative care support required was substantial. Her final days were comfortable and she remained alert. The patient passed away in February 2005 with her family in attendance.

Cancer Control In Tanzania[2]

Tanzania sits on the east coast of Africa, with Kenya to the north and Mozambique to the south. It is a large, diverse country of 37 million, and one of the poorest in the world. The economy is largely agricultural, accounting for half of the gross domestic product. The income per capita (purchasing power parity) is about $700. More than one-third of the population lives below the poverty line (Central Intelligence Agency, 2006).

Infant mortality in 2006 is estimated at 96 per 1,000 live births. Life expectancy at birth is 45 years for males and 46 years for females. This is heavily influenced by AIDS, the prevalence of which is 9 percent of adults. Adult literacy (over age 15) is 78 percent (Central Intelligence Agency, 2006).

A large proportion of the population has access to a variety of nutrients from small-scale farming. Animal protein, however, may be lacking in the diet of many because it must be purchased and most of the population is too poor. There is no evidence that dietary intake has changed much in recent years, although cardiovascular diseases and diabetes, generally associated with higher animal food and overall caloric intake, have begun to appear more frequently.

MAJOR HEALTH ISSUES

Communities are well informed about maternal and child health, including safe motherhood and utilization of family planning services at public clinics. The role of traditional birth attendants, who were the main practitioners in remote areas, is diminishing in many places due to provision of government health facilities near the communities. Other basic elements of primary health care have been implemented as the economic situation allows.

HIV/AIDS awareness is high, with an emphasis on the use of condoms

[2]This country profile is taken from a paper commissioned by the Institute of Medicine and prepared by Dr. Diwani Msemo and colleagues at the Ocean Road Cancer Institute in Dar es Salaam, Tanzania (Msemo et al., 2005).

and abstinence, or faithfulness for those who are married. Awareness programs have included the mass media, such as television plays. The government has urged all employers to form AIDS awareness committees in workplaces to sensitize workers. A nationwide program to provide antiretroviral therapy is being developed with the help of the Global Fund to Fight AIDS, Tuberculosis, and Malaria.

THE HEALTH CARE SYSTEM

The government or its agencies deliver most health care. Private-sector organizations, nongovernmental organizations (NGOs), and religious organizations contribute less than 20 percent of health services. Some hospitals are run jointly by the government and religious organizations, including some consultant hospitals and district hospitals. The relationship between the government and the religious organizations has always been cordial.

The distribution of health facilities has a heavy rural emphasis because more than 70 percent of the population lives in rural areas. The government referral system assumes the pyramid pattern recommended by health planners: from village health service at the lowest level to consultant hospital in cities.

Six of the nine universities in the country have medical and nursing faculties. However, this does not satisfy the country's needs because most graduates are posted to district and regional hospitals, while most people live in rural areas. Clinical officers, nursing officers, and assistants, the backbone of primary health care provision in the country, are trained at more than 70 nursing and clinical officers' training schools.

Health Care Financing

The government pays for health care in public facilities, where they exist. Certain services are funded entirely by donors, such as antiretroviral treatment for HIV/AIDS patients. Religious NGOs also provide services to the public. Patients contribute through cost sharing or through a national health insurance fund. Few Tanzanians are capable of meeting their health needs, however, due to low incomes and high unemployment.

CANCER CONTROL

Cancer is recognized by the government as a serious public health problem in Tanzania. Although much has been done to improve cancer services in the country, of the estimated 30,000 new patients each year, fewer than 10 percent are able to go for treatment at the Ocean Road Cancer Institute (ORCI), the only cancer institute in the country. Furthermore, about 80 percent of those who do come for treatment arrive when the cancer is far advanced and incurable. The government is also faced with other diseases such as HIV/AIDS, which has been declared a "national disaster," overshadowing other health needs. Furthermore, the public is not aware that cancer is a major problem. Most people do not know that smoking causes cancer.

The most commonly recorded cancers in adults are cancer of the cervix, Kaposi's sarcoma (related to AIDS), and cancers of the esophagus and breast. In children, Burkitt's lymphoma is the most commonly seen cancer, followed by retinoblastoma, nephroblastoma, and rhabdomyosarcoma.

Ocean Road Cancer Institute and the National Cancer Control Plan

Established by an Act of Parliament in 1996, ORCI, in the capital, Dar es Salaam, evolved from the radiotherapy department of the Muhimbili University teaching hospital. Surgical services, not available at ORCI, are offered at Muhimbili Hospital. ORCI was created based on the realization that the national cancer policy would require coordination and guidance by a designated institution in order for it to be effective. ORCI is the only designated cancer institute in sub-Saharan Africa outside of South Africa.

The ORCI management has prepared a National Cancer Control Programme (NCCP), which was endorsed by the Ministry of Health in 1997. A position paper on cancer services in Tanzania has also been reviewed and endorsed by the ORCI Board of Trustees. ORCI offers some aspects of palliative care, radiotherapy, chemotherapy, and cancer screening.

The Tanzania NCCP has seven objectives, each of which is defined by specific activities:

1. To establish reliable and sustainable sources of data on cancers in Tanzania through cancer surveys
2. To conduct educational and training programs for the identified target groups, including the public, primary health care workers, and students in health training at various levels
3. To conduct various types of research (epidemiological, clinical, anthropological) on cancers of particular importance, and to build capacity in research through international collaborations and other means
4. To foster cancer prevention initiatives for Tanzanian communities
5. To make early detection services more widely available in Tanzania
6. To establish cancer control networks within the country
7. To provide quality cancer treatment and palliative care to cancer patients

Work has begun on all of these objectives, but funding is not sufficient for much progress.

Prevention Activities

The magnitude of the tobacco problem is not well established. Major efforts in tobacco control have not been made, although some campaigns in newspapers and on television and radio have taken place. Alongside anti-tobacco messages, cigarette companies are targeting people of all ages, mostly in urban settings.

The hepatitis B vaccine was incorporated into routine childhood vaccinations in 2001, achieving reported coverage of 94 percent in 2004 (possibly an overestimate) for all three doses. The vaccine would be too expensive for Tanzania to afford on its own, so it is subsidized by the Global Alliance for Vaccines and Immunization.

Regarding secondary prevention, the only screening facilities are at ORCI in Dar es Salaam. Screening is directed toward breast cancer through clinical breast examination and mammography for those who are at risk and can afford to pay about $40 for the service. A cervical cancer screening project, using Pap smear and biopsy for those with a positive Pap smear, is also situated in Dar es Salaam. This project is donor funded with specific objectives and is time limited. Few individuals access the service; no exact figure is available on the number of patients screened annually.

Diagnosis and Treatment

Cancer therapy in Tanzania is available mainly at ORCI, where most patients are treated with radiation because they present too late for other treatments to be beneficial. ORCI has the only radiotherapy unit in the country. Surgery is rarely done in other hospitals, even if patients present early enough, due to lack of expertise or facilities or both. Poor nutritional status of most patients at the time of presentation also makes surgery riskier. Chemotherapy is given at ORCI for both solid and hematological malignancies, although a medical oncologist is not always on staff, which has been a recurrent problem.

About 2,500 new patients are seen annually at ORCI, a fraction of the people in the country with cancer. Those without access to diagnostic facilities are presumed to have died of unknown causes. Some people resort to traditional healers because they are easily accessible, living in the same communities. Others do so because they believe they have been bewitched. Others are diagnosed by referral hospitals, but fail to come to ORCI for treatment due to lack of funds. No national figures are available on the number of patients diagnosed and treated annually.

Palliative Care and Pain Control

Palliative care is in its infancy in Tanzania, with fewer than 10 percent of those who need palliative care having access. The number of patients who receive palliative care annually is not known. ORCI has practiced palliative care since its founding, and is the only hospital in the country that dispenses oral morphine. ORCI was instrumental in persuading the government to make the necessary arrangements to make oral morphine available for the first time. This involved making sure that staff members were trained in palliative care and the handling of morphine in order to meet the requirements of the pharmacy board. At ORCI, a month's supply of morphine syrup costs the equivalent of about two loaves of bread, so cost is not a barrier for most people.

Recently, services have been expanded to include some home-based care. With the growing numbers of HIV/AIDS patients, some NGOs have been established to offer palliative care. These NGOs get oral morphine from ORCI.

Regarding the World Health Organization (WHO) "Three-Step Analgesic Ladder," (see Chapter 7) Step 1 drugs are available in every health facility and over the counter in pharmacies at prices that are affordable for most people. Step 2 drugs (weak opioids) are not available in most hospitals, and even where they are available, they are too expensive for the average person. The only Step 3 drug available in most district, regional, and referral hospitals is injectable pethidine, which is not recommended for the chronic pain of late-stage cancer and AIDS patients.

A situation analysis and a needs assessment of palliative care, which was funded by WHO in 2002, revealed that the patients' biggest need was relief of pain with accessible and affordable drugs. The most common problem for patients and caregivers was the inability of patients to afford the drugs. In addition, most health professionals in Tanzania have had no training in pain control, so it is not surprising that they do not manage pain effectively. "Opioid phobia" is common among health professionals, as documented by the WHO situation analysis and needs assessment.

CANCER HEALTH CARE PROVIDERS

In 2005, there were six oncologists/radiotherapists in Tanzania, all working at ORCI. There were no formally trained oncology nurses, although most nurses working at ORCI had significant experience in cancer nursing. There was no laboratory technician with specialized cancer training.

No specialized training in oncology is available in the country. All six practicing oncologists have been trained outside the country and returned to render their service, despite a relative lack of incentive to do so compared with other specialties. Only one oncologist who left the country for training did not return.

CANCER ADVOCACY

With only one cancer institute for 37 million people, cancer awareness among Tanzanians is very low. Under these circumstances, advocacy is not only an option but a necessity. The Tanzania Cancer Association has begun initiatives to improve cancer care in the country, with the following objectives:

- Increase cancer awareness among Tanzanians
- Promote cancer prevention, early diagnosis treatment, and palliative care
- Improve treatment facilities for cancer patients
- Encourage research on cancer in Tanzania
- Utilize patients' voices to strengthen cancer care in Tanzania

It is not yet clear how effective the Cancer Association will be.

A CANCER PATIENT'S JOURNEY IN TANZANIA

Mrs. K. is a 42-year-old premenopausal lady who arrived at Ocean Road Cancer Institute in Dar es Salaam with a vesico-vaginal fistula secondary to cancer of the cervix.

She comes from a village called Ngulu in northern Tanzania. Four years ago she started having postcoital bleeding. Her closest friend Nzota told her that maybe her husband's penis is growing, which she called a normal occurrence. She shared that concern with her husband. But instead of empathizing with his wife, he was very happy because men believe that a man who makes a woman bleed after sex is a strong man. Two years later, when she developed a foul-smelling vaginal discharge, she asked another friend, Mrs. Makoko, who told her that it is normal for women to have vaginal discharge. She was not convinced by that explanation so she asked Namwaka, another friend, who told her that she may be bewitched and that she should not disclose this to her husband, because he would use it as an excuse for marrying a second wife. Namwaka arranged for Mrs. K. to see Kokoto—a well-known cancer witch doctor—in Nyumba ya mungu, about 20 kilometers away from Ngulu. Transport from Ngulu to Nyumba ya mungu is difficult due to poor infrastructure. Before traveling to see the witch doctor, she consulted a doctor in the village dispensary who, without doing a speculum examination, gave her ampicillin and Flagyl and assured her that she would be fine. She was never fine, and over the next year she visited the dispensary six times, each time being given similar antibiotics without relevant examinations. She later took a journey to Usangi district hospital, where similar antibiotics were given, again without appropriate examinations.

One of her daughters, who is in Moshi, was concerned with her mother's health and decided to take her to Mawenzi regional hospital, where the clinical diagnosis of cervical cancer was made after the patient pleaded with the doctor to inspect her vagina. The doctor otherwise did not suspect cancer. The diagnosis was terrifying information when told to the family. Most family members believed she was bewitched and should seek help from Kokoto, the cancer witch doctor. (Of note is that her eldest son was not informed because it is a cultural taboo for a son to hear that his mother is having vaginal discharge or bleeding, or is sexually active.)

She went to see Kokoto a week later. The cancer witch doctor confirmed that it was a cancer and said he was capable of curing it as long as she promised not to seek modern medicine. She started getting local herbs from Kokoto. During the first 3 months Mrs. K.'s general condition improved remarkably, but after that time, there was no further improvement. She continued to take local herbs for a year until she started leaking urine through her vagina. Her husband ran away from her at this point and married another woman because Mrs. K. came to be considered a social nuisance. At this point even Kokoto gave up and advised her to try modern medicine at Ocean Road Cancer Institute, where she presented with incurable Stage IVA cervical cancer.

REFERENCES

Central Intelligence Agency. 2006. Malaysia. In: *The World Fact Book 2006*. Washington, DC: Central Intelligence Agency.

Department of Statistics Malaysia. 1999. *Vital Statistics Malaysia 1999*. Kuala Lumpur, Malaysia: Department of Statistics Malaysia.

Department of Statistics Malaysia. 2006. *Department of Statistics Malaysia*. [Online]. Available: http://www.statistics.gov.my [accessed October 30, 2006].

Hamzah E. 2005. *Malaysian Case Study of Cancer Control*. Commissioned by the Institute of Medicine.

Hisham AN, Yip CH. 2004. Overview of breast cancer in Malaysian women: A problem with late diagnosis. *Asian Journal of Surgery* 27(2):130–133.

Lim GC. 2002. Overview of cancer in Malaysia. *Japanese Journal of Clinical Oncology* 32(Suppl):S37–S42. Ministry of Health Malaysia. 2003. *The First Report of the National Cancer Registry: Cancer Incidence in Malaysia 2002*. Kuala Lumpur, Malaysia: Ministry of Health Malaysia.

Ministry of Health Malaysia. 2006. *Ministry of Health (English version)*. [Online]. Available: http://www.moh.gov.my/MohPortal/index.jsp?lang=en [accessed October 30, 2006].

Ministry of Higher Education Malaysia. 2006. *Ministry of Higher Education*. [Online]. Available: http://www.mohe.gov.my/ [accessed October 30, 2006].

Msemo D. 2005. *Cancer Control in Tanzania*. Commissioned by the Institute of Medicine.

Pain and Policy Studies Group. 2003. Morphine consumption figures.
World Health Organization. 2006. *Core Health Indicators.* [Online]. Available: http://www3.who.int/whosis/core/core_select.cfm?strISO3_select=MYS&strIndicator_select=MortInfantBoth&intYear_select=latest&language=english [accessed July 10, 2006].
Yusoff H, Devaraj T, Rokiah M, Aishah K, Rafidah MN, Chan CK, Nor Asikin AK. 2003. *Penang Cancer Registry Report 1994–1998*. Penang, Malaysia: Penang Cancer Registry.

APPENDIX B

Acronyms and Abbreviations

AC	doxorubicin
ACCP	Alliance for Cervical Cancer Prevention
ACS	American Cancer Society
ACSU	American Cancer Society University
AIDS	acquired immunodeficiency syndrome
ALL	acute lymphoblastic leukemia
ASCO	American Society of Clinical Oncology
ASCUS	atypical cells of uncertain significance
ASH	Action on Smoking and Health
BHGI	Breast Health Global Initiative
BMI	body mass index
CBC	complete blood count
CBE	clinical breast examination
CDC	Centers for Disease Control and Prevention
CD-ROM	compact disc-read only memory
CIN	cervical intraepithelial neoplasia
CMF	cyclophosphamide, methotrexate, and 5-fluorouracil
CML	chronic myelogenous leukemia
CRS	creditor reporting system
CT	computed tomography
CTPR93	Control of Tobacco Products Regulation 1993
CTSU	Clinical Trial Service Unit

DALY	disability-adjusted life-year
DCIS	ductal carcinoma in situ
DES	diethylstilbestrol
DIRAC	Directory of Radiotherapy Centres
DTP	diphtheria, tetanus, polio
DVI	direct visual inspection
EC	epirubicin and cyclophosphamide
ED	Europa Donna
ER	estrogen receptor
ESMO	European Society for Medical Oncology
FAC	5-fluorouracil, doxorubicin, and cyclophosphamide
FCTC	Framework Convention on Tobacco Control
FDA	Food and Drug Administration
GAVI	Global Alliance for Vaccines and Immunization
GNI	gross national income
GSK	GlaxoSmithKline
HBsAg	hepatitis B surface antigen
HBV	hepatitis B virus
HC	hybrid capture
HCC	hepatocellular carcinoma
HCV	hepatitis C virus
HER-2/*neu*	Human epidermal growth factor receptor
HKL	Hospital Kuala Lumpur
HINARI	Health InterNetwork Access to Research Initiative
HIV/AIDS	human immunodeficiency virus/acquired immunodeficiency syndrome
HPV	human papillomavirus
HSIL	high-grade squamous intraepithelial lesion
HTLV-1	human T lymphotropic virus type 1
IAEA	International Atomic Energy Agency
IARC	International Agency for Research on Cancer
IHC	immunohistochemistry
ILO	International Labor Organization
INCB	International Narcotics Control Board
INCTR	International Network for Cancer Treatment and Research
INEN	Instituto Nacional de Enfermedades Neoplásicas (National Institute for Neoplastic Illnesses; Lima, Peru)
IOM	Institute of Medicine

IOP	International Outreach Program
KJ	kilojoules
LBC	liquid-based cytology
LEEP	loop electrosurgical excision procedure
LH-RH	luteinizing hormone-releasing hormone
LMCs	low- and middle-income countries
LSIL	low-grade squamous intraepithelial lesion
MBCC	Malaysian Breast Cancer Council
MECC	Middle East Cancer Consortium
MIC	medical information center
MISPHO	Monza International School of Pediatric Oncology
MOH	Ministry of Health
MRI	magnetic resonance imaging
NCCP	National Cancer Control Programme
NCD	noncommunicable disease
NCI	National Cancer Institute
NCR	National Cancer Registry
NGE	no global estimate
NGO	nongovernmental organizations
NIH	National Institutes of Health
NRT	nicotine replacement therapy
NSAID	non-steroidal anti-inflammatory drug
OC	oral contraceptive
OECD	Organization for Economic Cooperation and Development
ORCI	Ocean Road Cancer Institute
PACT	Programme of Action for Cancer Therapy
PAF	population attributable fraction
PATH	Program on Appropriate Technology for Health
PCR	polymerase chain reaction
PCU	pediatric cancer unit
PDA	personal digital assistant
PEPFAR	President's Emergency Plan for AIDS Relief
PET	positron emission tomography
POND	Pediatric Oncology Networked Database
PPSG	Pain and Policy Studies Group
PR	progesterone receptor
PSA	prostate specific antigen

QALY	quality-adjusted life-year
RRI	Reach to Recovery International
SIOP	International Society of Pediatric Oncology
SPECT	single photon emission computed tomography
STEPS	STEPwise Approach to Surveillance
STI	sexually transmitted infection
STM	specimen transport medium
TFI	Tobacco Free Initiative
TNM	tumor, nodes, metastases (cancer staging system)
UICC	International Union Against Cancer
UNICEF	United Nations Children's Fund
USAID	U.S. Agency for International Development
UV	ultraviolet
VIA	visual inspection with acetic acid
VILI	visual inspection with Lugol's iodine
YLL	years of life lost
WHA	World Health Assembly
WHF	World Heart Federation
WHO	World Health Organization
WHOCC	WHO Collaborating Center
WIA	Women's Indian Association (a designation for the Cancer Institute in Chennai)
WiRED	World Internet Resources for Education and Development